The SCD Athlete Cookbook

Over 250 Recipes and Meal Plans Following the
Specific Carbohydrate Diet That Are Gluten-Free and Grain-Free for
an Active Lifestyle

T.L. Wright

SPECIFIC
CULINARY
DESIGNS

Published by:
Specific Culinary Designs, LLC

ISBN: 979-8-218-74831-9

Library of Congress Cataloging-in-Publication Data is on file with the publisher.

Printed in the United States

10 9 8 7 6 5 4 3 2 1

Cover Design: Photography by T.L. Wright, cover designed and formatted by 100 Covers
Photographs: © T.L. Wright except page 329 author photo by photographer Brandon Trammel

Disclaimer - Important Note to Readers

To my family, friends, and fellow athletes who have taste-tested recipes, survived the mistakes, and supported me on this journey.

Contents

Preface

This book is for...

Athletes who want to fuel their athletic performance with whole foods.

Anyone who needs healthy alternatives and recipes for pre-packaged sports nutrition.

Anyone who wants to incorporate a whole food, scratch-made diet into their lifestyle.

Anyone who needs an organized meal prep system.

Anyone who wants delicious meals, following the Specific Carbohydrate Diet.

Even if you don't consider yourself an athlete, the recipes in The SCD Athelete Cookbook are designed to fuel a healthy and active lifestyle for anyone.

This cookbook is written for athletes who love to cook and especially eat.

However, the recipes are easy enough for a novice cook to follow and the gourmet chef to become inspired.

Within the landscape of social media today, it's not uncommon for recipes and meal plans to be generated by artificial intelligence. Unfortunately, many of these recipes and plans often lack testing. Thus the recipes become expensive experiments for the home cook, especially home cooks and athletes who must follow a restrictive diet for their health.

Every recipe in this cookbook has been tested by athletes, and regularly used by the author and her husband (who adamantly admits he is not a cook, but an exceptional dishwasher).

In fact, this book was designed specifically for the partner, parent or athlete who doesn't cook, and needs a "quick start" recipe collection based on the Specific Carbohydrate Diet.

Many people seek out the Specific Carbohydrate Diet due to a diagnosis. Hopefully as a reader, you have not found this book due to illness, but to improve your diet and learn new gut-friendly recipes. This cookbook will help you navigate some of the complexities of the diet, and provide guidance to reduce cooking fatigue. The cookbook offers a variety of recipes that fuel your active life and please the palate.

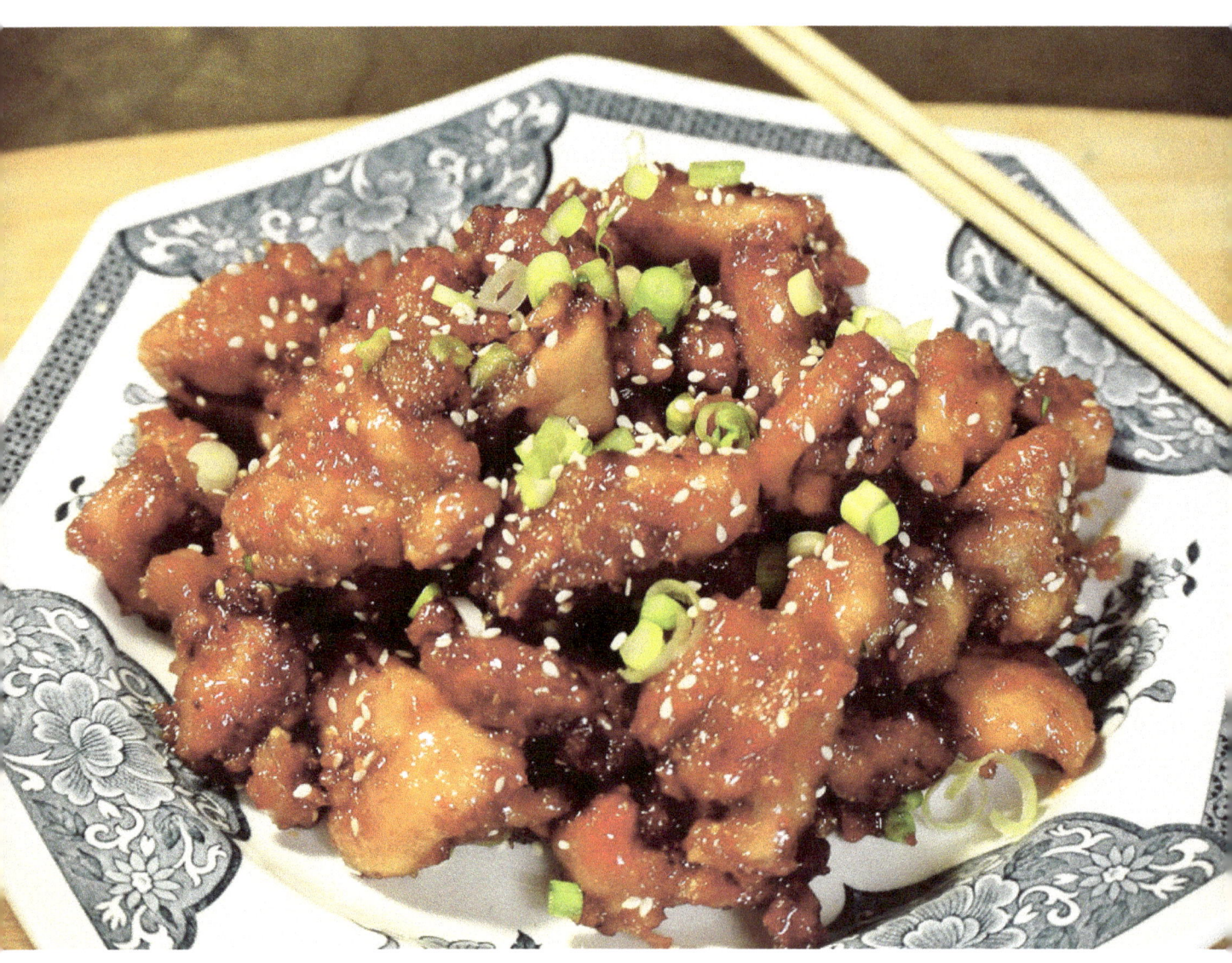

Orange Ginger Chicken

Author's Story

Food has always been my art medium of choice, and at one point considered becoming a professional chef.

Yet throughout my life I had a "weak stomach." Experiencing intense pain under my rib cage and along my left side during times of stress.
I was hospitalized.
I was tested.
I was misdiagnosed repeatedly for years.
Even though I loved to cook, eating food was a game of roulette.
Since some foods caused discomfort, a career as a chef seemed unlikely.

Although cooking was a creative outlet, my career path changed to sports and health sciences. Recipes became more focused on fueling athletic endeavors, such as long-distance triathlons and strength training. Yet I was still afflicted with mysterious pains and bowel ailments. Artificial sweeteners, even the "natural" ones, would tear my gut apart. Pre-packaged sports nutrition described as "easily digestible" or traditional "carb loading" recipes for athletes would send me running to restrooms.

Unfortunately, gastric distress among athletes is a common issue. Therefore, I spent years discounting serious symptoms and assuming they were a normal part of athletic training. Finally, a colonoscopy revealed I had been suffering from undiagnosed Crohn's Disease for over thirty years.

The one silver lining was that my active lifestyle and sports training was an outlet for stress. Since exercise is known to alleviate stress, exercise was helping my Crohn's Disease symptoms. However, the traditional "athlete's diet" does not. Shortly after my initial diagnosis, I started researching nutrition for inflammatory bowel disease. I found the Specific Carbohydrate Diet, and Elaine Gottschall's landmark book, *Breaking the Vicious Cycle: Intestinal Health Through Diet.*

Upon adopting the Specific Carbohydrate Diet, my symptoms greatly improved, and my inflammation markers decreased. Yet I still struggled fueling for my respective sports. Since many carbohydrates commonly consumed by athletes are considered illegal when following the diet. This challenge ignited my creativity in the kitchen and led to the creation of this cookbook.

I am incredibly grateful to Elaine Gottschall for her years of research and her landmark book. As a biochemist, her genius was her ability to simplify complex gastrointestinal processes and craft manageable recipes for a therapeutic diet. The Specific Carbohydrate Diet has helped millions of people around the world. My hope is that The SCD Athlete Cookbook will honor her great work and improve the overall health (and guts) of athletes.

Fuel right and fuel with real food, friends. ~T

The SCD Athlete Cookbook

Introduction

This cookbook was born because ALL athletes need REAL food.

Especially athletes battling inflammatory bowel disease (IBD) and other chronic illnesses. Currently there are minimal sport-nutrition products that are compliant with the Specific Carbohydrate Diet (SCD). There are even fewer cookbooks or meal plans specifically tailored to an athlete's unique nutritional needs. When first following any specialized diet, it can feel confusing and complex. Being an athlete, fueling for a sport adds a secondary layer of complexity.

This cookbook is designed to uncomplicate the complicated. It provides meal guidance and recipes for supporting an active life. You do not need an athletic goal to benefit from them. However, it's important to note, these plans and recipes have been tested in real life by real athletes. These recipes range from fuel for marathons and endurance events to year-long meal preparation for bodybuilding. It includes scratch-made recipes simplified for convenience, and meal systems to reduce the burden of cooking.

There are some amazing cookbooks that provide advice and recipe support for the Specific Carbohydrate Diet. I hope you explore them all and add to your growing cache of recipes. This book is just one tool in your toolbox for following SCD.

However, this cookbook is unique because it builds on the foundational information presented in *Breaking the Vicious Cycle: Intestinal Health Through Diet*. It delves into the details regarding athletic nutrition, simplifying some complex biological processes and assessing athletic performance. This book encourages readers to learn more about what impacts our health, weight, athletic performance, and digestion.

The recipes in this cookbook cover a wide range of cuisines and flavors. This allows variety in meal plans, so food doesn't bore you week after week. The book will also break down traditionally complex recipes into appetizing and easy to make meals. The general focus is to reduce your time in the kitchen so you can spend that time enjoying all your sports and activities. The goal of this book is to provide a simpler, sustainable whole food diet and introduce a new approach to athletic nutrition.

A Brief History of the Specific Carbohydrate Diet (SCD)

In the early 1900s, children died from malnutrition due to celiac disease and inflammatory bowel disease. Dr. Sidney Haas, a pediatrician in New York witnessed many cases of children "wasting" simply from malabsorption of foods and nutrients attributable to these diseases. In his practice, he was able to determine children afflicted with celiac disease could digest certain kinds of foods, and specifically certain carbohydrates. During his career he developed a specialized diet for the care and treatment of celiac disease. Publishing his findings in the medical book, *The Management of Celiac Disease*, which is still utilized in medical school curriculum and referenced today.

In the 1950s Elaine Gottschall was a desperate mother seeking treatment for her four-year-old daughter. Her daughter was afflicted with ulcerative colitis, a form of inflammatory bowel disease (IBD). Physicians at the time, gave her few treatment options with minimal hope for recovery. She sought Dr. Haas who despite his age, was still practicing as a physician, and treating patients. Over the course of two years working with Dr. Haas, Elaine's daughter was recovering from the disease and her health improved.

This new hope, and Dr. Haas's dedication to his patients, is what inspired Elaine to return to school at the age of forty-seven and eventually become a biochemist and cellular biologist. Her work was to reverse engineer the late Dr. Haas's diet, and give further insight into the complex biological systems and how different foods influence them.

She published her work in the book, *Food and Gut Reaction*, which simplified the biological explanation of how the diet works and provided compliant recipes. Elaine continued her research, helping desperate parents and patients use the diet to minimize symptoms and recover their health. The book was later republished under the name, *Breaking the Vicious Cycle; Intestinal Health Through Diet*, and Elaine's research remains the benchmark for the Specific Carbohydrate Diet (SCD), with millions of copies sold worldwide since her death in 2005.

If you are planning on starting the Specific Carbohydrate Diet or want to learn more, it is highly encouraged to read the book, *Breaking the Vicious Cycle* by Elaine Gottschall. This book is foundational for understanding how the diet works, what foods are considered illegal or legal, and why foods are prepared specific ways.

The Science of SCD Simplified

The theory of the Specific Carbohydrate Diet (SCD) is that not everyone's digestive system is able to process **all** types of carbohydrates efficiently. The word "specific" denotes certain types of carbohydrates are allowed based on their structure.

If you asked a person…

What is a monosaccharide, disaccharide, polysaccharide or oligosaccharide?

Chances are few people are familiar with these various molecular structures of carbohydrates.

Unlike many popular "low carb" or "no carb" diets, the Specific Carbohydrate Diet is based on the molecular composition of carbohydrates and how various foods digest in our bodies. For those following SCD, carbohydrates are limited to the type called a monosaccharide (a single-molecule carbohydrate). These molecules are the simplest form of a carbohydrate which can be absorbed directly into the bloodstream, and not the intestinal lining through enzymatic digestion.

Monosaccharides are generally found in fruit (with no added sugar), honey and certain vegetables. Whereas disaccharides, polysaccharides, and oligosaccharides are carbohydrates made up of multiple sugar molecules, requiring our bodies to use enzymes to break down the carbohydrates as part of digestion. [See diagrams for visual of carbohydrate molecular structures.]

ALL CARBOHYDRATES ARE DERIVED FROM SIMPLE SUGARS

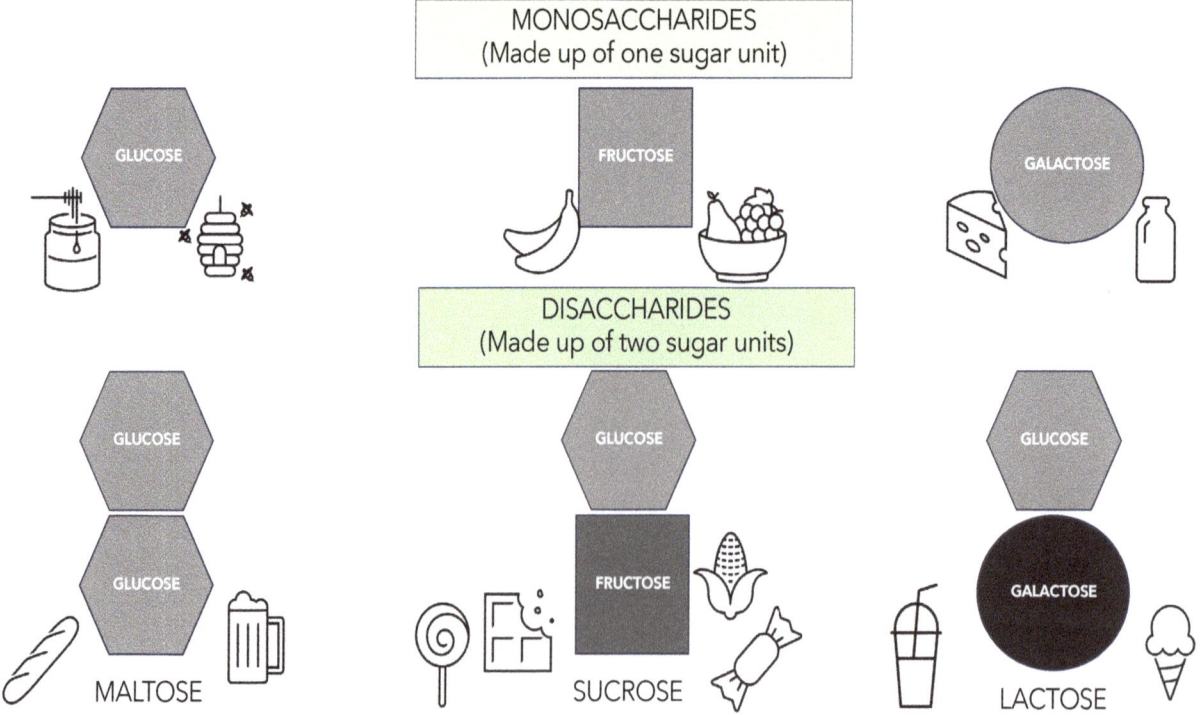

ALL CARBOHYDRATES ARE DERIVED FROM SIMPLE SUGARS

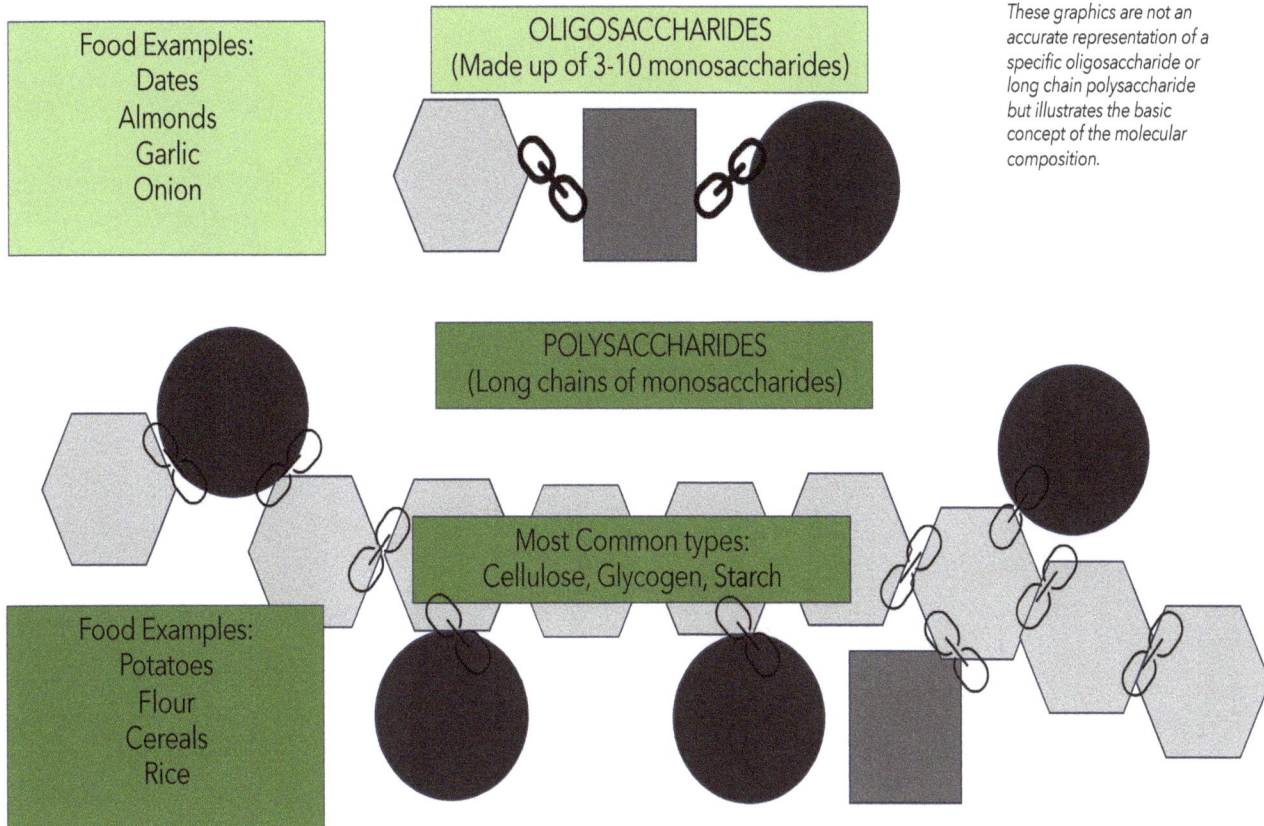

Food Examples:
Dates
Almonds
Garlic
Onion

OLIGOSACCHARIDES
(Made up of 3-10 monosaccharides)

These graphics are not an accurate representation of a specific oligosaccharide or long chain polysaccharide but illustrates the basic concept of the molecular composition.

POLYSACCHARIDES
(Long chains of monosaccharides)

Most Common types:
Cellulose, Glycogen, Starch

Food Examples:
Potatoes
Flour
Cereals
Rice

Some foods typically classified as oligosaccharides or polysaccharides may still be permitted on the Specific Carbohydrate Diet (SCD) because of their nutritional value, high fiber and/or water content. The book *Breaking the Vicious Cycle* explores these foods in detail, and many are categorized as advanced options within the diet.

At first glance, a diet centered around the molecular structure of carbohydrates for various foods may seem restrictive and intimidating. However the diet is well balanced and can be less restrictive than other recognizable diets (i.e. keto, vegan, etc.) The Specific Carbohydrate Diet has all the components of a balanced, whole food diet, including fats, protein, (specific) carbohydrates, and fiber.

The only major exclusions across all food groups are grains and certain high-starch, high-polysaccharide vegetables such as potatoes and corn. However, it's important to note that specific carbohydrates are restricted within all major food groups. For detailed guidance, it's recommended to consult *Breaking the Vicious Cycle* and the accompanying resource list provided in this book (see page 323).

What is Modified SCD (mSCD)?

Modified SCD (mSCD) is a variation of the Specific Carbohydrate Diet. There are some foods considered illegal and typically excluded under the Specific Carbohydrate Diet (SCD) but are often reintroduced in limited quantities after significant healing. In the book, *Breaking the Vicious Cycle*, it is mentioned some children can reintroduce illegal foods however this is not typically recommended. Generally, those who introduce these foods are asymptomatic or they've seen extensive biological recovery from their disease. Foods reintroduced are generally based on individual tolerance.

However here are a few examples of foods that were slowly reintroduced, but note they are not recommended when following SCD.

Unsweetened cocoa or cacao nibs
Green plantains
Various root vegetables
Legumes such as pinto beans
Feta cheese

Important Note: Introducing mSCD foods is not recommended in this cookbook. None of the recipes in the cookbook would be considered mSCD. Oftentimes recipes on social media or web searches promoted as SCD-compliant may include illegal or mSCD ingredients. When in doubt always check the SCD legal/illegal list from a reputable online source (see Resources page 323) or refer to the book *Breaking the Vicious Cycle; Intestinal Health Through Diet*, by Elaine Gottschall.

What Can I Eat Following SCD?

The Specific Carbohydrate Diet (SCD) uses a broad food reference guide for those following the diet. The good news is that it takes some of the thinking out of what you can and cannot eat. This extensive list categorizes foods as being legal or illegal. Foods identified as illegal are based on the molecular structure and carbohydrate content. For example, a sweet potato is considered illegal as it's a starchy vegetable with a polysaccharide composition. As someone once described the diet,

"It's like a 'painting by numbers' diet, instead of paint colors, its food and the foods on the list are what you can eat. If the food is illegal on the list, you don't eat it."

Those choosing to follow the Specific Carbohydrate Diet should also be prepared that not all the foods considered "legal" on the diet may work for them. Everyone has a different gastrointestinal tract, and a certain food tolerated by one person may not be tolerated by another person. (These details are discussed under Food Sensitivity page 10) Also not all recipes in this cookbook will be suitable for everyone, especially those experiencing moderate to severe symptoms.

For the foundational list of SCD foods, reference the book *Breaking the Vicious Cycle: Intestinal Health Through Diet*, by Elaine Gottschall. However, there are several SCD organizations and online resources that provide an updated list of foods. There are also many social media support groups available, but only a handful strictly adhere to the Specific Carbohydrate Diet. Please keep in mind that no grains (especially oatmeal or rice), sweet potatoes, potatoes, or corn are legal following SCD. These foods will always be considered illegal foods. Be cautious of any source, or group that says otherwise.

Since Elaine Gottschall passed away in 2005, for the last twenty years the food industry has been changing. People have been demanding less processed, more whole food products, tailored to special diets. Fortunately, companies have been producing foods customized to these diets and with fewer or no illegal ingredients.

In the last five years, there's been greater emphasis on less preservatives and additives in foods. However, those following SCD still need to take great caution when reading labels and verifying ingredients with manufacturers. Technically, under the guidelines of the Specific Carbohydrate Diet, all commercially made food is warned against. This is why no brand name foods are listed in the cookbook.

Unfortunately, manufacturers often change ingredient suppliers, and processing agents are not always labeled. When using this cookbook, you will see some manufactured ingredients labeled as "SCD legal" before the actual ingredient. This serves as a reminder to the reader of their personal responsibility to verify all the ingredients and manufacturing of various commercial foods.

Read more on page 12 where there is a complete reference section regarding ingredients and examples of reading food labels. Just because a product is advertised as "whole food" or "organic" doesn't always mean our bodies can tolerate the various ingredients companies use to extend shelf life or sustain texture.

It is important to note that this book does not provide a complete list of SCD legal and illegal foods. However, none of the recipes are made with SCD illegal ingredients as of date of publication. The recipes also follow the recommended cooking and preparation techniques, outlined in the book, *Breaking the Vicious Cycle* and the resources listed on page 323.

Food Sensitivity

For those new to the Specific Carbohydrate Diet (SCD), or experiencing symptoms related to various foods, it is essential to follow SCD guidelines for an extended period. Generally, the diet takes time, and not surprisingly the positive effects of the diet can take upwards to 2 years or longer. Even people in remission or asymptomatic will follow the diet indefinitely.

However not all SCD legal foods are tolerated by everyone. It's very important to identify which foods you may have a sensitivity to. You will want to be observant and learn how your body responds to different foods and what works best for you.

Consider common allergens among the general population such as…

Eggs
Nuts
Fish & shellfish
Soy
Wheat
Dairy

A food allergy is the immune system mistaking a food as a threat and producing antibodies to fight it, thus triggering an immunological reaction. Food allergies are very dangerous, and you should always avoid foods you are allergic to. Always follow medical directions from your physician regardless of whether the food is considered legal under SCD.

A food sensitivity generally occurs when the gastrointestinal system struggles to digest certain foods. This can be caused by, but not limited to an enzyme or other substance deficiency required for digestion. Normally, a food sensitivity does not cause a life-threatening or immunological response. However, avoiding common food allergens or eliminating certain foods is a step towards identifying food sensitivities.

Important to note when eliminating foods, all wheat is illegal under the Specific Carbohydrate Diet. Whereas dairy products are based on type. For example, dairy is allowed in certain aged cheeses and SCD legal yogurt (which is fermented for 24 hours and dripped to remove the lactose sugars). Soybeans are illegal as well, with the exception when fermented in tamari sauce and this exception is only based on individual tolerance and small quantities.

As for eggs, nuts, fish and shellfish, many people find they cannot tolerate these foods well. Which is where variations of the Specific Carbohydrate Diet originate, with some people eliminating certain legal foods on the list from their diet. For example, variations may include but are not limited to dairy-free SCD, Low-FODMAP SCD, Nut-free SCD, etc.

A simple way to find out if you have a food sensitivity is by eliminating a suspected food for a few weeks to a month and observing whether you feel better. Taking the time to figure out your food sensitivities is often worth the hassle as they can manifest over time with various symptoms or exacerbate existing inflammation.

An interesting aspect of food sensitivites are that people report changes as they age, and/or their gastrointestinal tract recovers. It is not uncommon for someone to have a food sensitivity for several years, then with slow and calculated reintroduction of a food they can eventually eat it. This process is commonly called a "Food Ladder" (*Source: NIH*). For example an "Egg Ladder" is used for eggs that are introduced slowly in various stages of preparation.

To illustrate, the first stage or rung of the ladder is introducing eggs in baked goods, such as a muffin, cookie or cupcake. The second stage or rung of the ladder, the egg is introduced in an item less baked such as a binder in meat loaf, pancake, popover or crepe. The third stage is trying a hard-boiled, or well-cooked scrambled egg. The final step is to try a less-cooked scrambled egg, soft-boiled or sunny side up. Generally, each stage is tested in small quantities, and you must be observant of reactions or symptoms. Always seek advice and/or directions from your physician before introducing foods with known sensitivities.

Essentially the same technique of slow introduction could be practiced with other food sensitivities such as dairy. However, it should always be followed within the guidelines of the Specific Carbohydrate Diet and under physician guidance. For example, forms of dairy are limited to specific types of cheeses and SCD legal yogurt. The book, *Breaking the Vicious Cycle* provides details and guidelines as to both.

"Safe" or "Flare" Foods Explained

As you delve into the Specific Carbohydrate Diet (SCD) resources or support groups you will often come across the common terms of "safe" or "flare foods". These phrases refer to foods that an individual has found easier to digest. When experiencing gastrointestinal (GI) distress, it is often recommended to choose foods that are well-tolerated and unlikely to worsen symptoms. No two tummies are alike. Therefore, a safe or flare food for one person may not be the same for another.

The common diet of bananas, rice, applesauce, and toast, known as (BRAT) diet during times of GI distress or illness may look slightly different following the Specific Carbohydrate Diet. Since those following SCD do not eat grains such as rice and toast made with flour. Alternatively, our diets may include pureed soups, homemade SCD yogurt, bone broth, ripe bananas and unsweetened apple sauce. Substitutions for store bought electrolytes are replaced with homemade ginger ale (using honey instead of sugar), and electrolyte drinks made with SCD legal ingredients.

However, a general rule of thumb is that safe or flare foods are minimally seasoned, and spice is usually avoided. Foods are also blended, pureed or well-cooked and cut into smaller pieces. Commonly high fiber fruits, nuts and vegetables may be altogether avoided, or peels and skins removed and cooked to aid in digestion. Also, people may avoid foods with a higher sugar content, such as honey or fruit juice as this may feed intestinal bacterial overgrowth. Generally, these safe foods are temporarily eaten until symptoms lessen or subside. If symptoms of GI distress are present always seek medical advice and treatment.

Scratch-Made Vs Packaged Foods

When you are following the Specific Carbohydrate Diet (SCD), making scratch-made foods, from fresh and whole food ingredients, is emphasized because you know the source of the food. Generally, most people first starting SCD avoid packaged food as they are eliminating ingredients which may trigger symptoms. Unfortunately, many packaged foods, can have trace amounts of ingredients or processing agents that the manufacturer does not need to disclose.

As a best practice of strictly following the Specific Carbohydrate Diet, it is best to avoid canned and prepackaged foods. Especially important if you're experiencing gastrointestinal distress or unresolved symptoms. Here are a few examples of ingredients or common phrases that are red flags (and often illegal foods) when reading labels.

Red Flags

- Concentrate *(of any kind)*
- Gums *(of any kind)*
- Sugar, including natural or organic *(all kinds of sugar are illegal except honey)*
- All natural sweeteners *(except honey)*
- Spices *(not clearly identified)*
- Anti-caking agents
- Alginate/Algae
- Corn meal
- Wheat
- Malt
- Barley
- Flavors, including natural or organic *(where the flavor ingredients are not clearly identified)*
- Yeast
- Rice
- Pectin
- Starch *(modified or starch of any kind)*
- Cellulose
- Flaxes and flax seed
- Dextrin and Maltodextrin
- Dextrose

It is important to note that when *Breaking the Vicious Cycle* was published the Specific Carbohydrate Diet considered canned vegetables illegal. This was due to potentially deceptive labeling which did not list additives or trace illegal ingredients in the canning process. Generally, this is still true, and frozen or fresh vegetables are always preferred over canned vegetables. However, labeling laws have changed over time and companies have improved manufacturing processes based on consumer demand.

There are several brands of certain canned or boxed vegetables that do not contain additives, artificial flavors or preservatives (even in the manufacturing process). Many of these product brands are used repeatedly by the SCD community and sold through Wellbees or other natural food stores. Note there are recipes in this cookbook that may include prepackaged ingredients however all of them can be substituted with fresh, frozen or scratch-made ingredients. Important to note, there are currently no brands of canned legumes that follow the preparation requirements of the Specific Carbohydrate Diet.

Here are some examples of common packaged foods comparing ingredients between different brands to help illustrate legal vs illegal ingredients (see below).

Are you able to spot the illegal ingredients and red flags in the list?

PACKAGED FOOD LABEL EXAMPLES	LEGAL	ILLEGAL
CANNED TOMATOES*	Crushed tomatoes, tomato puree, sea salt, basil leaf	Tomatoes, tomato juice, sugar, sea salt, citric acid, calcium chloride, spice.
BONE BROTH	Filtered water, organic chicken, organic carrots	Water, organic chicken bone broth, organic vegetable broth (organic carrot, organic celery root, organic onion juice concentrate) organic flavor, natural roasted flavor, salt, organic lemon juice concentrate, organic apple cider vinegar, organic rosemary extract, organic tumeric extract color
UNSWEETENED ALMOND MILK	Almonds, water	Almondmilk (filtered water, almonds), Contains 2% or less of: Vitamin and mineral blend (calcium carbonate, vitamin E acetate, vitamin A palmitate, vitamin D2), sunflower and/or almond and/or canola oil, sea salt, gellan gum, ascorbic acid (Vitamin C to protect freshness), natural flavor.
SPICE RUB	Sea salt, garlic, onion, black pepper, ground mustard, lemon peel, chili pepper, oregano & parsley.	Sea Salt, dehydrated onion, cane sugar, dextrose, maltodextrin, toasted onion, rice concentrate, yeast extract, natural flavor, spices, citric acid, tumeric, butter, sweet buttermilk.
FRUIT JUICE	Organic concord grape juice (not from concentrate)	Fruit juices from concentrate (water, concentrated juices of apples, pears, and grapes); natural flavor, ascorbic acid (Vitamin C)
SALAD DRESSING	Olive oil, distilled white vinegar, red wine vinegar, honey, basil, oregano, salt, pepper,	Vinegar, water, vegetable oil (soybean and/or canola oil), sugar, salt, garlic*, contains less than 2% of red bell peppers*, onions*, xanthan gum, spices, oleoresin paprika (color), potassium sorbate and calcium disodium edta (to protect flavor), *dried
KETCHUP	Tomato puree, apple cider vinegar, honey, salt, onion, cloves, garlic, cinnamon	Tomato concentrate, distilled vinegar, cane sugar, salt, onion powder, spice, natural flavorings
CANNED CHICKEN*	Chicken breast meat, water, salt	Chicken breast meat, water, seasoning (salt, modified food starch, sodium phosphates, chicken broth, and natural flavors)

See information about canned vegetables and foods above

When following SCD, many believe the only way to be certain if a packaged food is SCD-compliant is to confirm ingredients with a manufacturer. Normally this is done by letter (or email), detailing all the ingredients and preparation. However, the challenge is that a manufacturer can change their ingredients at any time without notification. Therefore, when in doubt, avoid packaged foods by using fresh foods or purchase prepared foods from an approved market such as Wellbee's (see Resources page 323).

Certain types of cheeses are allowed under the Specific Carbohydrate Diet, unfortunately many manufacturing processes include the use of cellulose, anticaking ingredients, and fillers in the processing of cheese. The general rule of legal cheeses are they need to be aged over three months, and contain zero carbohydrates or sugars, listed under the nutritional content. Avoid pre-sliced and pre-shredded cheese since many contain illegal ingredients to prevent cheese from sticking and prolong shelf life. It is always best to purchase blocks of cheese, then shred, grate, crumble or slice yourself.

Sauces and spices are two categories of foods that people do not consider when first starting the Specific Carbohydrate Diet. They realize that their favorite family recipe is not truly scratch made, and contains pre-packaged, store-bought sauces with illegal ingredients. For example, many popular commercially-made sauces in recipes such as sriracha sauce, ranch dressing, teriyaki sauce, Italian dressing, etc. are often full of illegal ingredients. Also, many people are not aware certain vinegars are made with added illegal sugars.

This can be a source of frustration for those who miss their favorite recipes because they can't mimic the exact flavor or loss of convenience. That is why the cookbook has designated sections for sauces and spice mixtures. It also includes common sauces that are adjusted to be SCD compliant. The recipes may not be the exact flavor, but some sauces and spices are comparable or may even taste better.

All in all, the simplest way to guarantee that food is SCD compliant is by using only fresh, whole food ingredients, scratch-made recipes, or buying pre-made foods from an approved store like Wellbees. (Please see the product source section page 323)

The Healthy Athlete

As athletes we get so caught up in chasing a personal record (PR), winning a championship, or earning a pro title. We are so focused on the athletic goal we oftentimes forget the purpose of training, which is our overall health, stress relief, and longevity. You don't have to be an elite athlete to be caught up in the rush of competition or let the athletic goal overtake your life.

Sometimes symptoms are an early warning sign that your nutrition and training plan need an overhaul. Essentially our bodies need a break. Your digestion is one of the first barometers of your overall health.

Are you eating appropriately for your physical output?
Are you meeting your necessary protein intake? Carbs? Fats?
Are you deficient in any nutrients?
Are your bowel movements normal?
Are you eating enough fiber?
Are you eating too much fiber?
Are you hydrated?
Are you having any symptoms of gastrointestinal distress?

These are just a few of the questions to ask yourself and assess how your athletic activities and nutrition may be impacting your health and how your body absorbs food.

Think of your body as a car. You can put top of the line gas or a battery in it, but if the engine can't use those energy sources properly, how efficient is it? How efficient will your body be?

When digestion is compromised it not only impacts our sports performance negatively, but also just general energy for life. Fatigue is a common symptom for those with inflammatory bowel disease, since the healthy surface area of the intestinal tract is generally diminished, and absorption is not efficient. Therefore, attention to food and hydration is incredibly necessary. As an athlete with inflammatory bowel disease (IBD) you will likely need to be monitored by your physician regularly for vitamin and mineral deficiencies.

Even without IBD, female athletes are more susceptible to iron and calcium deficiencies. They also need to consider their hormones, menstrual cycles, peri menopause and menopause-- how their cycle and life changes might impact their nutrition and performance. This may mean rotating in foods known for certain vitamins and minerals. However, when in doubt, common deficiencies that should be checked by your medical provider are iron, magnesium, calcium, B6, B12, vitamin D and hormone levels.

Recovery and sleep are often forgotten in pursuit of an athletic goal. If an athlete is training for a marathon and they go to bed late and get up early every day, this pattern could lead to poor recovery. In many cases, for those who have an autoimmune disease or IBD have the serious consequence of a flare. Flares can set back months of training within a matter of days. Don't allow poor recovery and sleep to lead to a flare. Oftentimes that extra day of rest is more valuable to your performance than that extra day of training. Long term consistency of short training sessions and good recovery often lead to better results, versus inconsistent long and intense training with sub-par recovery.

Consistency, Routine and Metabolic Adaptation

Athletes have the uncanny ability to tolerate boredom especially elite athletes. Both in training days and their diets. As athletes advance in their skills and abilities, they learn routines that work best for them. Whether that is a nine o'clock bedtime and four o'clock wake up or performing the same exercises day in and day out to maximize specific muscle groups. The routine is consistent which makes it effective.

Many routines center around foods and nutrition that maximizes their performance. However, this may lead to a boring palate. Elite athletes are generally very in tune with their bodies. They have learned what foods are easily digestible and which ones provide them maximum energy.

For those with long-term inflammatory bowel disease, many people identify which foods are safe. They also determine which foods are easiest to digest and don't cause them gastrointestinal (GI) distress. They are observant to symptoms and what gives them energy, very similar to how elite athletes are perceptive of their nutritional needs.

In both instances, routine and consistency in diet can be effective, but both diets and training routines need healthy variety. The body adapts to both training and nutrition, thus becoming less effective over time. This is where trainers, coaches and nutritionists may make small changes to an athlete's diet or routine to prevent metabolic or muscular adaptation.

Metabolic adaptation is our body's ability to adapt to its changing environment and a physiological response to caloric intake. Every person's body is unique and thus some people are more efficient at conserving energy than others. Basically, our body's metabolism adjusts to when and how to use the food we consume.

Metabolic adaptation is essentially a mechanism for perceived scarcity. When you reduce caloric consumption over long periods of time the body becomes more efficient at making energy with less. The downside to this is if a person wants to lose body fat it may be harder for them. The same is true for a person who wants to gain muscle mass. If your body has adapted based on scarcity or overconsumption, your body is going to figure out when and where to use those calories. This may not be healthy or benefit athletic performance.

The same concept is considered in training, with how muscles and our organs adapt and respond to exercise. The negative effects of muscle adaption are when our recovery capacity is stretched beyond its limits. Generally, this leads to decreased performance, overuse injuries, and decreased cardiovascular health.

For example, an endurance athlete or marathon runner has trained for a highly efficient cardiovascular system. However, without appropriate variety in exercise, the body becomes too adapted and thus overtime less efficient. Coaches will add in the appropriate strength and mobility training to reduce injuries, strengthen muscles, and increase metabolism. The same can be true for weightlifting centric sports such as powerlifting, bodybuilding, and functional fitness training. Coaches will add more cardiovascular training into the athlete's routine to improve heart and lung health and disrupt the negative effects of muscular and metabolic adaptation.

The general rule of athletic development and increased performance is consistency and routine. However, longevity in that sport and overall health is achieved when the appropriate variety of training and nutrition is applied.

For the average person seeking an athletic goal, consistency and routine is a struggle because generally they are trying to balance careers and life around their athletic pursuits. Therefore coaches, trainers, and nutritionists may hyperfocus on the consistency and routines. They do what has worked for them in the past, what is familiar and works for the majority. Unfortunately, their systems may not work for all athletes, especially an athlete with a chronic illness and special dietary needs.

This cookbook follows the Specific Carbohydrate Diet (SCD) guidelines, emphasizing nutrient-dense foods that support performance while offering a suitable variety within the diet's framework.

Sports Nutrition Simplified

How Much Food Do We Need to Eat?

In a sedentary society, it is common to overestimate the number of calories we need to consume. Even for active athletes its normal to miscalculate our calories. Presumptively people assume the fitter and more active the person, the more calories they need, versus the obese sedentary person. However the larger you are, the more calories you may require. Some of the fittest athletes in the world are hard-pressed to burn more than a thousand calories per hour. Whereas someone who is overweight performing the same exercise could easily burn beyond a thousand calories.

Important to note, caloric needs are highly individualized and specific to factors in an athlete's life. Factors such as age, gender, body composition, active exercise volume, intensity and non-exercise activity thermogenesis (NEAT). They all play a role in how much food to consume and what we should eat.

Today, technology such as fitness activity trackers or wearables, have helped us gain more insight. They approximate individual caloric needs centered around our activity level. However, these devices generally calculate based on weight and height only. They don't consider individual body composition, (i.e. the amount of muscle, or body fat a person has), or the efficiency of their metabolism. Another layer of complexity is whether the person is digesting and absorbing food appropriately. A person with a chronic illness may have different caloric needs than a person without.

This can debunk the standard, that if you eat calories in a surplus or deficit, you will gain or lose weight, and it doesn't matter which types of foods you eat. Unfortunately, this default position only scratches the surface when it comes to the complexities of auto-immune diseases, nutrition and their correlation with the gastrointestinal system. Asking the question, if your body can't properly digest and absorb those calories, are you really in a surplus or a deficit?

Luckily the Specific Carbohydrate Diet helps take some of the guesswork of which foods to eat and the athlete only need apply those foods appropriately for their individual needs. As noted before, not everyone can eat everything on the diet. Some people have existing food sensitivities and inflammation which can limit their nutrition. Therefore, it is very important to always consult with your physician before adopting any diet or regimen.

The Three F's: Food, Fuel, & Frequency

Food is fuel. But fuel is food applied appropriately to an exercise or an activity.

From the recreational to the elite athlete, all need to consider the importance of what, when and how they fuel. Being well-hydrated and well-fueled are both incredibly important before any physical activity or sport. The two main forms of energy our body needs during exercise are carbohydrates and fats. Protein is used, however more essential for recovery, repair and building of muscle, not necessarily a direct fuel source for activity.

Without diving into the details regarding anaerobic and aerobic metabolism, the general rule is that with low-intensity exercise we burn fat and with high-intensity exercise we burn mostly carbohydrates. Glycogen is stored in the muscles and is released when used for fuel during periods of intense exercise. Unlike fat stores, glycogen is in limited supply and once depleted, it is difficult to maintain a high level of intensity. (Usually described among athletes as "bonking"). Our bodies create glycogen through the consumption of carbohydrates.

Which may be challenging for athletes following a diet with restricted carbohydrates. However, the Specific Carbohydrate Diet (SCD) does not necessarily restrict carbs, just specifies the type of carbohydrates one can eat. The carbohydrate sources available under SCD include, specific vegetables, legumes, fruits, certain types of cheeses, legal SCD yogurt, honey, seeds and nuts. (This cookbook includes several recipes for fueling athletic activities.)

Frequency, by which an athlete eats is essential for performance. It is not surprising athletes eat multiple meals outside the standard of three times a day. Eating smaller meals frequently throughout the day allows them to optimize their training and recovery. They may have a caloric or macronutrient daily goal, but they divide their nutrition into smaller portions to prevent burdening the digestive system. Also, many athletes can attest (or have a personal story) where undigested foods during times of high intensity training was not a good thing.

Food is fuel, but it is also essential to recovery. Timing the right foods after training sessions or competitive events are key. Protein, carbohydrates and fats are necessary to help your muscles and body recover. Unfortunately, there is not a specific rule or guideline regarding timing macronutrient throughout the day because everyone's bodies are different. However, the general practice to consume carbohydrates and protein, post exercise restores glycogen and promotes muscle repair.

Calculating Caloric Deficits & Surplus

There are numerous tables and data to help athletes approximate the number of calories for an individual need. There are also tests, such as the resting metabolic rate test, which measures how many calories you burn while at rest. This is considered a baseline measurement and tool used to plan nutrition and exercise routines. Wearable fitness trackers also attempt to gauge caloric needs. This data is based on daily movement and energy exerted while performing the activity using heart and respiratory rates. However, there are also simple calculations to determine caloric needs as well.

Firstly, determine basal metabolic rate (BMR) and total daily energy expenditure (TDEE). These are the two basic calculations for establishing the number of calories you need to consume, to maintain weight and/or body composition. (Important to note there may be other factors influencing weight and body composition, however this is a basic calculation commonly used by certified training associations and dietary guidelines.)

Women
BMR = 655 + (4.3 x weight in lbs.) + (4.7 x height in in) - (4.7 x age)

Men
BMR = 66 + (6.3 x weight in lbs.) + (12.9 x height in in) - (6.8 x age)

Activity levels can be determined using the following scale:

Sedentary: BMR x 1.2
Lightly active: BMR x 1.375
Moderately active: BMR x 1.55
Very active: BMR x 1.725
Super active: BMR x 1.9

For example, a thirty-five-year-old man, who is 5 feet, 9 inches, and weighs 175 lbs. has an approximate BMR of 1821.

1,820.6 = 66 + (6.3 x 175lbs) + (12.9 x 69in) – (6.8 x 35)
1,820.6 = 66 + (1,102.5) + (890.1) - (238)

To measure the number of calories the example needed is based on his activity level (TDEE). If the example athlete is moderately active, then multiplying his BMR by 1.55 for an approximate total would be 2,822 calories.

2,821.93 = 1820.6 x 1.55

Source: NASM guidelines

If our baseline (BMR), are calories you need daily to sustain vital roles like cellular function, breathing, and heart rate, determining exertion and caloric burn is a bit more complex. The TDEE calculation is not one hundred percent accurate, however it is a helpful tool for providing an estimate. Fitness trackers tend to be a bit more exact, but not infallible for individual activity tracking. Let's assume the athlete wears a fitness tracker and has a high non-exercise activity thermogenesis (NEAT) rate and moderately exercises, the athlete would need enough calories to support their active lifestyle and athletic endeavors.

Tracking your calories and macronutrients will be the tool to determine if you are in a daily caloric surplus or deficit. Once BMR and TDEE are estimated, you can easily compare whether you are meeting caloric needs. There are several applications and food trackers available to help you record the foods eaten. Generally eating more than your maintenance calories may create a surplus. Not meeting your daily caloric goal may create a deficit. This, however, is determined by how well you are digesting and utilizing those calories. Following the Specific Carbohydrate Diet and logging your foods may help determine which foods digest well and reveal food sensitivities.

Macro Counting

Macronutrients are the nutrients that provide us energy in large quantities, commonly known as carbohydrates, proteins and fats. Micronutrients are the vitamins and minerals needed to keep bodily systems healthy and functioning, such as calcium, magnesium, sodium, fiber, etc. Micronutrients are derived from macronutrients and are based on the foods we eat. For example, eating a macronutrient protein source such as fish, provides the micronutrients of vitamin D, iron, vitamin B12 and vitamin E.

Nutrition is not just centered around calories in and calories out. The type of macronutrients matter. This means not eating enough carbohydrates can lead to poor sports performance, and not consuming enough protein can lead to poor muscle recovery.

A common tool in the toolbox of sports nutrition is macronutrient counting or "macro counting." Coaches, trainers, nutritionists, and athletes use macro counting to help them meet caloric and macronutrient needs. Using a food tracker that calculates the nutritional value of foods, the ratio of macros can be adjusted and individualized to the athlete. For example, an endurance athlete will likely have a higher carbohydrate macro goal, compared to a powerlifter with a higher protein macro goal.

Unfortunately, there are differing opinions and guidelines for macro ratios. The USDA recommends adults get 45-65% of calories from carbohydrates, 10-35% of calories from protein, and 20-35% from fat. (*Source: NIH News; The Dietary Guidelines of America USDA, August 2023*). However these ratios can vary greatly among athletes and an individual's specific needs.

Gastric Emptying

While we often focus on the heart, muscles, and lungs as the primary organs for athletic performance, the gastrointestinal (GI) tract plays a crucial role. The wrong foods, lack of calories, heat, hydration and overall stress of competition can drastically hinder athletic performance and cause GI distress. The rate by which food is consumed and digested in the small intestine is called the gastric emptying rate (GER). The small intestine is the primary organ of absorption and digestion.

The gastric emptying rate is important because it helps determine the ability to absorb food consumed during activity.

This rate can be influenced by the following:

- Food density
- Volume of food consumed
- Volume of liquid consumed
- Caloric density of a liquid
- Exercise intensity
- Body temperature
- Dehydration

Factors not commonly listed, but can impact GER are food sensitivities, IBS, IBD, and stress. For those athletes who run the risk of GI distress during exercise, being cognizant of their fuel and hydration is key. Any excess food or water not absorbed by the small intestine typically passes through the large intestine and exits out the "back door." Excessive emptying is generally a sign of poor absorption and digestion. Following and fueling based on the Specific Carbohydrate Diet may improve both.

Hydration

Hydration is critical for a healthy gastrointestinal system since water is needed in every step of digestion. Water is essential in the process of nutrient absorption, the osmolality of fluid, and the production of intestinal secretions. Hydration can be measured by sweat volume and gastric emptying rate. Fundamentally, if too much is going out than what is taken in, this is a possible sign of dehydration. There are specific medical tests for measuring sweat volume and gastric emptying rates. However, there are practical approaches to both for the athlete in training.

Sweating is a bodily function to regulate temperature and the primary way we lose fluid. The volume by which we sweat differs in rate. Determining this rate helps identify how much fluid we need during activity.

A basic way of calculating sweat rate is the following:

1. Ensure you are properly hydrated and have consumed enough food before exercising or training. Allow your body time to digest before starting any exercise.

2. Weigh yourself in the nude just before exercising and your bladder is empty.

3. Exercise for exactly one hour without eating or drinking anything. Choose an exercise that will mimic a typical training session or activity you do. For example, if you are training for a half marathon, run the same pace as you would for the half marathon during this hour.

4. Weigh yourself in the nude again and dry off all excess sweat.

5. Calculate your weight difference and convert it to kilograms. Subtract your weight after the workout from your weight before the workout. For example, if you lost 1 lb., then your loss in kilograms is approximately 0.45.

6. Multiply that number by 1,000 to find your sweat rate in milliliters per hour. For example, if your weight loss was 0.45 then sweat rate is 450 mL per hour.

(*Source: UCLA Health: Why athletes need to know how much they sweat*)

Essentially this sweat rate tells what ideally you should be drinking during activity. Temperature, humidity, fitness, and absorption can typically impact sweat rate. However, this calculation is another tool to gauge your body's hydration. Electrolytes help our bodies maintain and absorb necessary water, and sodium is the primary electrolyte lost in sweat. When doing high intensity workouts or in hot climates electrolytes are crucial for hydration.

For those following the Specific Carbohydrate Diet, there are some limitations to the type of electrolyte beverages. In this cookbook there are several recipes prioritizing electrolytes, both in food and drinks that follow the Specific Carbohydrate Diet guidelines.

Supplements

One of the major myths of sports nutrition is supplements are needed to improve athletic performance. However, this is not necessarily true for athletes following a healthy diet, who train properly and recover well. Supplements are generally not recommended under the Specific Carbohydrate Diet (SCD) unless specifically prescribed by a physician. If so, then the supplement ingredients should follow the guidelines of the diet and limit illegal ingredients.

Fortunately, there are whole foods that are legal under SCD that can either substitute or be an alternative to various supplements. Those would include the popular "protein shake," that you can make with SCD legal protein dense ingredients such as yogurt and pasteurized egg whites.

There are also animal-based products such as beef (bovine) or bone broth powder, dried egg white powder, and unflavored collagen to help supplement protein intake. However it is at the responsibility of the individual to verify the ingredients are legal under the Specific Carbohydrate Diet, and the manufacturing process does not include illegal additives not labeled. This cookbook does include several homemade protein shakes, and recipes. They also include some supplements that meet SCD requirements, but these can be omitted and/or replaced with alternative ingredients as needed.

As an important reminder, you should consult a doctor before taking any dietary supplement, especially if you have health conditions or take medications.

How to Use This Cookbook

Athletes may not have the time to prepare complicated, gourmet meals. As the priority is generally on work-life balance, training and recovery. This cookbook is designed to simplify meal prepping and planning. It is also designed with the novice home cook in mind. Therefore, minimal skills are needed to prepare the recipes, and the suggested kitchen gadgets will make preparation seem effortless.

Recipe Key

- Under the listed ingredients you will see preparation instructions for each ingredient. This is helpful because you will not need to read a lengthy preparation description in the body of the recipe while cooking. For example:

INGREDIENTS
1   minced shallot
2   cloves of grated garlic
2   cups of shredded, cooked chicken

- By preparing the ingredients ahead of time, ready for use, this will keep things organized, save time, and reduce mess at the end. It is inefficient to zest a lemon or peel garlic while in the middle of cooking a meal and trying to follow recipe instructions. If you are not familiar with various preparation terms and methods used throughout the book, such as sauteing, folding, mincing, etc. Please see the Common Culinary Terms Guide for reference (page 321).

- With each recipe there will be a list of recommended tools or kitchen gadgets. Some recipes require a specific gadget because many people may not have the culinary skills. Many novice cooks have not acquired the skill or patience for perfecting the thinness of a crepe. Nor is it to efficient to batch cook a large quantity. For example, the various wraps and tortilla recipes in this cookbook require a pizzelle or waffle cone maker to bake them evenly and quickly. These gadgets are also useful when avoiding fats, as minimal oil is needed for recipes. There is also a separate kitchen gadget guide on (page 29)

- You may see ingredients with an (*) next to them. This denotes a special instruction or dietary note is recommended. These notes may provide information, alternative ingredients, complementary recipes (with page numbers), or describe the type of legal ingredient needed. These notes are in the recipe, so you do not need to flip to a separate appendix or index page for details.

- Each recipe will include an approximate yield (serving). The number of servings differ per recipe and are oftentimes larger than needed for a given dish. This is purposely done to allow for leftovers to be frozen, dehydrated and stored for later use. Since SCD requires scratch-made sauces, and spices these multi-faceted recipes can be complicated. Therefore, storing extra servings will reduce time when the recipe is recommended in an accompanying meal plan.

- Estimated preparation (prep) times and total times are provided for time management. Most recipes don't require lengthy preparation (especially if an ingredient was previously cooked and stored for later use). However, some recipes require long marinating, soaking, slow cooking, dehydrating or refrigeration times. The estimated times allow you to plan appropriately.

- All recipes follow the imperial form of measurement commonly found in the US, which uses units such as teaspoons, tablespoons, and cups. However, liquid, frozen or a canned food may include weights in (oz) to help you determine the size needed.

- Within the recipe, tips and tricks may be suggested to improve preparation or flavor of the foods.

- More complex recipes may be broken into sections. For example, a cake may have a separate ingredient list and directions for the cake batter and the frosting. This keeps a recipe organized.

- All recipe directions are numbered in order and listed in short form writing, so you do not need to decipher important steps amid lengthy descriptions.

Levels of Cooking Experience

The recipes should all be approachable for the beginner to intermediate home cook, which is why several types of kitchen gadgets are recommended if someone lacks the necessary culinary skills. Also, there are reminders in the instructions to taste food as you go. Many people do not feel confident or lack experience in adding ingredients "to taste," which is why directions and listed ingredients will have prompts or reminders for the cook.

Estimated Macros

Each recipe includes an estimated macronutrient count; carbohydrates (C), proteins (P) and fats (F). Each are measured in grams and allows for easy entry in a nutrition tracker. However, since ingredients used may differ in nutrition, and the various nutrition trackers are not foolproof, they can only be an approximation.

Modular Meals

The recipes and meal prep are designed to be done in a modular system. This means you can enjoy a variety of unique dishes at each meal, even if they contain the same ingredients and nutritional content. This allows for variety and prevents boredom eating the same flavors over the course of three days. This is a common practice among athletes who need to follow a strict meal plan. For example, a bodybuilder may cook 2- 3 lbs. of ground beef as part of meal prep but divides the amount into three different flavors with seasoning or sauces: taco seasoning, Korean BBQ sauce, or a spaghetti sauce. This allows for different flavors but still maintains the original protein source and amounts.

"Recipe Stacking" and Using Leftovers

The term recipe stacking is a generic culinary term for serving foods in layers or stacking for presentation. However, this cookbook applies the term for meal planning, where the recipes in the cookbook can be used or "stacked" together to create variety and save time. This is different than modular meals because it doesn't rely on a sauce or spice for adding variety to an ingredient, but rather full recipes. For example, a protein bowl may require several ingredients that are leftovers from a prior meal. The recipes in this book are designed for large quantities and creating leftovers that can be frozen or used later. Also cooking in large quantities reduces the time needed per week for meal preparation. See Recipe "Stacking" Reference (page 315) for additional details.

Meal Planning

The recipes in this cookbook are designed around weekly and monthly meal planning. Chapters and recipes are organized to allow for flexibility based on nutritional and athletic performance needs. For example, an athlete who has an upcoming endurance race generally requires recipes with higher carbohydrate content. Therefore, he or she may want to create a meal plan around foods higher in specific carbohydrates such as squash, legumes, honey and fruits. The athlete may want to prepare recipes for that week to "carb load" such as Butternut Squash, Sage and Chicken White Lasagna (page 249), Best Mashed No-Tatoes (page 211), No Bake Lemon Coconut Cookie Dough (page 81) etc. For more information on strategies and simplifying meal planning review Meal Planning and Preparation page 35 for further details.

Time and Money Saving Tips and Tricks

Everyone is looking for ways to save time and money, especially an athlete who needs to balance, the responsibilities of work, home and training. Here are a list of tips and tricks to help ease the process of meal prepping based on recipes from this cookbook:

- Mirepoix is the culinary term for a mixture of diced vegetables commonly used in soups, and stews. The classic Mirepoix is made with equal parts onion, celery and carrots. Oftentimes you can find prepackaged fresh mirepoix in stores. However, buying these vegetables in bulk, dicing, and freezing in specified portions for later use will save you time and money in the long run.

- Making your own alternative flours is easier than you think. Generally, nut flours are convenient to buy in bulk these days. However vegetable and legume flours come in smaller portions and are not the most cost effective. You just need a few kitchen gadgets like a high-powered blender, an oven or dehydrator to make your own flour. There are recipes in this cookbook on how to make alternative flour.

- Buying fresh foods in bulk, especially fruits and vegetables when in season, i.e. squashes, peppers, tomatoes, apples etc. are often cost effective. Cooking, and/or freezing fruits and vegetables allow you to use them later. Just label and follow all long-term storage and canning instructions under the USDA guidelines.

- Portioning and storing citrus fruits are easy using silicone freezer trays. For example, a recipe may call for the zest and juice of one lemon. Zest one lemon and pour the juice over it in a freezer cube or ice tray. Remove the perfect portioned cubes and store in freezer bags for later use.

- Many of the recipes in this book freeze well such as casseroles or smoothies. When it is opportunistic during meal prep, either divide or double some of the recipes to be frozen and used for later.

- Freezing SCD yogurt is easy using silicone freezer trays or cubes. Once the yogurt is frozen into cubes, they can be removed, and the portions stored in freezer bag for later use in sauces and dishes. The higher the fat content the better they freeze and defrost.

- If you live with someone or share groceries, start a shared grocery list. You can easily add one to your phone either using an app or a shared notes function. Listing out common staples ahead of time helps create an organized checklist. As the week progresses and you find you are missing an ingredient, add it to the shared list so everyone can keep track.

- Several of the sauces in this cookbook freeze well. Generally, if there are leftover servings of sauce, they can be frozen for use in another recipe.

- Marinading in bulk is very useful for meal prep. For example, if you buy a large boneless pork shoulder it is easy to cut the meat into smaller portions and marinade it in freezer bags using different sauces or spices. Then you can freeze the different bags for another week of meals.

- Sheet pan meals have become very popular in recent years because preparation is generally easy, and clean-up is a breeze. There are several recipes in this cookbook that only require one sheet pan and the meals can be portioned out for eating or freezing throughout the week.

- For the certain training fuel or on the go recipes, it makes sense to dehydrate or freeze into smaller portions. Most athletes will likely not use an entire batch of gel fuel in one week. Note that some recipes with high fat content will not dehydrate well or reconstitute with the same texture.

- It is not uncommon when buying fresh herbs or chili peppers from the store to have extra amounts. By dehydrating and freezing leftover fresh herbs or chili peppers this helps to prevent waste and use for later. For example, a recipe generally does not need sixteen chili peppers, so by chopping up the extras, one can dehydrate them and grind to make chili powder. Please note there are specific storage instructions for various dehydrated foods. (Follow USDA guidelines for proper storage).

- For extra onions, radishes, daikon, and cabbage from a recipe, these can be quick pickled for use in other recipes. For food safety, quick pickled vegetables should be refrigerated and eaten within the week. For long term canning refer to the USDA guidelines on canning recommendations and instructions.

- Since nut milks and nuts are often a staple ingredient in the Specific Carbohydrate Diet, buying nuts in bulk and when on sale can be cost effective. Nuts can also be frozen dry in freezer bags to help prevent mold from forming.

- Certain desserts with higher fat content or made with honey often don't freeze solid, such as lemon curd. Therefore, they are perfect for freezing, and scooping out portions to be used as needed.

Kitchen Tools & Gadgets

Today there are many kitchen gadgets and tools to make cooking easier and faster. From programmable pressure cookers to multi-functional air fryers, there are tools to do it all. These tools are oftentimes essential to the novice home cook who hasn't mastered various cooking techniques, or the busy athlete who doesn't have hours to prepare meals. This following is a list of gadgets and kitchen tools that are suggested but not required. The tools annotated with an (*) asterisk are used in various recipes and without them you may require advanced culinary skills or alternative cooking methods. The **bold** items are necessary for several recipes in this cookbook and recommend adding to your kitchen.

- **Immersion or handheld blender with attachments***
- Food processor*
- Parchment paper
- **Pizzelle press or Waffle cone maker/ press***
- High powered blender*
- Dehydrator
- **Half gallon or (2) quart size fine mesh or cloth yogurt strainers with lids***
- Vacuum food sealer
- Heat resistant meat masher/mincing tool*
- Ice cream maker or high-powered ice cream blender (Ninja Creami) *
- **Multi-functional air fryer***
- Pots and pans of various sizes
- 4-5 Quart round enamel cast iron Dutch oven
- Sharp knives of assorted sizes
- Crockpot/Slow cooker*
- **Programmable multi-functional pressure cooker (Instant pot)***
- Standing mixer or electric hand mixer*
- **Freezer storage cubes or trays***
- Cooking tongs
- Cast iron skillet
- Nut milk maker
- Juicer
- Waffle iron*
- Muffin and bread tins or silicone baking trays (both standard and mini sized) *
- **3-4-inch diameter bun tins or silicone baking trays***
- Pizza stone

- Cutting board
- Baking sheets with edges*
- Flour sifter
- Rolling pin
- **Cheese grater with varying sizes (coarse to micro in size) ***
- Heat safe spatula and mixing spoons
- Colander both large and fine mesh*
- Airtight storage containers that are freezer, heat and dishwasher safe
- Plastic wrap
- Freezer or storage bags with zip-top
- Aluminum foil
- Vegetable peelers
- Popsicle freezer trays or molds
- Sparkling or carbonated water maker
- Vegetable spiral slicer*
- Panini press
- Electric churro, empanada or donut makers
- Crust cutter and pincher

Hygiene and General Food Safety

When following an elimination diet and watching for symptoms of gastric distress, it is important to practice good hygiene and follow general food safety guidelines. For example, if you experience gastric distress or other gastrointestinal symptoms, this could be due to cross contamination. Regrettably, in an elimination diet you might assume it was a specific type of food and not harmful bacteria that caused it.

Athletes may be at a slightly increased risk of food poisoning as high intensity training and travel impacts their immune system. There are countless stories of traveling athletes and teams succumbing to gastrointestinal distress either from unsafe food preparation, improperly stored foods and prepared meals. Also, many athletes travel with prepared food, packed in personal ice chests or insulated cooler backpacks. Unfortunately, this food can be compromised in checked luggage, vehicles or hot climates.

Basic hand washing is the first step in preventing food borne illnesses and cross contamination in the kitchen. Always wash hands before, during and after preparing foods, especially when handling raw poultry, meat and seafood, or any of their juices. Wash hands with warm water and a generous quantity of soap. Then lather and scrub for 20- 40 seconds, and rinse thoroughly under running water. Dry your hands with a clean towel or paper towel.

In this book you may see the use of food grade latex gloves suggested among the kitchen equipment for recipes with the direct handling of raw meat as a secondary precaution. There may also be directions to change out utensils or have ingredients ready in separate dishwasher safe ramekins or bowls. Instructions may include secondary reminders about cooking meat well. Using meat thermometers and water to help steam or cook foods thoroughly without losing moisture or flavor.

Knives, cutting boards, and other utensils used when preparing raw meats must be thoroughly washed with soapy hot water before using again. Avoid preparing vegetables in areas or with shared utensils where raw meat was handled. Professional kitchens will often color-code their boards and utensils to avoid cross-contamination.

In this book there are also notes and guidance suggesting long-term food storage. Frozen foods should always be labeled with the type of food, whether it is precooked or raw, and the date the food was prepared. This is important since many dishes use the leftovers or excess amounts for other recipes. Important to note, none of the recipes in this book follow pickling or canning guidelines for long term storage. All quick pickled food recipes should be refrigerated and consumed quickly within days of preparation.

Unfortunately, there are countless videos and cooking shows that do not follow safe food preparation practices and is often a disservice to novice cooks. It is especially important for those with underlying gastrointestinal issues to follow safe handling and food preparation guidelines. When in doubt always refer to the USDA and other government guidelines for best practices when preparing or storing food.

The SCD Athlete's Kitchen & Pantry

The ingredients in your kitchen and pantry are only limited based on the legal foods under the Specific Carbohydrate Diet. However, the legal food list has enormous variety and so the only other limiting factor is your personal tolerance to various legal foods. The list below is only an example, based on the various recipes in this cookbook and to help with shopping for ingredients. It is not limited to other SCD legal foods that you tolerate. Note, if an ingredient has an * this indicates special instructions or information.

Vegetables

Butternut squash
Pumpkin
Beets
Carrots
Green beans
Acorn squash
Tomatoes
Onion
Mushrooms
Leeks
Heart of palm
Artichoke hearts
Eggplant
Bell peppers
Cabbage
Zucchini
Yellow squash
Green peas
Snow peas

Brussel sprouts
Fresno or red chilis
Celery
Cucumber
Green onions
Daikon
Radishes
Lettuces
Ginger
Jalapenos
Snap peas
Broccoli
Cauliflower and cauliflower rice
Spaghetti squash
Garlic
Thai chili peppers
Shallots
*Any SCD legal vegetable not listed

Fruit

Bananas
Dates
Blueberries (frozen or fresh)
Cherries (frozen or fresh)
Lemons
Dried fruits (i.e. raisins, prunes, unsweetened cranberries, mangos)
Watermelon
Oranges
Apples
Pears

Grapes
Limes
Pineapple
Avocados
Prunes
Nectarines
Persimmons
Mandarins
Mango (frozen or fresh)
Peaches
*Any SCD legal fruit not listed

Sweetener
Honey
Date syrup with no added sweeteners

*Granulated honey

Pantry
Dried peas (yellow or green)
Dried black beans
Dried lentils (red)
Coconut flour
Almond flour
Hazelnut flour
Pecan flour
Walnut flour
Squash flour
*Canned pumpkin
*Canned butternut squash
*Canned tomatoes
*Tomato paste
*Vegetable flour
*SCD legal lentil or yellow pea pastas
Dried egg whites
Dried whole eggs
*Yellow split pea flour (see recipe)

Baking soda
Vanilla extract
Almond extract
Coconut extract
Fine ground (powdered)
espresso
Flaked unsweetened
coconut
Shredded unsweetened
coconut
* Unsweetened, unflavored
beef or bone broth
protein powder
*Unflavored, unsweetened
collagen
Vanilla beans
Unflavored gelatin
*Tamari sauce

Dairy/ Dairy Alternatives
Non-fat SCD Greek yogurt
Aged cheeses
(i.e. cheddar, parmesan cotija,
monterey jack) .

*Various nut milks

Protein
Lean ground beef
Lean ground bison
Chicken
Lean ground pork
Beef tri-tip trimmed of fat
Lean, no sugar bacon
Eggs
*Pasteurized SCD legal egg whites
Frozen or fresh, raw or cooked shrimp
Frozen or fresh cod filets
Frozen or fresh salmon filets
Ground Turkey

Fats
SCD legal nut butters
Nuts
Butter
Ghee
Full-fat SCD yogurt
Unsweetened coconut milk
Cacao butter
Coconut butter
Coconut oil
Coconut butter

Spices

Granulated garlic
Granulated onion
Dried minced onions
Dried minced garlic
Paprika
Cumin
Chinese five spice
Salt
Pepper
Curry powder
Cayenne powder
Cinnamon
Ground cardamon
Chili powder
Dried chives
Dried parsley
Dried Rosemary
Ground sage
Ground cloves
Allspice
Chipotle
Dried basil
Sesame seeds
Dried saffron

Ground turmeric
Dried cilantro
Dried thyme
Celery salt
Smoked paprika
Bay leaves
Poppy seeds
Mustard seed
Sumac
Ground nutmeg
Ground ginger
Dried dill weed
Ground white pepper
Dried oregano
Dried marjoram
Dried lemongrass
Ground mace
Caraway seeds
Coriander
Fennel seeds
Dill Seeds

*Unflavored beef (bovine) protein should only be beef or bone broth without any additives or other ingredients. Confirm ingredients and processing with manufacturer or make from scratch with a food dehydrator. If necessary omit and/or substitute in recipes.

*Unflavored collagen powders should be animal based, not contain seaweed, anti-caking agents, sweeteners, added probiotics, and/or cellulose. Always confirm ingredients with the manufacturer, or omit and/or substitute in recipes.

*Granulated honey, dried honey made with coconut flour. Does not contain cornstarch or illegal anti-caking ingredients.

*Vegetable flours are generally SCD legal vegetables dehydrated and ground to flour. These can be made at home with a dehydrator and high-powered blender. Or if commercially made the ingredients and processing need to be verified with the manufacturer.

*Be careful to read all ingredients for pasteurized liquid egg whites. This should be a mono ingredient, and not contain any preservatives or additional ingredients.

*Lentil or yellow pea pasta should be purchased from an SCD reputable company such as Wellbees, and/or verify ingredients and manufacturing follows SCD guidelines. Note these pastas can also be made at home.

*One of the main reasons canned tomatoes and other canned vegetables are considered illegal under the Specific Carbohydrate Diet is due to the possible deception in food labeling. However labeling laws have improved since the original publication of Elaine Gottschall's book Breaking the Vicious Cycle. For some countries (specifically Italy) there are labeling laws, requiring every ingredient is listed, even in trace amounts. However commonly canned vegetables such as pumpkin, butternut squash and tomatoes still require confirmation of ingredients and manufacturing processes before consuming. Substitute with fresh or frozen cooked vegetables as needed.

*Check the labels of the tamari, many will list rice wine vinegar and other ingredients which may be illegal when following SCD. Tamari should generally be gluten free, grain free, and sugar free. For example, tamari includes only water, organic soybeans, salt and/or organic alcohol (as part of fermentation process). Or see recipe for "No Soy Sauce" as a substitute.

Dehydrated Foods

Dried and dehydrated foods, not properly rehydrated before eating can cause gas, bloating and general gastrointestinal distress. In many of the recipes, especially using dried fruits, it is recommended to steep them in warm water. This is to prevent them from rehydrating and fermenting in your gut. Certain alternative flours, such as vegetable or pea flours are recommended in small quantities (i.e., cutting the amount of nut flours in baked goods, and used for dredging meats before frying or baking). It is also best to increase the moisture content in various recipes if lentil, pea or squash flour is used. If consuming dehydrated foods, avoid eating when performing physical activity unless the food is properly rehydrated. As they can be dehydrating to the gastrointestinal tract and digest too slowly.

Organizational Tips for the SCD Kitchen

When starting a new diet or regimen a best practice is to restock and refresh your refrigerator, pantry and freezer. Here are some tips for your kitchen:

- When checking your spice cabinet, look carefully at premade spice mixtures, many contain illegal ingredients under the Specific Carbohydrate Diet (SCD) such as sugars, and anti-caking ingredients. It is always best practice to buy single ingredient seasonings and create your own mixtures. This cookbook has a whole section of recipes dedicated to seasonings.

- Organizing a pantry based on type of staple prevents buying duplicates. It also helps keep track of foods soon to expire. For example, staples such as alternative (non-grain) flours can be grouped together, snacks, or other baking ingredients. Items soon to expire can be moved to the front of shelves so they are used first.

- Foods bought or prepared in bulk should be labeled and dated, along with any spice mixtures you make. Purchasing food grade silica gel desiccant packets for dried or dehydrated foods will help prevent spoilage due to moisture. Vacuum sealing foods will prolong shelf life and prevent freezer burn.

- It is helpful to dedicate an extra meal prep day per month for certain bulk food staples such as cooked legumes, pea flour, spice mixtures, and/or SCD yogurt. This will streamline and improve efficiency when cooking throughout the month.

- Organize kitchen by how often you use a tool or gadget. For example, if a programmable pressure cooker is used once a week for making yogurt, place it in a convenient spot. This may mean moving the juicer that you use once a month to another cabinet, closet or finished basement.

- If you have a dedicated freezer for storage, use large, color-coded bags or storage baskets to group different types of foods, as too often freezer foods become buried. For example, put all protein sources in a red storage basket, and all frozen vegetables in a green basket.

Meal Planning and Preparation

Meal planning is a strategy used by athletes to ensure their nutritional needs are met, save money and allow more time for training. Training for competitive sports, especially for adults balancing a career, or family life, it can feel like a second or third job for many. Parents of teen and young adult athletes may struggle with cooking for their athlete who has special dietary requirements. Therefore, meal planning is necessary to reduce time spent in the kitchen.

Since the Specific Carbohydrate Diet (SCD) is primarily based on fresh, whole foods with minimal additives or preservatives, there are few commercially available convenience foods. Even fewer for the competitive athlete. Therefore, preparing meals and foods from scratch is necessary. Meal planning reduces the amount of time in the kitchen and allows more time for training and recovery.

Meal Planning Made Simple

Once an athlete knows their nutritional macronutrient needs and training schedule, meal planning becomes simpler. For example, a male competitive athlete determined he needs 170 grams of protein, 226 grams of carbohydrates, and 76 grams of fat. His goal is to eat 6 meals a day, scheduled around his two sessions of training: 1 session for strength training, and 1 session for endurance or cardiovascular training per day. His plan is to eat an average of 28 grams of protein, 37 grams of carbohydrates and 12 grams of fat per meal. However, based on his training schedule he may want to increase his protein after strength training and increase carbohydrates before cardiovascular training.

The athlete's meal plan for a day may look like:

Meal 1 Aloha Bowl or Blender waffles with banana and nut butter
Meal 2 Butternut squash breakfast casserole
Meal 3 Lean flank steak, sautéed cabbage, and carrots
Meal 4 Apple slices, nut butter, and chicken bone broth soup
Meal 5 (SCD legal) Lentil pasta with baked chicken thighs and broccoli
Meal 6 (SCD legal) Non-fat Greek yogurt with berry compote and nut granola or nut butter

If he needs training fuel, then he may add a portable food or exercise fuel that meets his training needs. For example, if he has a long-distance run planned for the weekend, he may cook a batch of Peanut Butter Cookie Gel (see recipe page 79) and store for later use in the week.

The volume of each food will be based on his macro nutritional need and measured out ahead using a scale or measuring cups. Protein sources, main dishes, yogurt, baked goods, sauces and cooked vegetables can be prepared ahead. Fresh fruits or frozen vegetables can be quickly cut or cooked with minimal effort the day needed.

Generally, the athlete will prepare his meals Sunday and eat the same foods for a week. However, to add variety, he plans to use SCD legal sauces and various spice mixes to prevent meal monotony, such as cooking the flank steak with 2-3 different seasoning blends or low-fat marinades. He may also change the order of the meals during the day to trick his tastebuds, such as swapping Meal 1 for Meal 6. Or eating different fruits with the yogurt and protein pancakes.

These are just a couple strategies commonly used by athletes who need to follow a strict dietary regimen or for athletes who just don't want to spend time in the kitchen.

A Friday & Sunday Strategy

Some SCD foods or recipes require lengthier preparation. For example, SCD yogurt requires a 24-hour fermentation process, and SCD legal legumes require 12+ hours of soaking before cooking. Therefore, starting yogurt and soaking beans on Friday is ideal. Adopting a Friday and Sunday meal preparation routine helps relieve the cook and reduces preparation time. However, you are not limited to these specific days of the week. Instead select meal preparation days based on individual schedules and on training rest days. Fridays and Sundays are only suggested because many athletes use these days as training rest days. Especially if they have a competitive event scheduled for a Saturday.

Big Batches and Staples

When meal planning, it is not uncommon to select a specific day of the month to batch cook or prepare a large volume of food. Especially foods that are regular staples in one's diet, and store well long term in the freezer. There are several recipes in this cookbook annotated as "large batch" or "bulk" to reduce time in the kitchen throughout the month. For example, honey lemon curd, chewy peanut butter cookies, marshmallows, breads and buns, roasted chicken bone broth etc. All freeze well long term for use as needed.

There is also a chapter dedicated to freezer meals and slow cooker recipes. As a strategy, preparing freezer meals ahead of time will greatly reduce the amount of time in the kitchen on a weekly basis. Also, if you find yourself hosting guests or limited on time for weekly meal prep, these freezer and slow cooker meals can work in a pinch. However, carving out one day a month for batch cooking doesn't always work for everyone. Instead, some athletes select one large bulk recipe and prepare it along with their existing weekly meal plan. This ensures the athlete always has a freezer meal or staple food at the ready without spending an extra day in the kitchen.

10 Easy Strategies for Weekly Meal Preparation

Here are some easy strategies to follow when creating a meal plan and preparing foods on a weekly basis:

1. Make one sauce or dressing from scratch that can be used to flavor a variety of dishes.

2. Make one freezer meal or staple food; For example, chicken fajitas and pumpkin wraps both can be made in bulk and frozen for later use.

3. Refill or mix 1-2 spices or herb blends.

4. Cook your protein sources in bulk, such as roast chicken, ground beef, ground turkey etc., but divide them based on desired spices, marinades or sauces to create variety. (If you prefer freshly cooked meat throughout the week, then marinate and/or freeze in separate bags for easy day of preparation).

5. Keep a variety of frozen vegetables that can easily be steamed, air fried, sautéed or roasted throughout the week or day of preparation.

6. Soak legumes on a Friday or two days before meal prepping to cut preparation time.

7. Make SCD yogurt two days before a weekly meal preparation day to allow for 24-hour fermentation and dripping the yogurt. (See recipe on page 298 for more details)

8. Grate large batches of SCD legal blocks of cheese and freeze for later use.

9. Prepare two breakfast recipes, one sweeter and one savory to ensure variety.

10. Make one sweet treat or training fuel recipe a week, since many freeze well and make excellent portable foods in a pinch.

Another Athlete Example

Let's consider another example, this time with a female competitive athlete nearing her competition date. She needs to eat the same foods each day because she knows these are her "safe foods" and wants to stay consistent this week. She needs to consume 120 grams of protein, 160 grams of carbohydrates and 53 grams of fat. She trains 6 days a week (on a de-load strength training plan), one session per day so she does not need as many meals as the prior example of the male athlete.

Her meal plan for a day may look like:

Meal 1 SCD Grain-free protein pancakes with ripe banana and nut butter
Meal 2 Ground turkey sausage, egg white bake, and mashed lentils
Meal 3 SCD Chicken paella and roasted butternut squash
Meal 4 Non-fat or low fat SCD Greek yogurt with berry compote
Meal 5 Lean ground beef tacos with bell peppers and onions, served with pumpkin street tortillas and avocado

She will measure out the quantities for each meal with a scale and log in a tracker to ensure she is meeting her daily macronutrient goal. For her competition she will bring her meals with her and plans to have SCD Coconut Marshmallows, fruit, non-sweetened electrolyte water and salt on hand as a quick secondary source of fuel and electrolytes between competitive heats.

A Boring Palette = Easier Weekly Meal Preparation

One of the best attributes of competitive athletes is they can tolerate boredom well, both in training and their diet. For example, a powerlifter or swimmer is performing repetitive movements each day to perfect their technique, building either endurance and/or strength. Many athletes, especially ones with gastrointestinal issues, will use this same strategy for their nutrition.

They are highly focused on consistency and therefore not uncommon for them to eat the same foods each week, especially when leading up to a competition, as in the example of the female athlete. When you tolerate the same meals or foods every day well, then this makes meal preparation easier. If you truly need more variety but want to avoid a long day in the kitchen weekly, set aside one day in the month to prepare bulk freezer meals that can be easily cooked in a crockpot or baked. This will reduce the number of foods to prepare weekly and provide more variety.

See a few of the example meal plans for weekly inspiration and preparation.

Example 1

EXAMPLE MEAL PLAN		Monday	Tuesday	Wednesday	Thursday	Friday	Saturday	Sunday
*The volume of meals and types can be reduced, increased or changed as needed	Training Routine	Training	Training	Training	Training	Deload Training Day	Long Training Day, Race or Competition	Training Rest Day
	Volume of Cooking	Minimal or No Cooking	Minimal or No Cooking	Minimal or No Cooking	Minimal or No Cooking	Pre- Meal Prep Day	Minimal or No Cooking	Meal Prep Day
Number of Meals*	Types of Meals*							
Meal 1	Pre training Breakfast	Pumpkin Spice Protein Sheet Pan Pancakes with ripe banana and nut butter	Pumpkin Spice Protein Sheet Pan Pancakes with ripe banana and nut butter	Pumpkin Spice Protein Sheet Pan Pancakes with ripe banana and nut butter	Pumpkin Spice Protein Sheet Pan Pancakes with ripe banana and nut butter	Pumpkin Spice Protein Sheet Pan Pancakes with ripe banana and nut butter	Pumpkin Spice Protein Sheet Pan Pancakes with ripe banana and nut butter	Cauliflower Cream of No Wheat
Meal 2	Breakfast or Brunch	Sage & Turkey Breakfast sausage, and Green Eggs & "Ham" Sheet Pan Egg Bake	Sage & Turkey Breakfast sausage, and Green Eggs & "Ham" Sheet Pan Egg Bake	Sage & Turkey Breakfast sausage, and Green Eggs & "Ham" Sheet Pan Egg Bake	Sage & Turkey Breakfast sausage, and Green Eggs & "Ham" Sheet Pan Egg Bake	Sage & Turkey Breakfast sausage, and Green Eggs & "Ham" Sheet Pan Egg Bake	Sage & Turkey Breakfast sausage, and Green Eggs & "Ham" Sheet Pan Egg Bake	Butternut Choriz-No Mexican Breakfast Casserole
Meal 3	Lunch	SCD Chcken Paella with roasted butternut squash	SCD Chcken Paella with roasted butternut squash	SCD Chcken Paella with roasted butternut squash	SCD Chcken Paella with roasted butternut squash	SCD Chcken Paella with roasted butternut squash	SCD Chcken Paella with roasted butternut squash	Loaded Turkey and Veggie Spaghetti sauce with lentil pasta
Meal 4	Pre Training, Light Lunch or Snack	Non-fat SCD Greek Yogurt with Berry Compote	Non-fat SCD Greek Yogurt with Berry Compote	Non-fat SCD Greek Yogurt with Berry Compote	Non-fat SCD Greek Yogurt with Berry Compote	Non-fat SCD Greek Yogurt with Berry Compote	Non-fat SCD Greek Yogurt with Berry Compote	N/A (Non Training Day)
Meal 5	Dinner	Lean ground beef or bison Tacos with bell peppers and onion, and Pumpkin Street Tortillas with avocado	Lean ground beef or bison Tacos with bell peppers and onion, and Pumpkin Street Tortillas with avocado	Lean ground beef or bison Tacos with bell peppers and onion, and Pumpkin Street Tortillas with avocado	Lean ground beef or bison Tacos with bell peppers and onion, and Pumpkin Street Tortillas with avocado	Lean ground beef or bison Tacos with bell peppers and onion, and Pumpkin Street Tortillas with avocado	Lean ground beef or bison Tacos with bell peppers and onion, and Pumpkin Street Tortillas with avocado	Moo Shu Pork (or Chicken) with Plum Sauce
Training Fuel or Portable Foods						SCD Coconut Marshmallows	SCD Coconut Marshmallows	N/A (Non Training Day)
Batch Cooking/Pre-Prep						Soak Yellow Peas Start Non-Fat SCD Yogurt	Slow Cook Yellow Peas & Mash Drip Non-Fat SCD Yogurt	Asian Style Green Onion Wraps

PRIOR WEEK MEAL PREP	Preparation	PRIOR WEEK MEAL PREP	Preparation	PRIOR WEEK MEAL PREP	Preparation
Pumpkin Spice Protein Sheet Pan Pancakes	Once a week	SCD Coconut Marshmallows	Once a month	Roasted butternut squash (air fried)	Day of Meal
Sage & Turkey Breakfast sausage	Once a week	Pumpkin Street Tortillas	Once a month	Avocado	Day of Meal
Green Eggs & "Ham" Sheet Pan Egg Bake	Once a week			Fresh fruit	Day of Meal
Berry Compote	Once a week				
Lean Ground Beef Taco with onions and bell peppers	Once a week				
SCD Chcken Paella	Once a week				
SCD Non-Fat Yogurt	Once a week				

Example 2

EXAMPLE MEAL PLAN		Monday	Tuesday	Wednesday	Thursday	Friday	Saturday	Sunday
*The volume of meals and types can be reduced, increased or changed as needed	Training Routine	Training	Training	Training	Training	Deload Training Day	Long Training Day, Race or Competition	Training Rest Day
	Volume of Cooking	Minimal or No Cooking	Minimal or No Cooking	Minimal or No Cooking	Minimal or No Cooking	Pre- Meal Prep Day	Minimal or No Cooking	Meal Prep Day
Number of Meals*	Types of Meals*							
Meal 1	Pre training Breakfast	Pina Colada Protein Sheet Pan Pancakes	Cinnamon Bun Banana Muffins	Pina Colada Protein Sheet Pan Pancakes	Cinnamon Bun Banana Muffins	Pina Colada Protein Sheet Pan Pancakes	Cinnamon Bun Banana Muffins	Lemon Poppyseed Sheet Pan Protein Pancakes
Meal 2	Breakfast or Brunch	Sheet Pan "Combination" Sausage Egg Bake	Dad's Zucchini and Mushroom Frittata	Sheet Pan "Combination" Sausage Egg Bake	Dad's Zucchini and Mushroom Frittata	Sheet Pan "Combination" Sausage Egg Bake	Dad's Zucchini and Mushroom Frittata	Stuffed Breakfast Squash
Meal 3	Lunch	Sweet & Spicy Cowboy Chicken snd Air Fried Butternut Squash "Tots"	SCD Paleo Zuppa Toscano	Sweet & Spicy Cowboy Chicken snd Air Fried Butternut Squash "Tots"	SCD Paleo Zuppa Toscano	Sweet & Spicy Cowboy Chicken snd Air Fried Butternut Squash "Tots"	SCD Paleo Zuppa Toscano	Tandoori Chicken with Smoked Curry Pea Salad
Meal 4	Pre Training, Light Lunch or Snack	Savory Loaded No-Tato Chaffles	Ripe Banana and Nut Butter Wrapped in Stroopwaffel (Pumpkin Sweet Wraps)	Savory Loaded No-Tato Chaffles	Ripe Banana and Nut Butter Wrapped in Stroopwaffel (Pumpkin Sweet Wraps)	Savory Loaded No-Tato Chaffles	Ripe Banana and Nut Butter Wrapped in Stroopwaffel (Pumpkin Sweet Wraps)	N/A (Non Training Day)
Meal 5	Dinner	Yellow Pea Wraps, Gyro or Döner Meat, Döner Kebab White Garlic Sauce, Pickled Cabbage	Slow Cooker Chicken Tikka Masala	Yellow Pea Wraps, Gyro or Döner Meat, Döner Kebab White Garlic Sauce, Pickled Cabbage	Slow Cooker Chicken Tikka Masala	Yellow Pea Wraps, Gyro or Döner Meat, Döner Kebab White Garlic Sauce, Pickled Cabbage	Slow Cooker Chicken Tikka Masala	SCD Chicken Paella
Meal 6	Sweet Snack or Dessert	Vanilla Bean "Froyo" Tacos	SCD Coconut Marshmallows	Vanilla Bean "Froyo" Tacos	SCD Coconut Marshmallows	Vanilla Bean "Froyo" Tacos	SCD Coconut Marshmallows	Chewy and Soft Peanut Butter Cookies (Large Batch)
Training Fuel or Portable Foods						No Bake Lemon Coconut Cookie Dough	No Bake Lemon Coconut Cookie Dough	N/A (Non Training Day)
Batch Cooking/Pre-Prep						Soak Yellow Peas Start Non-Fat SCD Yogurt Cowboy Candy	Slow Cook Yellow Peas & Mash Drip Non-Fat SCD Yogurt	Yellow Pea Wraps

PRIOR WEEK MEAL PREP	Preparation	PRIOR WEEK MEAL PREP	Preparation	PRIOR WEEK MEAL PREP	Preparation
Pina Colada Protein Sheet Pan Pancakes	Once a week	Cinnamon Bun Banana Muffins	Once a month	Air Fried Butternut Squash "Tots"	Day of Meal
Sheet Pan "Combination" Sausage Egg Bake	Once a week	Savory Loaded No-Tato Chaffles	Once a month	Ripe Banana and Nut Butter	Day of Meal
Dad's Zucchini and Mushroom Frittata	Once a week	Stroopwaffels (Pumpkin Spice Sweet Wraps)	Once a month		
Sweet & Spicy Cowboy Chicken	Once a week	SCD Paleo Zuppa Toscano	Once a month		
Gyro or Döner Meat	Once a week	Yellow Pea Wraps	Once a month		
Döner Kebab White Garlic Sauce	Once a week	SCD Coconut Marshmallows	Once a month		
Pickled Cabbage	Once a week	No Bake Lemon Coconut Cookie Dough	Once a month		
SCD Yogurt (for Froyo)	Once a week				

Example 3

EXAMPLE MEAL PLAN		Monday	Tuesday	Wednesday	Thursday	Friday	Saturday	Sunday
The volume of meals and types can be reduced, increased or changed as needed	Training Routine	Training	Training	Training	Training	Deload Training Day	Long Training Day, Race or Competition	Training Rest Day
	Volume of Cooking	Minimal or No Cooking	Minimal or No Cooking	Minimal or No Cooking	Minimal or No Cooking	Pre- Meal Prep Day	Minimal or No Cooking	Meal Prep Day
Number of Meals*	Types of Meals*							
Meal 1	Pre training Breakfast	Banana Cinnamon Walnut Protein Sheet Pan Pancakes	Aloha Bowl	Banana Cinnamon Walnut Protein Sheet Pan Pancakes	Aloha Bowl	Banana Cinnamon Walnut Protein Sheet Pan Pancakes	Aloha Bowl	Pina Colada Protein Sheet Pan Pancakes
Meal 2	Breakfast or Brunch	Sage & Turkey Breakfast sausage, and Green Eggs & "Ham" Sheet Pan Egg Bake	Butternut Squash Breakfast Casserole	Sage & Turkey Breakfast sausage, and Green Eggs & "Ham" Sheet Pan Egg Bake	Butternut Squash Breakfast Casserole	Sage & Turkey Breakfast sausage, and Green Eggs & "Ham" Sheet Pan Egg Bake	Butternut Squash Breakfast Casserole	Dad's Zucchini and Mushroom Frittata
Meal 3	Lunch	Loaded Turkey and Veggie Spaghetti Sauce with SCD legal lentil noodles	Bison Fried Cauliflower Rice, and Air Fried Korean Sweet and Spicy Chicken Thighs	Loaded Turkey and Veggie Spaghetti Sauce with SCD legal lentil noodles	Bison Fried Cauliflower Rice, and Air Fried Korean Sweet and Spicy Chicken Thighs	Loaded Turkey and Veggie Spaghetti Sauce with SCD legal lentil noodles	Bison Fried Cauliflower Rice, and Air Fried Korean Sweet and Spicy Chicken Thighs	Sweet & Spicy Cowboy Chicken snd Air Fried Butternut Squash "Tots"
Meal 4	Pre Training, Light Lunch or Snack	Blender Beet Waffle with Choice of Nut Butter & Honey	Portable Baked Pasta	Blender Beet Waffle with Choice of Nut Butter & Honey	Portable Baked Pasta	Blender Beet Waffle with Choice of Nut Butter & Honey	Portable Baked Pasta	N/A (Non Training Day)
Meal 5	Dinner	Greek Lemon Butter Crockpot Chicken Roasted Greek Broccoli	SCD Enchilada Soup	Greek Lemon Butter Crockpot Chicken Roasted Greek Broccoli	SCD Enchilada Soup	Greek Lemon Butter Crockpot Chicken Roasted Greek Broccoli	SCD Enchilada Soup	Yellow Pea Wraps, Gyro or Döner Meat, Döner Kebab White Garlic Sauce, Pickled Cabbage
Meal 6	Sweet Snack or Dessert	Apples with Low Fat Caramel Apple Dip	Lemon Curd Froyo Pops	Apples with Low Fat Caramel Apple Dip	Lemon Curd Froyo Pops	Apples with Low Fat Caramel Apple Dip	Lemon Curd Froyo Pops	SCD Coconut Marshmallows
Training Fuel or Portable Foods						Peanut Butter Cookie Gel	Peanut Butter Cookie Gel	N/A (Non Training Day)
Batch Cooking/Pre-Prep						Soak Yellow Peas Start Non-Fat SCD Yogurt Cowboy Candy	Slow Cook Yellow Peas & Mash Drip Non-Fat SCD Yogurt	Yellow Pea Wraps

PRIOR WEEK MEAL PREP	Preparation	PRIOR WEEK MEAL PREP	Preparation	PRIOR WEEK MEAL PREP	Preparation
Banana Cinnamon Walnut Protein Sheet Pan Pancakes	Once a week	Loaded Turkey and Veggie Spaghetti Sauce	Once a month	SCD legal lentil noodles	Day of Meal
Sage & Turkey Breakfast sausage	Once a week	Blender Beet Waffle with Choice of Nut Butter & Honey	Once a month	Roasted Greek Broccoli	Day of Meal
Green Eggs & "Ham" Sheet Pan Egg Bake	Once a week	Greek Lemon Butter Crockpot Chicken	Once a month		
Apples with Low Fat Caramel Apple Dip	Once a week	Butternut Squash Breakfast Casserole	Once a month		
Aloha Bowl	Once a week	Lemon Curd Froyo Pops	Once a month		
Bison Fried Cauliflower Rice	Once a week	Peanut Butter Cookie Gel	Once a month		
Air Fried Korean Sweet and Spicy Chicken Thighs	Once a week	SCD Enchilada Soup	Once a month		
Portable Baked Pasta	Once a week				
SCD Non-Fat Yogurt	Once a week				

Socializing When Following SCD

Sports in general is socializing, and food is often a large part of that...

Brunch after long training runs.

Beers with fellow competitors after celebrating a victory.

Dinners to commemorate a long preparatory season.

Coffees and chatting after exercise classes.

Championship wins include popping champagne bottles.

All are examples of how food and athletic achievements go hand in hand. However, if an athlete is following any restrictive diet for health or performance, sometimes it can be lonely. These post sport activities can pose a particular challenge. Especially if many foods at social events do not follow the diet.

The Specific Carbohydrate Diet (SCD) is not necessarily limited by the athlete, but rather limited by the outside world. Restaurants and even the average food product can have ingredients that the athlete can't eat. In social situations centered on sport, this can feel isolating. Here are some ways to enjoy socializing with fellow competitors, friends and family centered around food.

Pack your own desserts.
Bring celebratory desserts or provide enough servings to share with the group.

Plan for restaurants.
If you know where you'll be celebrating after an event or training, contact the restaurant and confirm legal menu items ahead of time.

Savor your sauces.
Make SCD legal sauces and bring them to an event. Oftentimes you can request for plain or unseasoned meat or vegetables at most events. Not expecting the host to cater to your dietary needs and by having flavorful sauces available make plain foods enjoyable. A best practice is to inform the host as needed.

Common coffee hacks.
When going to coffee, bring a refillable thermos or travel coffee cup with SCD legal flavored nut milk or creamers. Many places will just pour the coffee, tea or espresso directly into the cup or thermos. You can also bring honey sticks or packets to add to sweeten coffees once purchased. Oftentimes unflavored SCD legal collagen can be stored in small to go containers or plastic zip top bags for an added source of protein.

No beer breweries.
Since beer is illegal under SCD, an athlete may suggest breweries and bars that offer non-alcoholic options such as carbonated water and fresh squeezed juice. Or find ones that offer SCD legal alcohol if enjoying a drink with fellow athletes to celebrate a victory.

Socializing with similar athletes.
Some athletes may need to lean out or make weight for their sport. Socializing with other athletes, even competitors, in the same situation helps with loneliness. Oftentimes the Specific Carbohydrate Diet works for many other athletes who are trying to meet the same performance goals. Providing healthy food options, sharing your meals or recipes when socializing may be welcomed by your fellow athletes.

SCD Cooking & Basic Preparation Guidelines to Follow

Yogurt: Ferment for 24 hours at a stable temperature (100–110°F) to remove lactose. (see SCD Instapot Yogurt recipe page 298)

Legumes: Soak for at least 10–12 hours, then drain and boil until tender. Baking soda can be used in the soaking process to break down the skins for digestibility. (see Easy SCD Crockpot Yellow Peas and Beans recipe page 304)

Broths & Stocks: There are very few SCD legal broths and stocks, therefore homemade is ideal. This is to prevent any additives, starches, or MSG. (see Roasted Chicken and Bone Broth recipe page 255)

Fruit Juice: Freshly squeezed juice from SCD legal fruits are allowed, however store-bought juice is often non-compliant since concentrates, sugars and/or possible additives are illegal under SCD food guidelines.

Cheese: Many prepackaged grated and sliced cheeses may contain cellulose, anticaking ingredients, and fillers in the processing of cheese or to extend shelf life. The general rule of legal cheeses are they need to be aged over 3 months, and contain zero carbohydrates or sugars, regarding nutritional content. It is always best to purchase blocks of cheese, and shred or slice yourself.

Canned vegetables: There are several brands of certain canned vegetables that do not contain additives, artificial flavors or preservatives (even in the manufacturing process). Many of these canned product brands are used repeatedly by the SCD community and sold through Wellbees or other natural food stores. However, as a best practice use fresh or frozen vegetables.

Nut Butters & Nut Flours: Must come from SCD-legal nuts (i.e. almonds, cashews, walnuts, and coconuts, etc.). Ensure no additives, preservatives or starches are used in the ingredients or manufacturing process. Recipes vary for homemade nut butters; however, they cannot contain any SCD illegal ingredients or sweeteners other than honey.

The SCD Athlete Cookbook
Recipes

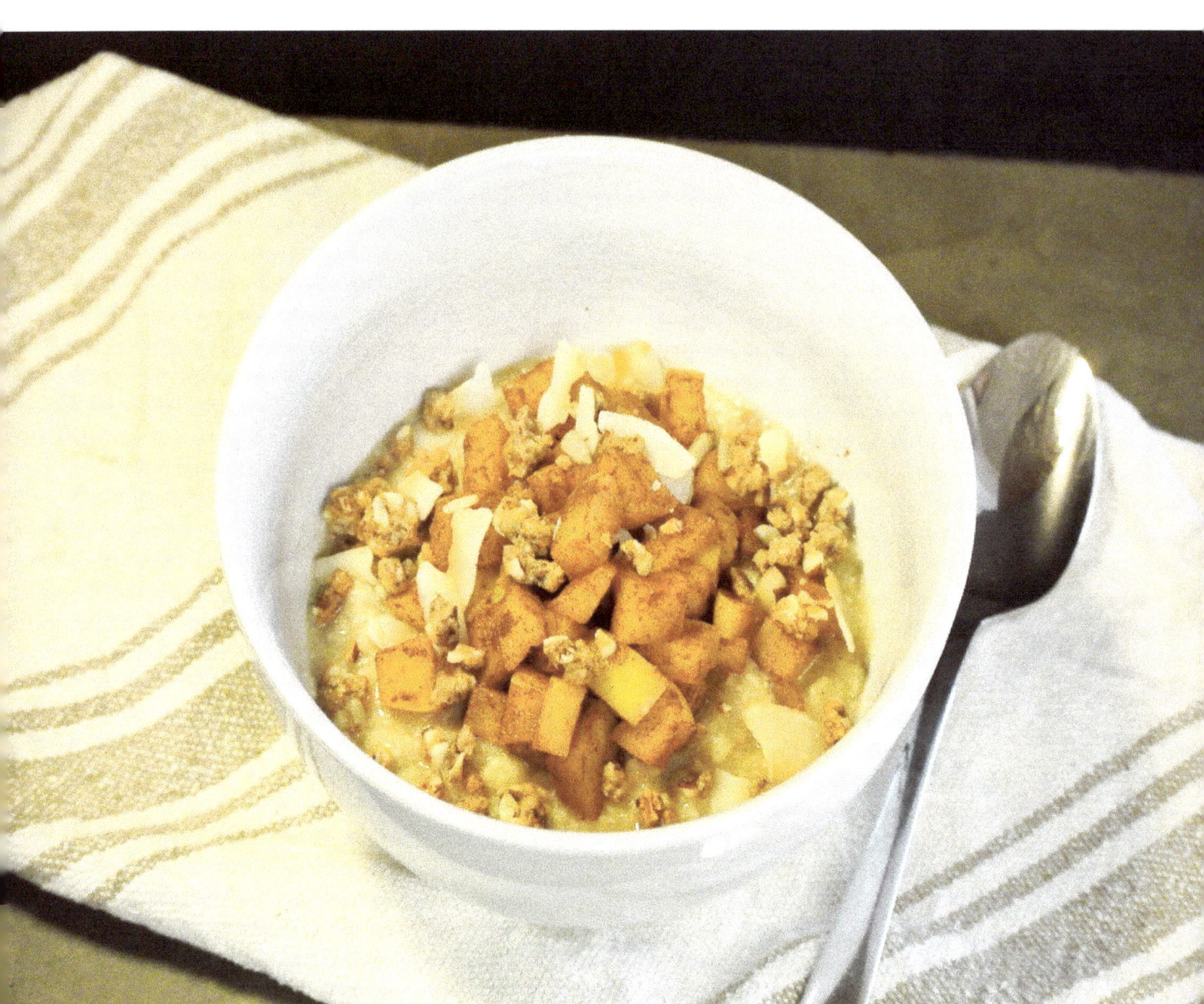

Apple Cinnamon Paleo Porridge

Breakfasts & Baked Goods

Breakfast has always been considered the most important meal of the day because it is the first meal after a night of sleep and by nature fasting. Eating a nutritious breakfast provides the fuel to perform your best, both physically and mentally. Generally, breakfast should include the three macronutrients of protein, carbohydrates, and healthy fats. SCD legal fiber should also be considered as part of a morning meal to promote digestion, increase satiety and regulate blood sugar.

Many breakfasts consist of baked goods, which is convenient since they are portable and quick fuel sources. It is not uncommon for athletes to pair a muffin or bread along with fruit for healthy on-the-go sources of glycogen, especially when early morning training sessions are on their schedule.

Athletes commonly eat two smaller meals for breakfast to ensure they meet their nutritional needs and avoid having to catch up on macronutrients later in the day. Oftentimes breakfast plays the crucial role of a pre-training or post-training recovery meal (if they had trained in a fasted state). This section contains a variety of breakfast, and baked goods recipes focused on macronutrient balance.

Pumpkin Spice Protein Sheet Pan Pancakes

Approximate Yield	Prep Time 20 min	Estimated Macronutrients
10 servings	**Total Time 55 min**	**14 g P • 13 g C • 1 g F**

INGREDIENTS

2 mashed bananas
1 can of pureed pumpkin (15 oz or 2 cups) or butternut squash
1 cup of dried egg white powder or legal egg white protein*
4 teaspoons of honey
2 teaspoons of vanilla extract
3-4 teaspoons of Pumpkin Pie Spice (see recipe page 144)
½ teaspoon baking soda
Pinch of sea salt
1 ½ cups of pasteurized liquid egg whites*
Optional: ¼ cup of unsweetened, unflavored beef or bone broth protein powder*

KITCHEN EQUIPMENT

Immersion blender
Large mixing bowl
Measuring spoons & measuring cups
Spatula or large spoon
Baking sheet/pan or cookie sheet with raised edges
(approximately 9.5 in x 13 in)
Aluminum foil

SPECIAL INSTRUCTIONS/ DIET INFORMATION

*If you are unable to eat the different protein powders, replace with dried egg white powder.
*If you are unable to eat or source dried egg white powder you can replace with almond flour. However it will not rise as high, the texture will be different, and there will be higher fat and less protein for the macronutrients.
*Be careful to read all ingredients for liquid egg whites. This should be a mono ingredient, and not contain any preservatives or additional ingredients. Regular separated egg whites can be used but the batter will be thicker and require many eggs.
*Unflavored beef (bovine) protein should only be beef or bone broth without any additives or other ingredients. Confirm ingredients and processing with manufacturer.

DIRECTIONS

1. Preheat oven to 350 degrees F. Line the baking sheet with aluminum foil ensuring it covers the edges (one large continuous piece is best to prevent leaks). Be careful not to poke any holes or rip the foil. Spray or brush the foil with cooking oil very well, including the sides of the pan covered in foil.
2. In the large mixing bowl, mash the banana and pumpkin together with an immersion blender. Add the remaining ingredients and continue to mix with the blender until all clumps are gone.
3. Pour the batter into the greased pan and place in oven. Bake for 30-35 min. Insert a toothpick or knife into the center and if it comes out clean the pancakes are done. Immediately cut into 10 rectangle pancakes, and remove from the pan while still warm to prevent the foil from sticking to the pancakes. Either serve while warm or store in the refrigerator in an airtight container.

Apple Cinnamon Paleo Porridge

Approximate Yield	**Prep Time 15 min**	**Estimated Macronutrients**
4 (1 cup) servings	**Total Time 20 min**	**11 g P • 18 g C • 1 g F**

INGREDIENTS

Apple Compote
1 honey crisp, fuji or green apple (washed, cored and diced)
½ tablespoon cinnamon
1 tablespoon lemon juice

Paleo Porridge
1 12 oz package or 1½ cups of frozen rice cauliflower*
2 tablespoon honey
½ cup unsweetened cashew milk or other unsweetened nut milk*
½ tablespoon vanilla extract
Pinch of sea salt
¼ teaspoon nutmeg
¼ teaspoon cinnamon
¼ teaspoon cloves
½ cup of pasteurized liquid egg whites

Choose an optional added protein or thickening ingredients:
(Please note, your choice may be based on your individualized food tolerances and/or nutrition goals. For this recipe's macros I utilized egg white protein powder and unsweetened, unflavored beef bone broth protein powder.)

¼ cup of dried egg whites or egg white protein powder*
¼ cup of unsweetened, unflavored beef or bone broth protein powder *
¼ cup SCD Nonfat Greek Yogurt (see recipe page 298)
2 tablespoon coconut flour
¼ cup almond flour

KITCHEN EQUIPMENT

Medium pot
Immersion blender
Measuring cups & spoons
Large spoon or spatula

SPECIAL INSTRUCTIONS/DIET INFORMATION

*Fresh steamed cauliflower can be riced and used; however, the different texture of fresh cauliflower can often vary and may affect the texture of the dish.

*Any nut milks should only consist of nuts, water, or salt. No emulsifiers, gums, sweeteners or additives should be in the ingredient list. If you are unable to source a SCD legal nut milk you can make them easily at home (see recipe page 299).

*Unflavored beef (bovine) protein should only be beef or bone broth without any additives or other ingredients. Confirm ingredients and processing with manufacturer.

*If you are unable to eat the different protein powders, replace with ¼ cup of dried egg white powder.

*If you are unable to eat or source dried egg white powder you can replace with almond flour. However it will not rise as high, the texture will be different, and there will be higher fat and less protein for the macronutrients.

*There are very few commercially available protein powders that meet the guidelines of Specific Carbohydrate Diet. They should be labeled as unflavored and have only 1-3 SCD legal ingredients. It is recommended that all consumers reach out to a company in writing to confirm ingredients, since manufacturers can change ingredients without notification. Consumers should confirm the manufacturing process does not require the use of SCD illegal ingredients or unlisted additives.

DIRECTIONS

1. Steam the cauliflower rice per the package instructions or in a microwavable glass container with lid.
2. On medium heat combine the apples, lemon juice and cinnamon in the small pot. Cook the apples until tender and stirring to prevent burning. When the apples are tender pierced with a fork, set aside in a separate bowl.
3. Combine the cauliflower rice to the pot, and all other ingredients (except the apples, protein/thickening ingredients) and liquid egg whites (you will add these later). Using the immersion blender pulse until the porridge is smooth.
4. Add in the liquid egg whites slowly and stirring to prevent the eggs from scrambling. To thicken the porridge to your liking, add in the listed powders or nut flours, stirring until desired thickness. Keep stirring until all ingredients are thoroughly mixed and simmering. Remove from heat when ready to serve.
5. Serve the porridge warm in bowls and top with apple compote. The servings can be separated into glass containers with lids to consume later.

Cauliflower Cream of No Wheat

Approximate Yield	Prep Time 15 min	Estimated Macronutrients
4 servings	Total Time 30 min	2 g P • 21 g C • 3 g F

INGREDIENTS

2 cups of frozen cauliflower rice*
1 cup coconut or unsweetened cashew milk*
4 tablespoons honey
1 teaspoon vanilla extract
Dash of ground cinnamon
Pinch of sea salt

KITCHEN EQUIPMENT

Handheld immersion blender
Measuring spoons & measuring cups
Heat-resistant spoon or spatula
Medium pot
Plastic storage containers with lids or silicone cups with lids to freeze

SPECIAL INSTRUCTIONS/DIET INFORMATION

*Fresh steamed cauliflower can be riced and used; however, the different texture of fresh cauliflower can often vary and may affect the texture of the dish.

*Any nut milks should only consist of nuts, water, or salt. No emulsifiers, gums, sweeteners or additives should be in the ingredient list. If you are unable to source a SCD legal nut milk you can make them easily at home (see recipe page 299).

DIRECTIONS

1. Using the microwave or stovetop to steam the cauliflower rice (per package instructions). Add all the other ingredients and cauliflower to pot.
2. Using the immersion blender puree the cauliflower mix.
3. Cook until light simmer and then remove to cool. Store in freezer safe storage container or silicone cups for freezing.

Blueberry Blender English Muffins

Approximate Yield **12 servings**	**Prep Time 20 min** **Total Time 90 min**	**Estimated Macronutrients** **11 g P • 19 g C • 16 g F**

INGREDIENTS

Wet
4 eggs
¾ cup of SCD Nonfat Greek Yogurt (see recipe page 298)
¼ cup honey
3 tablespoons melted butter or ghee
1 ½ tablespoons apple cider vinegar

Dry
2 cups of almond flour
¼ cup of dried egg white powder*
3 tablespoons coconut flour
1 teaspoon baking soda
Pinch of sea salt

1 cup of defrosted frozen blueberries
Neutral oil or butter for greasing the pan
Optional: 1 tablespoon coarsely ground Yellow Split Pea
Flour (see recipe page 304)

KITCHEN EQUIPMENT

Food processor or blender
Measuring spoons & measuring cups
Spatula or large spoon
Oven
3–4-inch diameter 6 bun silicone or non-stick pan

SPECIAL INSTRUCTIONS/DIET INFORMATION

*If you are unable to eat or source dried egg white powder you can replace with almond flour. However it will not rise as high, the texture will be different, and there will be higher fat and less protein for the macronutrients.

DIRECTIONS

1. Preheat oven to 350 degrees F. Grease the bun pan, and optionally dust the bottoms of each bun round with a light sprinkling of pea flour and set aside.
2. Mix all the dry ingredients in a small mixing bowl and set aside.
3. In the blender or food processor, add all the wet ingredients and pulse until mixed well.
4. Add in the remaining dry ingredients until a wet dough has formed. Then add in the blueberries. Give the batter a single pulse, and do not over blend the blueberries into the batter.
5. Pour batter into the greased bun pan and bake for 18-22 minutes.
6. Do not open the oven until 15 minutes has passed, as the buns need a chance to rise. When an inserted knife comes out clean, the buns are fully baked. Remove from oven and allow to cool on wire baking racks.

Breakfast Aloha Bowl

Approximate Yield	Prep Time 15 min	Estimated Macronutrients
4-5 servings	Total Time 15 min	5 g P • 28 g C • 8 g F

INGREDIENTS
1 cup of SCD Non-Fat Greek Yogurt (see recipe page 298 and notes) *
1 ½ cup of frozen pineapple chunks
2 medium ripe bananas (frozen and cut into chunks)
½ cup of unsweetened cashew milk, reduced fat unsweetened coconut milk or nut milk*
Optional:
3-4 tablespoons of honey (optional to taste)
1 teaspoon coconut or vanilla extract

Garnishes
¼ cup of chopped toasted macadamia nuts
¼ cup of toasted unsweetened coconut chips
Diced tropical fruit of choice

KITCHEN EQUIPMENT
Blender
Measuring spoons & measuring cups
Spatula or large spoon
Silicone ice cube freezer trays

SPECIAL INSTRUCTIONS/DIET INFORMATION
*SCD Yogurt can be substituted with non-dairy coconut yogurt prepared following SCD preparation guidelines and yogurt cultures.
*Any nut milks should only consist of nuts, water, or salt. No emulsifiers, gums, sweeteners or additives should be in the ingredient list. If you are unable to source a SCD legal nut milk you can make them easily at home (see recipe page 299).

DIRECTIONS
1. Place all ingredients in a blender, following the same order provided in the ingredient list above.
2. Blend until smooth consistency, serve cold in a bowl with garnishes.
3. Note, the smoothie portion can be frozen in silicone freezer ice cube trays and defrosted and re-blended for later use.

Pina Colada Protein Sheet Pan Pancakes

Approximate Yield
10 servings

Prep Time 20 min
Total Time 55 min

Estimated Macronutrients
13 g P • 23 g C • 4 g F

INGREDIENTS

4 mashed ripe bananas
1 ¼ cup of crushed pineapple
3 tablespoons of honey
1 teaspoon of vanilla extract
⅓ cup almond flour
1 cup of egg white protein powder or dried egg white powder*
1 tablespoon coconut flour
¼ cup finely shredded unsweetened coconut
1 teaspoon baking soda
Pinch of sea salt
¾ cup -1 cup of pasteurized liquid egg whites*
Optional: ½ cup of unsweetened coconut flakes

KITCHEN EQUIPMENT

Immersion blender
Large mixing bowl
Measuring spoons & measuring cups
Spatula or large spoon
Baking sheet/pan or cookie sheet with raised edges
(approximately 9.5 in x 13 in)
Aluminum foil

SPECIAL INSTRUCTIONS/DIET INFORMATION

*If you are unable to eat the different protein powders, replace with dried egg white powder.
*If you are unable to eat or source dried egg white powder you can replace with almond flour. However it will not rise as high, the texture will be different, and there will be higher fat and less protein for the macronutrients.
*Use less liquid egg whites if taking the protein pancakes to go and need to be eaten cold.
*Be careful to read all ingredients for liquid egg whites. This should be a mono ingredient, and not contain any preservatives or additional ingredients. Regular separated egg whites can be used but the batter will be thicker and require many eggs.

DIRECTIONS

1. Preheat oven to 350 degrees F. Line the baking sheet with aluminum foil ensuring it covers the edges (one large continuous piece is best to prevent leaks). Be careful not to poke any holes or rip the foil. Spray or brush the foil with cooking oil very well, including the sides of the pan covered in foil.
2. In a large mixing bowl, puree the banana and pineapple together with an immersion blender. Add the remaining ingredients and continue to mix with the blender until all clumps are gone.
3. Pour the batter into the greased pan and place in oven. Optional to sprinkle the toasted unsweetened coconut flakes on top before baking.
4. Bake for 30-35 min. Insert a toothpick or knife into the center and if it comes out clean the pancakes are done. Immediately cut into 10 rectangle pancakes and remove from the pan while still warm (to prevent the foil from sticking to the pancakes). Either serve while warm or store in the refrigerator in an airtight container.

Hulk Mint Protein Shake

Approximate Yield	Prep Time 15 min	Estimated Macronutrients
4 servings	**Total Time 15 min**	**22 g P • 24 g C • 1 g F**

INGREDIENTS

1 cup of ice cubes
1 cup of baby spinach
1 frozen banana
¼ teaspoon peppermint extract
1 tablespoon vanilla extract
1 tablespoon of honey or honey simple syrup
1 cup SCD Nonfat Greek yogurt (see recipe page 298 and notes) *
¼ - ½ cup of unsweetened cashew or coconut milk*
Optional: ½ cup of unsweetened, unflavored beef or bone broth protein powder*

KITCHEN EQUIPMENT

Blender
Measuring spoons & measuring cups
Silicone ice cube freezer trays

SPECIAL INSTRUCTIONS/DIET INFORMATION

*SCD Yogurt can be substituted with non-dairy coconut yogurt prepared following SCD preparation guidelines and yogurt cultures. Important to note macronutrients will change.
*Any nut milks should only consist of nuts, water, or salt. No emulsifiers, gums, sweeteners or additives should be in the ingredient list. If you are unable to source a SCD legal nut milk you can make them easily at home (see recipe page 299).
*Unflavored beef (bovine) protein should only be beef or bone broth without any additives or other ingredients. Confirm ingredients and processing with manufacturer.

DIRECTIONS

1. Place all ingredients in a blender, following the same order provided in the ingredient list above.
2. Blend until smooth consistency and serve cold.
3. Note, the smoothie can be frozen in silicone ice cube freezer trays and defrosted and blended for later use.

Black Cherry Protein Smoothie

Approximate Yield	Prep Time 15 min	Estimated Macronutrients
10 servings	**Total Time 15 min**	**14 g P • 13 g C • 1 g F**

INGREDIENTS

1 cup of ice cubes
1 cup of frozen sweet cherries (pitted and destemmed)
1 cup of SCD Nonfat Greek Yogurt (see recipe page 298 and notes) *
1 tablespoon of honey
½ cup tart red cherry juice
½ cup of unsweetened nut milk of choice (for thinning as needed) *
Optional:
Add in cooked Cherry Compote for added flavor or substituting cherry juice (see recipe page 108)
½ cup of unsweetened, unflavored beef or bone broth protein powder*

KITCHEN EQUIPMENT

Measuring spoons & measuring cups
Spatula or large spoon
Blender
Silicone ice cube freezer trays

SPECIAL INSTRUCTIONS/DIET INFORMATION

*SCD Yogurt can be substituted with non-dairy coconut yogurt prepared following SCD preparation guidelines and yogurt cultures.
*Unflavored beef (bovine) protein should only be beef or bone broth without any additives or other ingredients. Confirm ingredients and processing with manufacturer.
*Any nut milks should only consist of nuts, water, or salt. No emulsifiers, gums, sweeteners or additives should be in the ingredient list. If you are unable to source a SCD legal nut milk you can make them easily at home (see recipe page 299).

DIRECTIONS

1. Place all ingredients in a blender, following the same order provided in the ingredient list above.
2. Blend until smooth consistency and serve cold.
3. Note, the smoothie can be frozen in silicone ice cube freezer trays and defrosted and blended for later use.

Carrot Cake Smoothie

Approximate Yield	Prep Time 15 min	Estimated Macronutrients
4-5 servings	Total Time 15 min	14 g P • 27 g C • 1 g F

INGREDIENTS

1 cup of SCD Nonfat Greek Yogurt (see recipe page 298)
½ cup ice cubes
¼ cup of frozen or cold carrot puree*
1 frozen banana
2 dried pitted medjool dates (Steeped and softened in ¼ cup hot water is preferred. The steeping water can be added to the smoothie once cooled)
¼ teaspoon cinnamon
½ teaspoon vanilla extract
¼ teaspoon ground ginger
⅛ teaspoon or pinch of ground nutmeg
1 tablespoon of honey
½ cup of unsweetened nut milk of choice*
Optional:
½ cup unsweetened, unflavored beef or bone broth protein powder*

KITCHEN EQUIPMENT

Measuring spoons & measuring cups
Spatula or large spoon
Blender
Silicone ice cube freezer trays

SPECIAL INSTRUCTIONS/DIET INFORMATION

*SCD Yogurt can be substituted with non-dairy coconut yogurt prepared following SCD preparation guidelines and yogurt cultures.
*A bag of frozen carrots steamed and pureed with an immersion blender and then frozen in ¼ cup cubes.
*Unflavored beef (bovine) protein should only be beef or bone broth without any additives or other ingredients. Confirm ingredients and processing with manufacturer.
*Any nut milks should only consist of nuts, water, or salt. No emulsifiers, gums, sweeteners or additives should be in the ingredient list. If you are unable to source a SCD legal nut milk you can make them easily at home (see recipe page 299).

DIRECTIONS

1. Place all ingredients in a blender, following the same order provided in the ingredient list above.
2. Blend until smooth consistency and serve cold.
3. Note, the smoothie can be frozen in silicone ice cube freezer trays and defrosted and blended for later use.

Carrot Cake Sheet Pan Pancakes

Approximate Yield	**Prep Time 20 min**	**Estimated Macronutrients**
10 servings	**Total Time 55 min**	**14 g P • 13 g C • 1 g F**

INGREDIENTS

8 oz (approximately 1 cup) of frozen carrots, steamed and pureed

3.2 oz of pineapple sauce or ⅔ cup of crushed pineapple

2 mashed bananas

¼ cup egg white protein powder or ¼ cup dried egg white powder*

Optional: ¼ cup of unsweetened, unflavored beef or bone broth protein powder *

4 tablespoons of honey

1 tablespoon vanilla extract

2 ½ teaspoons ground cinnamon

1 teaspoon ground ginger

1 teaspoon baking soda

¼ teaspoon nutmeg

Pinch of sea salt

1 ¾ cups of pasteurized liquid egg whites*

KITCHEN EQUIPMENT

Immersion blender

Measuring spoons & cups

Spatula

Baking sheet/pan or cookie sheet with raised edges (approximately 9.5 in x 13 in)

Aluminum foil

SPECIAL INSTRUCTIONS/DIET INFORMATION

*If you are unable to eat the different protein powders, replace with 1/3 cup of dried egg white powder.

*If you are unable to eat or source dried egg white powder you can replace with almond flour. However it will not rise as high, the texture will be different, and there will be higher fat and less protein for the macronutrients.

*Unflavored beef (bovine) protein should only be beef or bone broth without any additives or other ingredients. Confirm processing with manufacturer.

*Be careful to read all ingredients for liquid egg whites. This should be a mono ingredient, and not contain any preservatives or additional ingredients. Regular separated egg whites can be used but the batter will be thicker and require many eggs.

DIRECTIONS

1. Preheat oven to 350 degrees F. Line the baking sheet with aluminum foil ensuring it covers the edges (one large continuous piece is best to prevent leaks). Be careful not to poke any holes or rip the foil. Spray or brush the foil with cooking oil very well, including the sides of the pan covered in foil.

2. In a large mixing bowl, mash the banana, carrots and pineapple together with an immersion blender. Add the remaining ingredients and continue to mix with the blender until all clumps are gone.

3. Pour the batter into the greased pan and place in oven.

4. Bake for 30-35 min. Insert a toothpick or knife into the center and if it comes out clean the pancakes are done. Immediately cut into 10 rectangle pancakes and remove from the pan while still warm to prevent the foil from sticking to the pancakes. Either serve while warm or store in the refrigerator in an airtight container.

Lemon Blueberry Sheet Pan Protein Pancakes

Approximate Yield	Prep Time 20 min	Estimated Macronutrients
10 servings	**Total Time 55 min**	**24 g P • 22 g C • 9 g F**

INGREDIENTS

3 mashed ripe bananas
1 whole lemon zested and ¼ cup of juice
3 whole eggs
¼ cup of honey
1 teaspoon of vanilla extract
1 cup of egg white protein powder or dried egg white powder*
2 tablespoons coconut flour
1 teaspoon baking soda
Pinch of sea salt
1 ½ cup of pasteurized liquid egg whites*
Optional: ¼ cup of unsweetened, unflavored beef or bone broth protein powder*

1 cup of Blueberry Compote (see recipe page 108)

KITCHEN EQUIPMENT

Immersion blender
Large mixing bowl
Measuring spoons & measuring cups
Spatula or large spoon
Baking sheet/pan or cookie sheet with raised edges
(approximately 9.5 in x 13 in)
Aluminum foil

SPECIAL INSTRUCTIONS/DIET INFORMATION

*If you are unable to eat the different protein powders, replace with dried egg white powder.
*If you are unable to eat or source dried egg white powder you can replace with almond flour. However it will not rise as high, the texture will be different, and there will be higher fat and less protein for the macronutrients.
*Use less liquid egg whites if taking the protein pancakes to go and need to be eaten cold.
*Be careful to read all ingredients for liquid egg whites. This should be a mono ingredient, and not contain any preservatives or additional ingredients. Regular separated egg whites can be used but the batter will be thicker and require many eggs.
*Unflavored beef (bovine) protein should only be beef or bone broth without any additives or other ingredients. Confirm ingredients and processing with manufacturer.

DIRECTIONS

1. Preheat oven to 350 degrees F. Line the baking sheet with aluminum foil ensuring it covers the edges (one large continuous piece is best to prevent leaks). Be careful not to poke any holes or rip the foil. Spray or brush the foil with cooking oil very well, including the sides of the pan covered in foil.
2. In a large mixing bowl, puree the banana, lemon juice and lemon zest, together with an immersion blender. Add the remaining ingredients, adding the egg whites last and continue to mix with the blender until all clumps are gone.
3. Pour the batter into the greased foiled lined baking sheet. Drizzle and pour the blueberry compote evenly over the top of the batter and using a spoon knife make shallow swirls along the surface. Place in oven to bake.
4. Bake for 30-35 min. Insert a toothpick or knife into the center and if it comes out clean the pancakes are done. Immediately cut into 10 rectangle pancakes and remove from the pan while still warm to prevent the foil from sticking to the pancakes. Either serve while warm or store in the refrigerator in an airtight container.

Cream Cheese Pumpkin Protein Sheet Pan Pancakes

Approximate Yield	Prep Time 20 min	Estimated Macronutrients
10 servings	Total Time 55 min	14 g P • 13 g C • 1 g F

INGREDIENTS

Pumpkin pancake batter

2 mashed bananas
1 can of pureed pumpkin (15 oz or 2 cups) or butternut squash
1 cup of dried egg white powder or SCD legal egg white protein
¼ cup of almond flour
4 teaspoons of honey
2 teaspoons of vanilla extract
3-4 teaspoons of Pumpkin Spice Seasoning (see recipe page 144)
½ teaspoon baking soda
Pinch of sea salt
1 ½ cups of pasteurized liquid egg whites*
Optional: ¼ cup unsweetened, unflavored beef or bone broth protein powder*

"Cream Cheese" batter

2 tablespoons honey
1 cup of dripped Nonfat SCD Greek Yogurt (see recipe page 298)
1 teaspoon vanilla
1 whole egg
1 tablespoon dried egg white powder*
½ teaspoon of unflavored gelatin

KITCHEN EQUIPMENT

Immersion blender
Measuring spoons & measuring cups
Spatula or large spoon
Baking sheet/pan or cookie sheet with raised edges (approximately 9.5 in x 13 in)
Aluminum foil

SPECIAL INSTRUCTIONS/DIET INFORMATION

*If you are unable to source or eat the different protein powders, replace with dried egg white powder and increase the amount by 1 tablespoon.

*If you are unable to eat or source dried egg white powder you can replace with almond flour. However it will not rise as high, the texture will be different, and there will be higher fat and less protein for the macronutrients.

*Be careful to read all ingredients for liquid egg whites. This should be a mono ingredient, and not contain any preservatives or additional ingredients. Regular separated egg whites can be used but the batter will be thicker and require many eggs.

*Unflavored beef (bovine) protein should only be beef or bone broth without any additives or other ingredients. Confirm ingredients and processing with manufacturer.

DIRECTIONS

1. Preheat oven to 350 degrees F. Line the baking sheet with aluminum foil ensuring it covers the sides and edges (one large continuous piece is best to prevent leaks). Be careful not to poke any holes or rip the foil. Spray or brush the foil with cooking oil very well, including the sides of the pan covered in foil.
2. In a large mixing bowl, mash the banana and pumpkin together with an immersion blender. Add the remaining ingredients and continue to mix with the blender until all clumps are gone.
3. Pour the pumpkin batter into the greased pan. Then add the cream cheese filling in dollops onto the pumpkin batter and, using a knife, to swirl lightly and place in oven.
4. Bake for 30-35 min. Insert a toothpick or knife into the center and if it comes out clean the pancakes are done. Immediately cut into 10 rectangle pancakes and remove from the pan while still warm to prevent the foil from sticking to the pancakes. Either serve while warm or store in the refrigerator in an airtight container.

Apple Cinnamon Sheet Pan Protein Pancakes

Approximate Yield	Prep Time 20 min	Estimated Macronutrients
10 servings	**Total Time 55 min**	**12 g P • 21 g C • 2 g F**

INGREDIENTS

2 mashed bananas
1 cup of unsweetened apple sauce
¼ cup egg white protein powder or ¼ cup dried egg white powder*
4 tablespoons of honey
1 tablespoon vanilla extract
1 teaspoon baking soda
Pinch of sea salt
1 ½ cups of pasteurized liquid egg whites*
Optional: ¼ cup of unsweetened, unflavored beef (bovine) or bone broth protein powder *
¼ cup dried apples
¼ cup chopped walnuts

KITCHEN EQUIPMENT

Immersion blender
Measuring spoons & measuring cups
Spatula or large spoon
Large mixing bowl
Baking sheet/pan or cookie sheet with raised edges
(approximately 9.5 in x 13 in)
Aluminum foil

SPECIAL INSTRUCTIONS/DIET INFORMATION

*If you are unable to eat the different protein powders, replace with ⅓ cup of dried egg white powder
*If you are unable to eat or source dried egg white powder you can replace with almond flour. However it will not rise as high, the texture will be different, and there will be higher fat and less protein for the macronutrients.
*Be careful to read all ingredients for liquid egg whites. This should be a mono ingredient, and not contain any preservatives or additional ingredients. Regular separated egg whites can be used but the batter will be thicker and require many eggs.

DIRECTIONS

1. Preheat oven to 350 degrees F. Line the baking sheet with aluminum foil ensuring it covers the edges (one large continuous piece is best to prevent leaks). Be careful not to poke any holes or rip the foil. Spray or brush the foil with cooking oil very well, including the sides of the pan covered in foil.
2. In a large mixing bowl, mash the bananas, and apple sauce together with an immersion blender. Add the remaining ingredients and continue to mix with the blender until all clumps are gone.
3. Pour the batter into the greased pan, sprinkle the dried apples and chopped walnuts along the top of the batter, then place in oven.
4. Bake for 30-35 min. Insert a toothpick or knife into the center and if it comes out clean the pancakes are done. Immediately cut into 10 rectangle pancakes and remove from the pan while still warm to prevent the foil from sticking to the pancakes. Either serve while warm or store in the refrigerator in an airtight container.

Lemon Poppyseed Sheet Pan Protein Pancakes

Approximate Yield	**Prep Time 20 min**	**Estimated Macronutrients**
10 servings	**Total Time 55 min**	**25 g P • 22 g C • 9 g F**

INGREDIENTS

3 mashed ripe bananas
1 whole lemon zested and ¼ cup of juice
3 whole eggs
¼ cup of honey
1 teaspoon of vanilla extract
1 cup of egg white protein powder or dried egg white powder*
2 tablespoons coconut flour
1 teaspoon baking soda
Pinch of sea salt
1 ½ cup of pasteurized liquid egg whites*
1 ½ tablespoon poppy seeds
Optional:
¼ cup of unsweetened, unflavored beef or bone broth protein powder*
¼ cup Honey Lemon Curd (see recipe page 278)

KITCHEN EQUIPMENT

Immersion blender
Large mixing bowl
Measuring spoons & measuring cups
Spatula or large spoon
Baking sheet/pan or cookie sheet with raised edges
(approximately 9.5 in x 13 in)
Aluminum foil

SPECIAL INSTRUCTIONS/DIET INFORMATION

*If you are unable to eat the different protein powders, replace with dried egg white powder.
*If you are unable to eat or source dried egg white powder you can replace with almond flour. However it will not rise as high, the texture will be different, and there will be higher fat and less protein for the macronutrients.
*Use less liquid egg whites if taking the protein pancakes to go and need to be eaten cold.
*Be careful to read all ingredients for liquid egg whites. This should be a mono ingredient, and not contain any preservatives or additional ingredients. Regular separated egg whites can be used but the batter will be thicker and require many eggs.
*Unflavored beef (bovine) protein should only be beef or bone broth without any additives or other ingredients. Confirm ingredients and processing with manufacturer.

DIRECTIONS

1. Preheat oven to 350 degrees F. Line the baking sheet with aluminum foil, ensuring it covers the edges (one large continuous piece is best to prevent leaks). Be careful not to poke any holes or rip the foil. Spray or brush the foil with cooking oil very well, including the sides of the pan covered in foil.
2. In a large mixing bowl, puree the banana, lemon juice and lemon zest, together with an immersion blender. Add the remaining ingredients and continue to mix with the blender until all clumps are gone.
3. Pour the batter into the greased pan and place in oven.
4. Bake for 30-35 min. Insert a toothpick or knife into the center and if it comes out clean the pancakes are done. Immediately cut into 10 rectangle pancakes and remove from the pan while still warm to prevent the foil from sticking to the pancakes. Either serve while warm or store in the refrigerator in an airtight container.

Banana Cinnamon Walnut Protein Sheet Pan Pancakes

Approximate Yield	Prep Time 20 min	Estimated Macronutrients
10 servings	Total Time 55 min	14 g P • 15 g C • 2 g F

INGREDIENTS

5 mashed bananas
1 cup egg whites protein powder or dried egg white powder*
1 ½ cups of pasteurized liquid egg whites*
½ cup of chopped walnuts
2 tablespoons of cinnamon (reserve 1 tablespoon for topping)
2 teaspoons of honey (+ 1 tablespoon to reserve for topping)
2 teaspoons of vanilla extract
½ teaspoon baking soda
Pinch of sea salt
Optional: ¼ cup of unsweetened, unflavored beef or bone broth protein powder

KITCHEN EQUIPMENT

Immersion blender
Mixing bowl
Measuring spoons & measuring cups
Spatula or large spoon
Baking sheet/pan or cookie sheet with raised edges
(approximately 9.5 in x 13 in)
Aluminum foil

SPECIAL INSTRUCTIONS/DIET INFORMATION

*If you are unable to eat the different protein powders, replace with 1 ¼ cup of dried egg white powder
*If you are unable to eat or source dried egg white powder you can replace with almond flour. However it will not rise as high, the texture will be different, and there will be higher fat and less protein for the macronutrients.
*Unflavored beef (bovine) protein should only be beef or bone broth without any additives or other ingredients. Confirm ingredients and processing with manufacturer.
*Be careful to read all ingredients for pasteurized liquid egg whites. This should be a mono ingredient, and not contain any preservatives or additional ingredients. Regular separated egg whites can be used but the batter will be thicker and require many eggs.

DIRECTIONS

1. Preheat oven to 350 degrees F. Line the baking sheet with aluminum foil ensuring it covers the edges (one large continuous piece is best to prevent leaks). Be careful not to poke any holes or rip the foil. Spray or brush the foil with cooking oil very well, including the sides of the pan covered in foil.

2. In a large mixing bowl, mash the banana with an immersion blender. Add the remaining ingredients and continue to mix with the blender until all clumps are gone.

3. Pour the batter into the greased pan and place in oven. Sprinkle the remaining cinnamon evenly over the batter. Followed by drizzling honey. Using a toothpick swirl the honey and cinnamon together. Sprinkle the chopped walnuts evenly over the top.

4. Bake for 30-35 min. Insert a toothpick or knife into the center and if it comes out clean the pancakes are done. Immediately cut into 10 rectangle pancakes and remove from the pan while still warm to prevent the foil from sticking to the pancakes. Either serve while warm or store in the refrigerator in an airtight container.

Protein Banana Bread

Approximate Yield	Prep Time 20 min	Estimated Macronutrients
12 servings	**Total Time 90 min**	**16 g P • 27 g C • 11 g F**

INGREDIENTS

Wet

4 ripe bananas

¾ cup SCD Nonfat Greek Yogurt (see recipe page 298)

2 eggs

¼ cup of honey

2 tablespoons melted butter or olive oil

1 tablespoon vanilla extract

Dry

¼ cup of coconut flour

½ cup almond flour

½ cup dried egg white powder or egg white protein powder*

1 teaspoon baking soda

¼ teaspoon sea salt

KITCHEN EQUIPMENT

Mixer and beaters

Measuring spoons & measuring cups

Mixing bowls

Immersion blender

Oven

Standard bread loaf pan (approximately 8 ½ x 4 ½ in.)

Spatula for stirring

Baking parchment paper

SPECIAL INSTRUCTIONS/DIET INFORMATION

*If you are unable to eat or source an egg white protein powder with legal ingredients, or dried powdered egg whites, you can substitute with more almond flour. However, it will not rise as high, the texture will be different, and there will be higher fat and less protein when counting macros.

DIRECTIONS

1. Preheat oven to 350 degrees F. Line the bread loaf pan with parchment paper and set aside.
2. Mix all the bread's dry ingredients in a small mixing bowl and set aside
3. In a large mixing bowl, mash the bananas with the immersion blender, beat in the eggs and combine all the wet ingredients.
4. Slowly add in the dry ingredients until a wet dough has formed.
5. Pour the batter into the bread loaf pan, and bake for 50-70 minutes, until tops are golden, and a knife or toothpick inserted in the center comes out clean.
6. You may need to lightly tent with foil to prevent the top from browning too dark. When cooked through remove from oven and set aside to cool.

Loaded Pumpkin Bread

Approximate Yield	Prep Time 20 min	Estimated Macronutrients
12 servings	Total Time 90 min	16 g P • 35 g C • 18 g F

INGREDIENTS

Wet
1 (15 oz) can of pumpkin puree or 1 ½ cups pureed pumpkin
½ teaspoon vanilla extract
3 eggs
2 tablespoons of butter or coconut oil
⅓ cup honey

Dry
¾ teaspoon baking soda
¼ teaspoon sea salt
¼ cup coconut flour
⅓ cup dried egg white powder*
¾ cup almond flour
1 tablespoon Pumpkin Pie Spice (see recipe page 144)

½ cup hot water
½ cup of raisins finely chopped
7 pitted and dried medjool dates finely chopped
½ cup of chopped raw walnuts
½ teaspoon ground cinnamon
1 tablespoon honey

KITCHEN EQUIPMENT
Mixer and beaters
Measuring spoons & measuring cups
Spatula or large spoon
Mixing bowls
Oven
Standard bread loaf pan (approximately 8 ½ x 4 ½ in.)
Baking parchment paper

SPECIAL INSTRUCTIONS/DIET INFORMATION
*If you are unable to eat or source dried egg white powder you can replace with almond flour. However it will not rise as high, the texture will be different, and there will be higher fat and less protein for the macronutrients.

DIRECTIONS
1. Preheat oven to 350 degrees F. Line the bread loaf pan with parchment paper ensuring all sides are covered.
2. Check the dates for any pits or hard remnants. Remove and discard any before mincing. Soak the minced raisins and dates together in warm water for 10 minutes, when saturated drain the water.
3. Chop the walnuts finely then add into a small bowl with the raisins and dates. Mix in the cinnamon and honey until well coated.
4. Mix all the bread's dry ingredients in a small mixing bowl and set aside.
5. In a large mixing bowl, beat the egg and add in the remaining wet ingredients mixing well together. Slowly add in the dry ingredients until a wet dough has formed.
6. Fold in the steeped raisins, dates or chopped walnuts mixture.
7. Pour the dough into the bread loaf pan.
8. Bake for 50-70 minutes until top is crusty and dark gold. Test for doneness with knife or toothpick by inserting in the center and it comes out clean. Important to note, do not open the oven until 40 minutes has passed. When fully baked remove from oven and set aside to cool.

Apple Cinnamon Muffins

Approximate Yield	**Prep Time 20 min**	**Estimated Macronutrients**
12 servings	**Total Time 45 min**	**10 g P • 20 g C • 10 g F**

INGREDIENTS

Wet

1 large apple shredded (approximately ¾ – 1 cup)
1 tablespoon lemon juice
¼ cup honey
2 eggs
⅓ cup pasteurized liquid egg whites*
1 tablespoon vanilla extract
2 tablespoons butter (melted)

Dry

3 tablespoons coconut flour
¼ cup dried egg white powder*
1 ½ teaspoon ground cinnamon
½ teaspoon nutmeg
¼ teaspoon cloves
½ teaspoon sea salt
½ teaspoon baking soda

Optional Mix ins or Topping

¼ cup chopped walnuts
¼- ½ cup dried apples

KITCHEN EQUIPMENT

Mixer and beaters
Immersion blender
Mixing bowls
Oven
Standard muffin pan (12-24 muffins)
Baking parchment paper muffin/cupcake liners

SPECIAL INSTRUCTIONS/DIET INFORMATION

*If you are unable to eat or source dried egg white powder you can replace with almond flour. However it will not rise as high, the texture will be different, and there will be higher fat and less protein for the macronutrients.

* If using pasteurized liquid egg whites, be careful to read all ingredients. This should be a mono ingredient, and not contain any preservatives or additives, other than pasteurized egg whites. Regular separated egg whites can be used but the batter will be thicker and require many eggs. Note the conversion is 2 tablespoons of liquid eggs to 1 egg white.

DIRECTIONS

1. Preheat oven to 350 degrees F. Line the muffin pan with parchment paper liners.
2. In a small mixing bowl stir in all the topping ingredients and set aside.
3. Mix all the dry ingredients in a small mixing bowl and set aside.
4. In a large mixing bowl, mash the bananas with the immersion blender and combine all the wet ingredients together.
5. Slowly add in the dry ingredients until a wet dough has formed.
6. Pour the batter halfway into each lined muffin tin.
7. Place a sprinkle of topping on each muffin and then swirl it with a knife or toothpick.
8. Bake for 15-20 minutes or until an inserted knife or toothpick in the center comes out clean. Serve warm.

Walnut and Cranberry Bread

Approximate Yield	Prep Time 20 min	Estimated Macronutrients
12 servings	Total Time 90 min	18 g P • 19 g C • 24 g F

INGREDIENTS

Wet
4 egg yolks + 4 egg whites (separated)
1 cup of walnut and cashew butter*
¼ cup unsweetened cashew milk or other nut milk*
2 tablespoons honey
1 tablespoon apple cider vinegar

Dry
¼ cup of coconut flour
¼ cup dried egg white powder or egg white protein powder*
1 teaspoon baking soda
½ teaspoon sea salt

¼ cup halved or chopped walnuts
¼ cup of unsweetened dried cranberries

KITCHEN EQUIPMENT

Mixer and beaters
Measuring spoons & measuring cups
Spatula
Oven
Standard bread loaf pan (approximately 8 ½ x 4 ½ in.)
or 3–4-inch diameter 6 bun silicone or non-stick pan
Baking parchment paper

SPECIAL INSTRUCTIONS/DIET INFORMATION

*Egg whites need to be separated and not liquid in a carton as they will not whip into peaks
*If you are unable to eat the different protein powders, replace with dried egg white powder and increase the amount by ½ -1 tablespoon.
*If you are unable to eat or source dried egg white powder you can replace with almond flour. However it will not rise as high, the texture will be different, and there will be higher fat and less protein for the macronutrients.
*Any nut milks should only consist of nuts, water, or salt. No emulsifiers, gums, sweeteners or additives should be in the ingredient list. If you are unable to source a SCD legal nut milk you can make them easily at home (see recipe page 299).
*Nut butters that are SCD legal should only include the nut and possibly a legal oil and/or salt. For example, peanut butter is generally roasted peanuts and salt. There are some brands that will sweeten with honey but there are very few commercially available.

DIRECTIONS

1. Preheat oven to 325 degrees F. Line the bread loaf pan with parchment paper or grease the bun pan and set aside.
2. Boil 1 cup of filtered water and add the cranberries. Steep the cranberries for 30 minutes. (You can also mix in honey for some added sweetness.)
3. Mix all the dry ingredients in a small mixing bowl and set aside
4. In a large mixing bowl, beat the egg whites until stiff peaks form (a standing mixer is recommended as this can take time).
5. Add in the remaining wet ingredients and beat together with the egg whites. Slowly add in the dry ingredients until a wet dough has formed.
6. Strain the cranberries of liquid and set aside with the halved walnuts.
7. Pour half the batter into the bread loaf pan, and sprinkle with half the cranberries and walnuts. Then pour the remaining half of the batter and the last of the cranberries and walnuts.
8. Bake for 50-60 minutes until tops are golden and when a knife or toothpick inserted in the center comes out clean. Do not open the oven until 40 minutes has passed, although buns may be done baking after 40 minutes. However, the bread will need the full time to bake and will not rise if the oven is opened too early.
9. Remove from oven, allow to cool, slice and serve.

Cinnamon Bun Banana Muffins

Approximate Yield
12 servings

Prep Time 20 min
Total Time 90 min

Estimated Macronutrients
12 g P • 44 g C • 10 g F

INGREDIENTS

Wet
3 ripe bananas
1 cup pasteurized liquid egg whites*
½ cup honey
1 tablespoon vanilla extract

Dry
½ cup of coconut flour
½ cup dried egg white powder*
¼ teaspoon sea salt
½ teaspoon baking soda

Topping
½ cup chopped walnuts
¼ cup honey
2 tablespoons unsalted butter
2 tablespoons ground cinnamon

KITCHEN EQUIPMENT
Mixer and beaters
Immersion blender
Mixing bowls of various sizes
Oven
Standard size 12- 24 muffin pan
Baking parchment paper muffin/cupcake liners

SPECIAL INSTRUCTIONS/DIET INFORMATION
* When using pasteurized liquid egg whites, be careful to read all ingredients. This should be a mono ingredient, and not contain any preservatives or additives, other than pasteurized egg whites. Regular separated egg whites can be used but the batter will be thicker and require many eggs. Note the conversion is 2 tablespoons of liquid eggs to 1 egg white.
*If you are unable to eat or source dried egg white powder you can replace with almond flour. However it will not rise as high, the texture will be different, and there will be higher fat and less protein for the macronutrients.

DIRECTIONS
1. Preheat oven to 350 degrees F. Line the muffin pan with parchment paper liners.
2. In a small mixing bowl stir in all the topping ingredients, mixing well and set aside.
3. Mix all the dry ingredients in a small bowl and set aside
4. In a large mixing bowl, mash the bananas with the immersion blender and combine all the wet ingredients
5. Slowly add in the dry ingredients until a wet dough has formed.
6. Pour the batter halfway into each lined muffin tin.
7. Place a dollop of topping on each muffin and then swirl it with a knife or toothpick.
8. Bale for 15-20 minutes or until a knife or toothpick inserted in the center comes out clean. Serve warm.

Cinnamon Raisin Bread

Approximate Yield	Prep Time 20 min	Estimated Macronutrients
12 servings	Total Time 90 min	16 g P • 44 g C • 24 g F

INGREDIENTS

Wet
4 eggs (whites and yolks divided)
10 oz (1 ¼ cup) of raw cashew butter*
6 tablespoons honey (or ⅓ cup approximately)
2 teaspoons vanilla extract
2 teaspoons apple cider vinegar
½ cup unsweetened cashew milk or other nut milk*

Dry
¼ cup of coconut flour
2 tablespoons dried egg white powder*
½ teaspoon sea salt
1 teaspoon baking soda

Cinnamon Raisin Mixture
3 tablespoons honey
1 tablespoon cinnamon
⅔ cups of raisins (soaked in warm water for 30 min, drained and then chopped fine)
2 tablespoons coconut butter melted

Frosting
1 ½ tablespoons honey
¾ cup coconut butter crumbles (melted)
½ teaspoon vanilla extract
3 tablespoons unsweetened cashew milk

KITCHEN EQUIPMENT
Mixer and beaters
Mixing bowls
Measuring spoons & measuring cups
Oven
Standard bread loaf pan (approximately 8 ½ x 4 ½ in.)
Spatula or large spoon
Small spatula
Baking parchment paper

SPECIAL INSTRUCTIONS/DIET INFORMATION
*Egg whites need to be separated and not liquid in a carton as they will not whip into peaks.
*If you are unable to eat or source dried egg white powder you can replace with almond flour. However it will not rise as high, the texture will be different, and there will be higher fat and less protein for the macronutrients.
*Nut butters that are SCD legal should only include the nut and possibly a legal oil and/or salt.
For example, peanut butter is generally roasted peanuts and salt. There are some brands that will sweeten with honey but there are very few commercially available.
*Any nut milks should only consist of nuts, water, or salt. No emulsifiers, gums, sweeteners or additives should be in the ingredient list. If you are unable to source a SCD legal nut milk you can make them easily at home (see recipe page 299).

DIRECTIONS
1. Preheat oven to 325 degrees F. Line the bread loaf pan with parchment paper and grease the bun pan and set aside.
2. Soak raisins in warm water for 30 min, when saturated drain and start preparing the Cinnamon Raisin mixture. If the raisins expanded, then chop into smaller pieces. Stir the raisins in with the coconut butter, cinnamon, and honey. Set aside.
3. Mix all the bread's dry ingredients in a small mixing bowl and set aside
4. In a large mixing bowl, beat the egg whites until stiff peaks form (a standing mixer is recommended as this can take time).
5. Add in the remaining wet ingredients until mixed together with egg whites. Slowly add in the dry ingredients until a wet dough has formed.
6. Beat gently until everything is mixed well.
7. Pour half of the dough into the bread loaf pan, then add in half of the cinnamon raisin mixture on top. Use a knife to create swirls and even out the raisin mixture in the bread.
8. Pour the rest of the bread batter and top it with the cinnamon raisin mixture. Use the same knife to swirl the raisins into the dough evenly.

DIRECTIONS (continued)

9. Bake for 50-60 minutes, do not open the oven until 40 minutes has passed. When a knife or toothpick inserted in the center comes out clean remove from oven and set aside to cool.

10. In a separate small bowl, add all the frosting ingredients and mix well. Ensuring there aren't any lumps. Using a small spatula, spread over the top of the bread when still a bit warm. Allow to cool and harden a bit before slicing and serving.

Dad's Zucchini Bread Recipe

Approximate Yield	**Prep Time 20 min**	**Estimated Macronutrients**
12 servings	**Total Time 90 min**	**13 g P • 11 g C • 17 g F**

INGREDIENTS

Wet
¼ cup unsweetened apple sauce
¼ cup of honey
2 eggs
2 tablespoons melted butter or avocado oil
1 teaspoon vanilla extract

Dry
2 cups of almond flour
½ cup dried egg white powder*
1 ½ teaspoon ground cinnamon
½ teaspoon baking soda
½ teaspoon sea salt
¼ teaspoon ground ginger powder

2 cups of shredded zucchini (approximately 1 large zucchini)
½ cup of chopped walnuts

KITCHEN EQUIPMENT

Mixer and beaters
Measuring spoons & measuring cups
Small bowl
Large mixing bowl
Spatula
Oven
Standard bread loaf pan (approximately 8 ½ x 4 ½ in.)
Baking parchment paper

SPECIAL INSTRUCTIONS/DIET INFORMATION

*If you are unable to eat or source dried egg white powder you can replace with almond flour. However it will not rise as high, the texture will be different, and there will be higher fat and less protein for the macronutrients.

DIRECTIONS

1. Preheat oven to 325 degrees F. Line the bread loaf pan with parchment paper, covering all sides, and be careful not to tear or rip a hole.
2. Combine all the dry ingredients in a small mixing bowl and set aside.
3. In a large mixing bowl, beat the eggs and combine all the wet ingredients together.
4. Slowly add in the dry ingredients until a wet dough has formed. Then fold in the shredded zucchini and chopped walnuts.
5. Pour the batter into the bread loaf pan, and bake for 50-70 minutes, until the top is golden, and an inserted knife or toothpick in the center of the bread comes out clean. You may need to lightly tent with foil to prevent the top from browning too dark. When baked through remove from oven and set aside to cool.

Dad's Zucchini and Mushroom Frittata

Approximate Yield 8-10 servings	Prep Time 20 min Total Time 45 min	Estimated Macronutrients 11 g P • 7 g C • 11 g F

INGREDIENTS

1 large (2 cups) shredded zucchini
6 large mushrooms (washed, destemmed and caps sliced lengthwise and thinly)
2 tablespoons finely minced red onion or shallots
8 eggs*
½ cup unsweetened cashew milk or other nut milk*
½ cup almond flour
½ cup grated aged parmesan*
1 ¼ teaspoon seasoned salt

Spray olive or avocado oil for greasing the baking dish

KITCHEN EQUIPMENT

Glass or ceramic baking dish 9 x 13
(Using an 8x8 baking dish or seasoned cast iron pan may require a longer baking time and serving sizes will differ)
Measuring spoons & measuring cups
Spatula or large spoon
Large mixing bowl

SPECIAL INSTRUCTIONS/DIET INFORMATION

*If you need to reduce fat you can substitute 8 whole eggs, with 4 whole eggs and 4 egg whites.
* You can also reduce the parmesan cheese by ¼ cup, and add ¼ cup of dried powdered egg whites.
*Any nut milks should only consist of nuts, water, or salt. No emulsifiers, gums, sweeteners or additives should be in the ingredient list. If you are unable to source a SCD legal nut milk you can make them easily at home (see recipe page 299).
*Cheeses should be aged over 3 months, and contain zero carbohydrates or sugars, regarding nutritional content. Pre-sliced and pre-shredded cheese will likely contain illegal ingredients to prevent the cheese from sticking and prolong shelf life. It is always best to purchase blocks of cheese, then shred, grate, crumble or slice yourself.

DIRECTIONS

1. Preheat oven to 350 degrees F and grease the baking dish with the spray oil and set aside.
2. In a large mixing bowl, beat the eggs, cashew milk and spices. Then whisk in the almond flour and parmesan.
3. Fold in the zucchini, mushroom and minced onion.
4. In the greased baking dish, pour the egg, cheese and vegetable mixture.
5. Place the baking dish in the oven and bake for 20-25 minutes.
6. Remove from oven when a knife inserted in the center comes out clean, then allow to cool.
7. The frittata can be cut into squares and served either warm or eaten cold.

Green Eggs & "Ham" Sheet Pan Bake

Approximate Yield	Prep Time 20 min	Estimated Macronutrients
10 servings	Total Time 55 min	9 g P • 6 g C • 3 g F

Commercially made ham is generally not legal, due to the brining process and many of the ingredients do not meet the guidelines of the Specific Carbohydrate Diet. As a substitute prosciutto or no sugar bacon is recommended for this recipe

INGREDIENTS
8 oz-10oz of frozen spinach
½ cup diced (no sugar or added sweeteners) bacon or prosciutto*
½ red onion diced or ¼ cup minced dried onion
1 ½-2 cups of pasteurized liquid egg whites*
¼ teaspoon salt
¼ teaspoon granulated garlic
¼ teaspoon pepper

Optional: ½ cup of shredded monterey jack or cheddar cheese*

Spray olive or avocado oil for greasing the baking sheet/jelly roll sheet

KITCHEN EQUIPMENT
Large baking sheet with raised edge or baking jelly roll sheet
Measuring spoons & measuring cups
Medium mixing bowl
Non-stick large skillet
Heat-resistant spoon or spatula
Aluminum foil

SPECIAL INSTRUCTIONS/DIET INFORMATION
* If using pasteurized liquid egg whites, be careful to read all ingredients. This should be a mono ingredient, and not contain any preservatives or additives, other than pasteurized egg whites. Regular separated egg whites can be used but the batter will be thicker and require many eggs. Note the conversion is 2 tablespoons of liquid eggs to 1 egg white.
*Always read labels carefully verify ingredients with manufacturers for prepackaged bacon.
*Be very careful to read and verify the ingredients for prosciutto, many brands have extra additives and illegal ingredients used in processing. Generally, prosciutto directly from Italy should only include salt and pork listed as ingredients.
* Cheeses should be aged over 3 months, and contain zero carbohydrates or sugars, regarding nutritional content. Pre-sliced and pre-shredded cheese will likely contain illegal ingredients to prevent the cheese from sticking and prolong shelf life. It is always best to purchase blocks of cheese, then shred, grate, crumble or slice yourself.

DIRECTIONS
1. Preheat oven to 350 degrees F and cover the baking sheet with a continuous sheet of foil. (Be careful not to rip or create a hole in the foil) Then grease the foil lined baking sheet with the spray oil and set aside.
2. In a large non-stick skillet on medium to high heat, sauté the onion and bacon. (If using prosciutto you do not need to saute it) Once the bacon starts to brown and crisp, add in the frozen spinach, and spices. (Note: reduce the amount of salt if using prosciutto) Continue to sauté and all ingredients are cooked. Remove the mixture from heat and allow to cool.
3. On the greased foil lined baking sheet, spread the meat and vegetable mixture out evenly. If using prosciutto, just lay the pieces on the top of the onions and spinach. Then pour the egg whites all over it, and the vegetables are well covered.
4. Place the baking sheet in the oven and bake for 30-35 minutes.
5. Remove the egg bake from oven and cut immediately into 10 squares. Remove the squares with a spatula before it cools so they do not stick to the aluminum foil. Store in an airtight container in the refrigerator as premade breakfast egg bake.

Sheet Pan Combination Sausage Egg Bake

Approximate Yield	Prep Time 20 min	Estimated Macronutrients
10 servings	Total Time 55 min	18 g P • 36 g C • 9 g F

INGREDIENTS

1 cup of crumbled, cooked Sage Turkey Sausage (see recipe page 72)
8 oz-10 oz (2 cups) frozen spinach
½ red onion diced or ¼ cup minced dried onion
4 large mushrooms (washed, destemmed and sliced)
4-5 baby red, yellow and orange bell peppers, stems removed, deseeded and chopped
8 egg whites or 1 cup of pasteurized liquid egg whites*
2 whole eggs
½ cup unsweetened cashew milk or other nut milk*
1-2 tablespoons olive oil
2 teaspoons dried parsley
1 teaspoon Dijon or yellow mustard*
¼ teaspoon salt
¼ teaspoon granulated garlic
¼ teaspoon pepper
Optional: ½ cup shredded aged gruyere or cheddar cheese*

Spray olive or avocado oil for greasing the baking sheet/jelly roll sheet

KITCHEN EQUIPMENT

Large baking sheet with raised edge or baking jelly roll sheet
Medium mixing bowl
Heat-resistant spoon or spatula
Measuring spoons & measuring cups
Non-stick large skillet
Aluminum foil

SPECIAL INSTRUCTIONS/DIET INFORMATION

* If using liquid egg whites, be careful to read all ingredients. This should be a mono ingredient, and not contain any preservatives or additives, other than pasteurized egg whites. Regular separated egg whites can be used but the batter will be thicker and require many eggs. Note the conversion is 2 tablespoons of liquid eggs to 1 egg white.

*Any nut milks should only consist of nuts, water, or salt. No emulsifiers, gums, sweeteners or additives should be in the ingredient list. If you are unable to source a SCD legal nut milk you can make them easily at home (see recipe page 299).

*There are a few commercial brands of mustard made with SCD legal ingredients. However always check ingredients carefully. Confirm with the company and determine unlisted ingredients are not being used in the manufacturing process.

* Cheeses should be aged over 3 months, and contain zero carbohydrates or sugars, regarding nutritional content. Pre-sliced and pre-shredded cheese will likely contain illegal ingredients to prevent the cheese from sticking and prolong shelf life. It is always best to purchase blocks of cheese, then shred, grate, crumble or slice yourself.

DIRECTIONS

1. Preheat oven to 350 degrees F and grease the baking sheet with the spray oil and set aside.
2. In a non-stick large skillet, spray the skillet with oil and cook the onion, bell peppers, and mushrooms. Halfway through the cooking process add frozen spinach and the sausage. Continue to sauté and ingredients are cooked. Remove from heat and allow to cool.
3. In a medium mixing bowl, combine the eggs, liquid egg whites, cashew milk, mustard, and spices. Whisk well and set aside.
4. In the greased baking sheet, spread out the meat and vegetable mixture evenly.
5. Pour the egg mixture over it all. If using cheese in the dish, sprinkle shredded cheese all over the top.
6. Place the baking sheet in the oven and bake for 30-35 minutes.
7. Remove the egg bake from oven and cut immediately into 10 squares. Remove the squares with a spatula from the foil, before it cools and doesn't stick. Store in an airtight container in the refrigerator as premade breakfasts.

Sage and Turkey Breakfast Sausage

Approximate Yield	Prep Time 10 min	Estimated Macronutrients
10-12 servings	Total Time 30 min	14 g P • 6 g C • 7 g F

INGREDIENTS
20 oz ground turkey or lean ground pork
4 tablespoons dehydrated minced onion flakes or ½ cup fresh minced onion
¼ cup bone broth or filtered water
2- 3 tablespoons Italian Sage Spice Rub (see recipe page 145)
¼ cup honey
Sea salt to taste
Olive oil

KITCHEN EQUIPMENT
Large non-stick skillet
Measuring spoons & cups
Handheld meat chopper, mincer or heat-resistant spatula
Large heat-resistant spoon or spatula

SPECIAL INSTRUCTIONS/DIET INFORMATION
*Add honey to taste, use more to offset the spice.

DIRECTIONS
1. Heat the olive oil in the skillet on medium heat, then add the ground turkey or ground pork, onion and water (or bone broth).
2. Continue to sauté and break up the turkey until cooked in the water. Add in the spices and honey, stirring well and the meat is well-coated.
3. Continuing cooking until the moisture is reduced, and both meat and onions are well cooked. Lower the heat on the stovetop to warm when done.
4. Remove the ground turkey from heat and serve or use the sausage crumbles in other recipes or meals.

Stuffed Breakfast Squash

Approximate Yield	Prep Time 20 min	Estimated Macronutrients
4 servings	Total Time 55 min	24 g P • 31 g C • 12 g F

INGREDIENTS

2 acorn squashes
2 cups of leftover cooked Sage Turkey Breakfast Sausage (see recipe page 72)
1 green apple cored and diced thinly
¾ cup of chopped walnuts
1 minced shallot
2 teaspoons olive oil
¼ teaspoon of cinnamon
¼ teaspoon salt
¼ teaspoon ground dried sage
Salt and pepper to taste
Optional:
1 cup of minced mushrooms for stuffing*
¼ cup cooked and crumbled (no sugar or added sweeteners) bacon*
honey*

KITCHEN EQUIPMENT

Baking sheet pan
Measuring spoons & measuring cups
Large skillet
Handheld meat chopper, mincer or heat-resistant spatula
Baking parchment paper

SPECIAL INSTRUCTIONS/DIET INFORMATION

*Note mushrooms overwhelm the subtle flavors of the dish and therefore optional.
*Always read labels carefully verify ingredients with manufacturers for prepackaged bacon.
*Some may not prefer a sweeter flavor profile so omit as needed.

DIRECTIONS

1. Preheat oven to 400 degrees F. Line the sheet pan with parchment paper
2. To prepare the squash, use a sharp chef's knife to slice through it from the tip to the stem. Its easiest to pierce the squash in the center along a depression line, then cut through the tip. Finish by slicing through the top portion just next to the stem.
3. Drizzle the olive oil over the squash, and sprinkle with the salt. Place the acorn squash halves cut side down. (You do not need to clean out the pulp and seeds before roasting)
4. Place the acorn squashes in the oven and bake until the squash flesh is very easily pierced through by a fork, approximately 30 to 45 minutes (depending on the size of your squash). Remove the squash from the oven and allow to cool. When the squash is cool enough to touch, use a large spoon scoop and discard the middle pulp and seeds.
5. Heating the olive oil sauté the (optional) mushrooms, shallot, apples, walnuts and spices. When the shallots and apples are both tender, add in the turkey sausage and (optional) bacon. Sauté until both are heated through.
6. Scoop the stuffing into each half of the acorn squashes, drizzle with the (optional) honey and sprinkle with salt and pepper. Serve warm and cut in quarters.
7. Important to note you may have extra stuffing. The leftovers can be tossed with roasted butternut squash for a breakfast bowl or eaten as a side with eggs.

Butternut Squash Breakfast Casserole

Approximate Yield	Prep Time 20 min	Estimated Macronutrients
8-12 servings	Total Time 90 min	16 g P • 12 g C • 9 g F

INGREDIENTS

1-2 long neck butternut squash (seeded, peeled and shredded)

¾ cup of diced (no sugar or added sweeteners) bacon*

½ small onion chopped or ¼ cup of dried onion

2 eggs

1 ½ cup pasteurized liquid egg whites or egg whites*

1 tablespoon Dijon or yellow mustard*

½ teaspoon granulated garlic

½ teaspoon granulated onion

8 oz-10oz (1 ¼ cup) frozen spinach

1 ½ cups shredded cheddar cheese*

Spray olive or avocado oil for greasing casserole/baking dish and skillet

KITCHEN EQUIPMENT

8 x 10 or 9x 13 glass baking dish depending on depth

Medium mixing bowl

Non-stick medium skillet

Coarse cheese grater

Aluminum foil

SPECIAL INSTRUCTIONS/DIET INFORMATION

*If using pasteurized liquid egg whites, be careful to read all ingredients. This should be a mono ingredient, and not contain any preservatives or additives, other than pasteurized egg whites. Separated egg whites can be used but the batter will be thicker and require many eggs. Note the approximate conversion is 2 tablespoons of liquid eggs to 1 egg white.

*Always read labels carefully verify ingredients with manufacturers for prepackaged bacon.

*There are a few commercial brands of mustard made with SCD legal ingredients. However always check ingredients carefully. Confirm with the company and determine unlisted ingredients are not being used in the manufacturing process.

* Cheeses should be aged over 3 months, and contain zero carbohydrates or sugars, regarding nutritional content. Pre-sliced and pre-shredded cheese will likely contain illegal ingredients to prevent the cheese from sticking and prolong shelf life. It is always best to purchase blocks of cheese, then shred, grate, crumble or slice yourself.

DIRECTIONS

1. In a non-stick medium skillet, spray the skillet with oil and cook the diced bacon and the onion. Halfway through the cooking process add frozen spinach. Continue to sauté until all ingredients are cooked. Remove from heat and allow to cool.

2. For the butternut squash, peel the skin off and shred the long neck of the butternut squash using a grater. (Avoiding the portion with the seeds). Set aside the grated butternut squash.

3. Preheat oven to 350 degrees F and grease the baking dish with the olive oil then set aside.

4. In a medium mixing bowl, combine the eggs, liquid egg whites, mustard, and spices. Whisk all ingredients together well and set aside.

5. In the greased baking dish, layer the bottom of the dish with a thin layer of shredded butternut squash. Followed by a layer of the spinach, bacon and onion. Then sprinkle with shredded cheese and pour some of the egg mixture over it all. Follow the same layering pattern until the final two layers are the egg mixture and topping it with shredded cheese. Be careful to leave space between the top of the baking dish and cheese.

6. Cover with foil loosely to prevent the cheese from sticking to it and bake the casserole for 60 min. Remove the foil and return the casserole to the oven. Bake for another 10 minutes until the sides of the casserole are crusty and the cheese turns golden.

7. If you find the cheese is getting too brown, then loosely cover with foil during the baking process as needed. The butternut squash should be tender when sliced with a knife.

8. Remove from oven and allow to cool for 10 minutes before serving.

Butternut Choriz-No Mexican Breakfast Casserole

Approximate Yield	Prep Time 20 min	Estimated Macronutrients
8-12 servings	Total Time 55 min	32g P • 8 g C • 18 g F

INGREDIENTS

1-2 long neck butternut squash (peeled and shredded)
1 ½ cup of ground pork or beef (approximately 1 lb.)
¼-½ cup of filtered water
2 tablespoons SCD Taco Seasoning (see recipe page 147)
½ cup favorite salsa or Restaurant- Style Salsa (see recipe page 137)
½ small onion chopped or ¼ cup of dried onion
2 eggs
1 ½ cup pasteurized liquid egg whites or egg whites*
½ cup shredded cheddar cheese*
½ cup of shredded monterey jack cheese*
2- 3 tablespoons dried chives

Spray olive or avocado oil for greasing casserole/baking dish and skillet

KITCHEN EQUIPMENT

8 x 10 or 9x 13 glass baking dish depending on depth
Medium mixing bowl
Non-stick medium skillet
Coarse cheese grater
Aluminum foil

SPECIAL INSTRUCTIONS/DIET INFORMATION

* If using pasteurized liquid egg whites, be careful to read all ingredients. This should be a mono ingredient, and not contain any preservatives or additives, other than pasteurized egg whites. Separated egg whites can be used but the batter will be thicker and require many eggs. Note the approximate conversion is 2 tablespoons of liquid eggs to 1 egg white.
* Cheeses should be aged over 3 months, and contain zero carbohydrates or sugars, regarding nutritional content. Pre-sliced and pre-shredded cheese will likely contain illegal ingredients to prevent the cheese from sticking and prolong shelf life. It is always best to purchase blocks of cheese, then shred, grate, crumble or slice yourself.

DIRECTIONS

1. In a non-stick medium skillet, spray the skillet with oil and cook the ground pork or beef. Add the taco seasoning, some filtered water and the onion halfway through the cooking process.
2. Continue to sauté until all ingredients are cooked. Remove from heat and allow to cool.
3. For the butternut squash, peel the skin off and shred the long neck of the butternut squash using a grater. (Avoiding the portion with the seeds). Set aside the grated butternut squash.
4. Preheat oven to 350 degrees F, grease the baking dish with the olive oil and set aside.
5. In a medium mixing bowl, combine the eggs, liquid egg whites, and spices (except chives 1 tablespoon chives and salsa). Whisk well and set aside.
6. In the greased baking dish, layer the bottom of the dish with shredded butternut squash. Followed by the ground pork or beef. Then sprinkle with shredded cheese, dollops of salsa and pour some of the egg mixture over it all.
7. Follow the same layering pattern until the final layer is the egg mixture, topped with shredded cheese and dried chives.
8. Cover with foil loosely to prevent the cheese from sticking to it and bake the casserole for 60 min. Remove the foil and return the casserole to the oven. Bake for another 10 minutes until the sides of the casserole are crusty and the cheese turns golden.
9. If you find the cheese is getting too brown, then loosely cover with foil during the baking process as needed. The butternut squash should be tender when sliced with a knife.
10. Remove from oven and allow to cool for 10 minutes before serving.

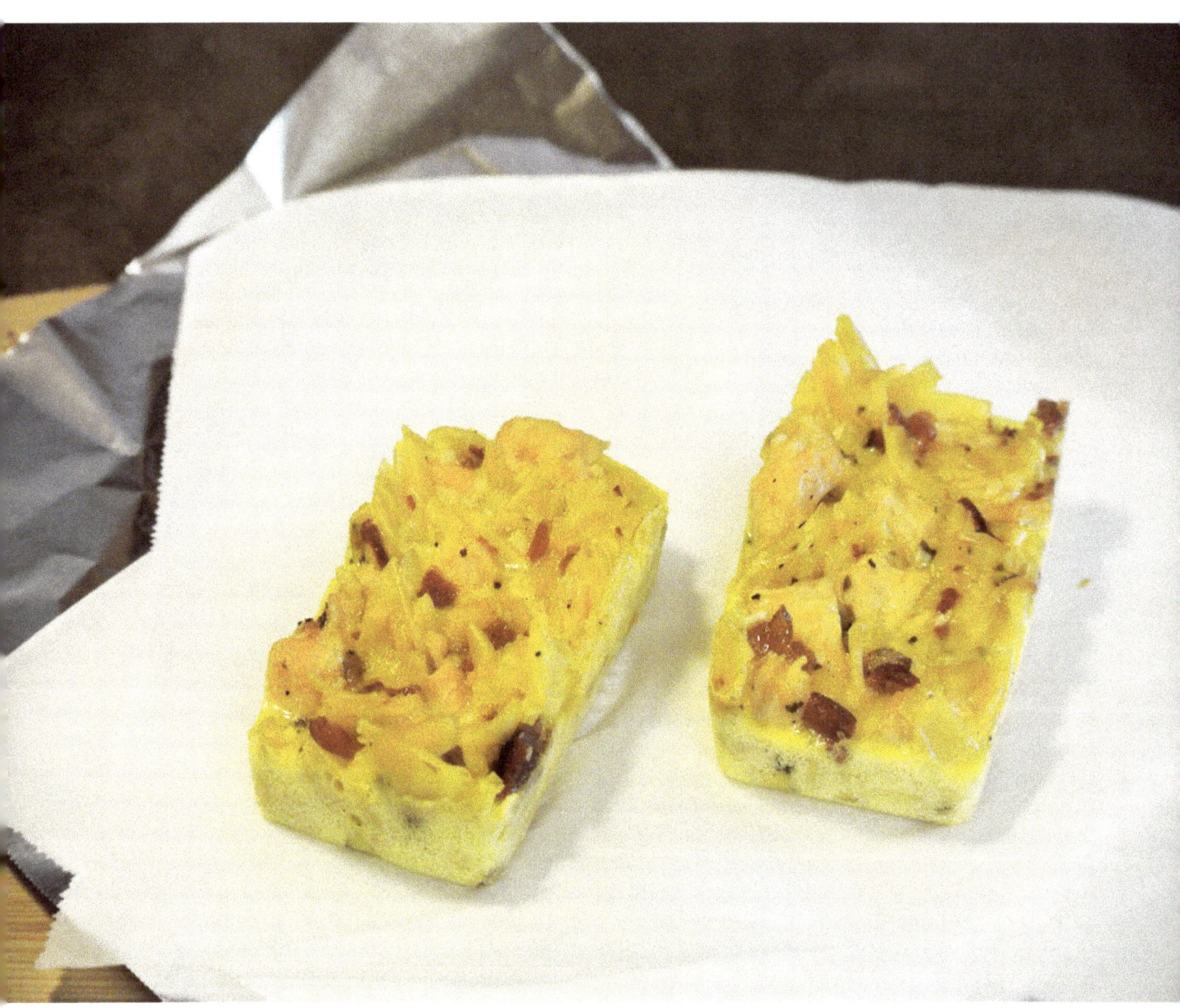

Bacon & Chicken Portable Baked Pasta

Exercise Fuels & Portable Foods

Athletes need nutritious, convenient and real food when travelling, training or competing. Long distance runners, triathletes, and cyclists need portable whole foods to fuel them. Especially if that training takes them into remote areas where convenient food is limited.

During competition, athletes require high glucose foods to prevent "bonking" and provide energy to muscles when needed. This collection of recipes has been tested through endurance events and weightlifting competitions. Not every recipe may work for the specific dietary needs of an athlete. As a good technique, athletes should practice with their fuel and food, well before a competitive event. This collection of recipes offers enough variety to help you find what works best for you.

It is important to note that athletes are not limited in fuel and portable food choices. Many baked goods, such as breads, cookies, muffins, and even soups can be great portable options and fuel sources. Additionally, the recipes in this section use fewer seasonings and spices, as the stomach tends to be more sensitive before, during, and after physical activity. This cookbook contains a variety of recipes in different sections that can support athletic training and activities.

Wild Berry Gel

Approximate Yield	**Prep Time 15 min**	**Estimated Macronutrients**
6 servings	**Total Time 30 min**	**0 g P • 26 g C • 0 g F**

INGREDIENTS

½ cup of honey
1 bag of mixed frozen berries
¼ cup of unflavored, unsweetened collagen powder*
¼ teaspoon baking soda
½ cup unflavored and unsweetened alkaline/electrolyte water (divided)
1 teaspoon salt or 2 teaspoons of unflavored, unsweetened electrolyte salts or (see recipe in special instructions) *
Optional: ½ teaspoon gelatin

KITCHEN EQUIPMENT

Electric juicer or fine mesh colander/strainer
Handheld immersion blender
Reusable baby food pouches
Measuring spoons & measuring cups
Small saucepot
Airtight medium storage container
Heat-resistant spoon or spatula

SPECIAL INSTRUCTIONS/DIET INFORMATION

*Collagen powders should be animal based, not contain seaweed, anti-caking agents, sweeteners, added probiotics, and/or cellulose. Always confirm ingredients with the manufacturer.
*To make unflavored electrolytes packets at home, measure out on a scale: 2500mg sodium chloride, 385 mg potassium chloride, 390 mg magnesium malate or 265 mg dimagnesium malate. (*Source LMNT raw unflavored electrolyte recipe*)

DIRECTIONS

1. In the small saucepot place the frozen berries and ¼ cup of the alkaline/electrolyte water. Cook the water and berries while stirring regularly until tender and simmering.
2. Remove from heat and allow to cool. Puree with an immersion blender or food processor.
3. To remove seeds, place the berries in the electric juicer or strain the juice using a fine mesh metal colander. Place the strained juice in the refrigerator for later.
4. In the saucepan heat the honey, then 6-8 tablespoons pureed berry juice, ¼ cup of electrolyte water, baking soda, collagen, and electrolyte salts.
5. Stirring the mixture continuously until everything is dissolved. Reduce the liquid until the gel is smooth and thicker consistency. Stir in the optional gelatin if a more solid gel is needed.
6. Remove from heat and allow to cool. Pour the gel into the storage container and/or reusable baby food pouches.
7. Store in airtight containers in the refrigerator. For 3-5 days. For long term storage the pouches may need to be stored frozen to prevent molding. Defrost as needed for events and training fuel. Note, its recommended to double bag with a zip top plastic bag during training to prevent any leaks or spills.

Peanut Butter Cookie Gel

Approximate Yield	Prep Time 15 min	Estimated Macronutrients
6-8 servings	**Total Time 30 min**	**5 g P • 18 g C • 3 g F**

INGREDIENTS
½ cup of honey
3 tablespoons peanut butter (heaping)*
¼ cup of unflavored, unsweetened collagen powder*
Optional: 1 tablespoon unsweetened, unflavored beef or bone broth protein powder*
¼ cup unflavored and unsweetened alkaline/electrolyte water
1 teaspoon baking soda
1 teaspoon salt or 1-2 teaspoons of electrolyte salts (see recipe in special instructions) *

KITCHEN EQUIPMENT
Reusable baby food pouches
Small saucepot
Measuring spoons & measuring cups
Airtight medium storage container
Heat-resistant spoon or spatula

SPECIAL INSTRUCTIONS/DIET INFORMATION
* Nut butters that are SCD legal should only include the nut and possibly a legal oil and/or salt. For example, peanut butter is generally roasted peanuts and salt. There are some brands that will sweeten with honey but there are very few commercially available.
*Collagen powders should be animal based, not contain seaweed, anti-caking agents, sweeteners, added probiotics, and/or cellulose. Always confirm ingredients with the manufacturer.
*Unflavored beef (bovine) protein should only be beef or bone broth without any additives or other ingredients. Confirm ingredients and processing with manufacturer.
*To make unflavored electrolytes packets at home, measure out on a scale: 2500mg sodium chloride, 385 mg potassium chloride, 390 mg magnesium malate or 265 mg dimagnesium malate. (*Source LMNT raw unflavored electrolyte recipe*)

DIRECTIONS
1. In the small saucepot on low to medium heat add all ingredients in order.
2. Stirring continuously until everything is dissolved and the gel is a smooth texture.
3. Remove from heat and allow to cool. Pour into the storage container and/or reusable baby food pouches.
4. Store in airtight containers in the refrigerator, up to 3-5 days. For long term storage the pouches may need to be stored frozen to prevent molding. Defrost as needed for events and training fuel.
5. Important tip: When using the reusable baby food pouches, place them in zip top plastic pouches when on your person as training fuel. Reusable pouches are prone to leak when squeezed too hard or not properly sealed.

No Bake Snickerdoodle Cookie Dough

Approximate Yield	Prep Time 15 min	Estimated Macronutrients
6-8 servings	Total Time 30 min	8 g P • 31 g C • 7 g F

No bake lentil or yellow split pea dough makes a great source of training fuel as well as a dessert or snack.

INGREDIENTS

1 cup cooked and cooled yellow split peas (see recipe page 304)
⅓ cup of honey
¼ cup cashew butter (heaping) *
2 teaspoons vanilla extract
2 teaspoons ground cinnamon
¼ teaspoon baking soda
¼ teaspoon sea salt
6 tablespoons almond flour (this is based on desired thickness) *
Optional fuel add-ins:
Add favorite unflavored electrolyte salt to taste or as needed.
For caffeine add ¼ teaspoon espresso powder per 1 tablespoon of no bake cookie dough

Note: If using as fuel, mixing in an add-in may not be recommended for consuming with a squeezable pouch.

Optional add-ins:
Choice of chopped nuts
Chopped dried and pitted dates

KITCHEN EQUIPMENT

Food processor of handheld immersion blender
Mixing bowl
Measuring spoons & measuring cups
Spatula or large spoon
Airtight container for storage or reusable squeeze pouch

SPECIAL INSTRUCTIONS/DIET INFORMATION

*Nut butters that are SCD legal should only include the nut and possibly a legal oil and/or salt. For example, peanut butter is generally roasted peanuts and salt. There are some brands that will sweeten with honey but there are very few commercially available.
*You can substitute the almond flour with 1-3 tablespoons of coconut flour

DIRECTIONS

1. In a food processor or using a handheld immersion blender and mixing bowl, blend the yellow peas.
2. Combine the remaining ingredients until reaching the desired thickness of cookie dough.
3. You can also fold in various add-ins like chopped nuts, toasted coconuts, etc.
4. Store in an airtight container. You can also freeze it into little balls and add to SCD ice cream to make cookie dough ice cream.
5. Freeze into larger balls that will fit in the opening of a reusable pouch. When needed place the frozen dough in the pouch and allow to defrost for use as training fuel.

No Bake Lemon Coconut Cookie Dough

Approximate Yield **6-8 servings**	**Prep Time 15 min** **Total Time 30 min**	**Estimated Macronutrients** **7 g P • 27 g C • 9 g F**

No bake lentil or yellow split pea dough makes a great source of training fuel as well as a dessert or snack.

INGREDIENTS

¾ cup cooked and cooled Yellow Split Peas (see recipe page 304)
⅓ cup of honey
1 lemon juiced and zested
3 tablespoons cashew butter (heaping)*
¼ teaspoon baking soda
1 teaspoon vanilla extract
¼ teaspoon sea salt
½ tablespoon lemon zest
⅛ teaspoon ground ginger*
3 tablespoons finely shredded unsweetened coconut
8 tablespoons of almond flour (this is based on desired thickness) *

Optional fuel add-ins:
Add favorite unflavored electrolyte salt to taste or as needed.
Note: If using as fuel, mixing in an add-in may not be recommended for consuming with a squeezable pouch.

Optional add-ins:
Toasted unsweetened coconut flakes

KITCHEN EQUIPMENT

Food processor of handheld immersion blender
Measuring spoons & measuring cups
Spatula or large spoon
Mixing bowl
Airtight container
Optional: Reusable baby food pouch

SPECIAL INSTRUCTIONS/DIET INFORMATION

*Nut butters that are SCD legal should only include the nut and possibly a legal oil and/or salt. For example, peanut butter is generally roasted peanuts and salt. There are some brands that will sweeten with honey but there are very few commercially available.
*You can substitute the almond flour with 1-3 tablespoon of coconut flour
*Ginger can sometimes overpower the lemon.

DIRECTIONS

1. In a food processor or using a handheld immersion blender and mixing bowl, pulse until yellow peas are smooth.
2. Combine the remaining ingredients until the dough reaches the desired thickness, and similar in texture to other chewy cookies.
3. You can also fold in various add-ins like chopped nuts, toasted coconut flakes, etc.
4. Store in an airtight container. You can also freeze the dough into little balls, and add to SCD legal ice cream to make cookie dough ice cream.

Electrolyte Gummies

Approximate Yield **60-80 servings**	**Prep Time 15 min** **Total Time 30 min**	**Estimated Macronutrients** **1 g P • 3 g C • 0 g F**

INGREDIENTS

3 tablespoons unflavored gelatin
3 tablespoons honey (heaping)
½ cup of SCD legal fruit juice (see notes) *
½ cup water
1 teaspoon salt or 2 teaspoons legal electrolyte salt (see recipe in special instructions) *

KITCHEN EQUIPMENT

Silicone gelatin candy/gummy molds
Measuring spoons & measuring cups
Wire or silicone whisk
Small saucepot
Candy or gummy dropper

SPECIAL INSTRUCTIONS/DIET INFORMATION

*SCD legal fruit juice does not contain added sugars, sweeteners or made from concentrate. Recommended flavors of juice include lemon, lime, tart cherry, grape, pineapple, and mango.

*To make unflavored electrolytes packets at home, measure out on a scale: 2500mg sodium chloride, 385 mg potassium chloride, 390 mg magnesium malate or 265 mg dimagnesium malate. (*Source LMNT raw unflavored electrolyte recipe*)

DIRECTIONS

1. In the small saucepot add juice and water. Bring to light simmer on low heat
2. Add honey and salt (or electrolyte salt).
3. Add gelatin to the pot very slowly and keep stirring 60-90 seconds with each tablespoon of gelatin.
4. Mix all ingredients very well for another 30 seconds or until all the gelatin has dissolved.
5. Remove from the pot from the heat and allow to cool for 2- 5 minutes.
6. Take the gummy dropper, pipette the gelatin mixture and fill each of the gummy/candy molds. (It helps to have the molds on a flat surface such as a baking sheet, to easily place them in the freezer without spills.)
7. Place the gummy/candy molds in the freezer to set for 10 minutes. Once the gummies are set, you can pop them out of the molds.
8. Store in an airtight container in the refrigerator, for 3-5 days. For long term storage they will need to be stored frozen to prevent molding. Defrost as needed for events and training fuel.
9. Important to note, these gummies may melt and become a gelatinous in warm conditions so always double bag or store in baby food pouch for training sessions.

Electrolyte Juice

Approximate Yield
6 servings

Prep Time 15 min
Total Time 2 hours
(To allow for refrigeration)

Estimated Macronutrients
1 g P • 33 g C • 0 g F

INGREDIENTS

4-6 tablespoons honey
1 cup filtered water
1 cup cranberry or tart cherry juice*
1 ½ cups of pineapple juice*
1 ½ orange or mango juice*
1 cup of apple juice*
¼ cup lime juice
3 teaspoons salt or 3 teaspoons legal electrolyte salt (see recipe in special instructions) *
Optional: ⅛- ¼ teaspoon baking soda
Filtered water as needed

KITCHEN EQUIPMENT

Small pot or saucepan
Heat resistant spatula or spoon
Large (36-48 oz) leak free bottle with lid or mason jar

SPECIAL INSTRUCTIONS/DIET INFORMATION

*SCD legal fruit juice does not contain added sugars, sweeteners or made from concentrate. Recommended flavors of juice include lemon, lime, tart cherry, grape, pineapple, and mango.
*To make unflavored electrolytes packets at home, measure out on a scale: 2500mg sodium chloride, 385 mg potassium chloride, 390 mg magnesium malate or 265 mg dimagnesium malate. (*Source LMNT raw unflavored electrolyte recipe*)

DIRECTIONS

1. In the small saucepot add the honey and water. Bring to light simmer while stirring on medium heat to create a simple syrup. Remove from heat and allow to cool.
2. Pour all juices in a large jar, bottle or container. Stir and mix the juices well or place lid on the container and shake up the juice.
3. Add in salt or electrolytes, cooled simple honey syrup, and filtered water as needed. Note this is all to taste and based on personal preference. The goal is to balance the sweetness with the saltiness. Also, the baking soda will change the taste of the juice.
4. Store in the refrigerator, for 3-5 days.

Electrolyte Vegetable Juice

Approximate Yield
6-8 servings

Prep Time 20 min
Total Time 90 min
(To allow for refrigeration)

Estimated Macronutrients
4 g P • 30 g C • 2 g F

INGREDIENTS

2 lbs. tomatoes, chopped
2 carrots, peeled and chopped
2 persian cucumbers, peeled and chopped
2 green bell peppers, chopped (seeds and stems removed)
1 red bell pepper, chopped (seeds and stems removed)
1 yellow onion, chopped
1 cup of celery stalks chopped
½ cup of peeled and cooked beets
2 cloves garlic
2 cups of filtered water
1 cup of tomato juice or sauce*
1 lemon juiced (approximately 2- 2 ½ tablespoons juice)
2 tablespoon honey
2 ½ teaspoon sea salt
1 teaspoon grated horseradish
1 teaspoon Worcestershire sauce (see recipe page 120)
¼ teaspoon ground white pepper
¼ teaspoon granulated garlic
Salt and honey to taste
Optional: Cayenne pepper for spice
Optional: ¼ cup of fresh parsley chopped

KITCHEN EQUIPMENT

Electric juicer
2 Large bowls
Large pot
Food processor or handheld immersion blender
Measuring spoons & measuring cups
Heat resistant spoon or spatula
Sterilized large mason jars with lids
Optional: Sieve or fine mesh colander
Silicone freezer cubes/containers

SPECIAL INSTRUCTIONS/DIET INFORMATION

*If you cannot source SCD legal tomato sauce, drain a large can of crushed or finely diced tomatoes over a fine mesh sieve or colander over another bowl to catch the juice. Pressing down the tomatoes to extract more juice as needed.

*Adding honey is to taste, and more can be added after the sauce is blended well.

*Canned tomatoes are typically not allowed under SCD. However, there are Italian brands of canned tomatoes and tomato pastes with no artificial flavors, preservatives or additives listed as ingredients, nor used in the manufacturing process. These brands are generally sold through Wellbees and a few other stores. Read store bought canned tomato and tomato paste labels carefully. If necessary, you can make your own tomato sauce or paste using fresh tomatoes or canned tomato juice (if salt is the only other ingredient).

DIRECTIONS

1. Rinse, peel and chop ingredients for vegetable juice and place in a large bowl.
2. Juice the vegetables per the electric juicer's instructions, catching the vegetable juice in another bowl.
3. In a large pot on medium heat, pour in the vegetable juice and tomato juice. Stirring to blend the juices.
4. Add all the remaining ingredients to the pot, stirring as the pot simmers. Taste the juice whether additional salt, cayenne or honey may be needed.
5. Transfer the juice into a sterilized glass container or mason jar with lid and refrigerate for an hour. However, it can also be frozen in silicone cubes or ice trays and thawed later if needed. Ideally for long term storage, the juice can be canned following USDA guidelines.
6. For the leftover vegetable pulp and tomatoes, use in the Gazpacho recipe or Slow Cooker Tomato Vegetable Pot Roast. (see recipes page 167 & 268)

Cauliflower Yellow Pea Mini Muffins

Approximate Yield **12-36 servings**	**Prep Time 15 min** **Total Time 55 min**	**Estimated Macronutrients** **7 g P • 4 g C • 4 g F**

INGREDIENTS

1 cup cooked, Yellow Pea Mash (see recipe page 304)
1 (12 oz) package or approximately 2 cups of frozen rice cauliflower (cooked)*
½ cup dried minced onion or ¾ cup finely grated fresh onion*
3 egg whites
2 beaten whole eggs
2 tablespoons olive oil
2 tablespoons Parmesan- No Seasoning (see recipe page 152)
1 teaspoon dried parsley

Optional add-ins
¼ cup of cooked diced (no sugar or added sweeteners) bacon* or cooked shredded chicken
1 tablespoon dried or fresh minced chives

Neutral oil for greasing the muffin baking tin

KITCHEN EQUIPMENT

Large mixing bowl
Measuring spoons & measuring cups
Spatula or large spoon
24 count mini muffin baking tin or silicone tray*

SPECIAL INSTRUCTIONS/DIET INFORMATION

*Fresh steamed cauliflower can be riced and used; however, the different texture of fresh cauliflower can often vary and may affect the texture of the dish.
*A 12-count standard size muffin tray will work; however, you may need to bake the muffins/tots longer.
*Note the freshly grated onion will produce more moisture and have a stronger taste. You may need to bake longer to reduce the moisture from the raw onion.
*Always read labels carefully verify ingredients with manufacturers for prepackaged bacon.

DIRECTIONS

1. Preheat the oven for 375 degrees F and grease the muffin baking tin.
2. In a large bowl, mix all the ingredients with a spatula until well combined.
3. Spoon the batter into the muffin tins or silicone baking tray and bake for 30-35 minutes.
4. Remove from the oven when the muffins are done, and an inserted knife comes out clean.
5. These muffins freeze well. Once cooled and removed from the baking trays they can be stored in gallon zip top freezer bags for later use.
6. If you prefer a crispier version, the muffins can also be reheated in the oven or air fryer, spray with a bit of neutral oil and air fry or bake at 375 degrees F. Baking and air frying times may vary based on whether they are defrosted or frozen.

Cauliflower Butternut Squash Mini Muffins

Approximate Yield	Prep Time 15 min	Estimated Macronutrients
12-36 servings	**Total Time 55 min**	**3 g P • 4 g C • 5 g F**

This recipe has both a sweet and savory variation.

INGREDIENTS

Savory Variation
1 can of butternut squash (15 oz) or cooked, pureed butternut squash 2 cups
12 oz package or 3 cups of frozen rice cauliflower (cooked)*
½ cup dried minced onion or ¾ cup finely grated fresh onion*
½ cup almond flour
2 large eggs
2 tablespoons olive oil
1 ½ tablespoons Parmesan-No Seasoning (see recipe page 152)
1 tablespoon dried parsley

Sweet Variation
1 can of butternut squash (15 oz) or cooked, pureed butternut squash 2 cups
1 (12 oz) package or approximately 2 cups of frozen rice cauliflower (cooked)
⅔ cup almond flour
2 large eggs
2 tablespoons honey
1 ½ tablespoons Pumpkin Spice (see recipe page 144)
1 tablespoon olive oil

Neutral oil for greasing the muffin baking tin

KITCHEN EQUIPMENT
Large mixing bowl
Measuring spoons & measuring cups
Spatula or large spoon
24 count mini muffin baking tin or silicone baking tray*
Optional microwavable dish with lid

SPECIAL INSTRUCTIONS/DIET INFORMATION
*Fresh steamed cauliflower can be riced and used; however, the different texture of fresh cauliflower can often vary and may affect the texture of the dish.
*A 12-count standard size muffin tray will work, however you may need to bake the muffins/tots longer.
*Note the freshly grated onion will produce more moisture and have a stronger taste. You may need to bake longer to reduce the moisture from the raw onion.

DIRECTIONS
1. Preheat the oven for 375 degrees F and grease the muffin baking tin.
2. In a large bowl mix all the ingredients with a spatula until well combined.
3. Spoon the batter into the muffin tins or silicone baking tray and bake for 30-35 minutes.
4. Remove from the oven when the muffins are done, and an inserted knife comes out clean.
5. These muffins freeze well. Once cooled and removed from the baking tray they can be stored in gallon zip top freezer bags for later use.
6. If you prefer a crispier version, the muffins can also be reheated in the oven or air fryer, spray with a bit of neutral oil and air fry or bake at 375 degrees F. Baking and air frying times may vary based on whether they are defrosted or frozen.

Savory Loaded No-Tato Chaffles

Approximate Yield	**Prep Time 15 min**	**Estimated Macronutrients**
6 servings	**Total Time 30 min**	**23 g P • 12 g C • 19 g F**

INGREDIENTS

1 cup of Best Mashed No-Tatos (see recipe page 211)
3 eggs, beaten
¼ cup of diced, cooked (no sugar or added sweeteners) bacon*
½ tablespoon dried or fresh minced chives
Optional: ¼ cup of shredded cheddar cheese*

Neutral spray or avocado oil to grease waffle maker

KITCHEN EQUIPMENT

Waffle maker/iron
Small to medium mixing bowl
Measuring spoons & measuring cups
Spatula or large spoon

SPECIAL INSTRUCTION/DIET INFORMATION

*Always read labels carefully verify ingredients with manufacturers for prepackaged bacon.
*Cheese is recommended if taking packing the chaffle to go or when training since the cheese helps bind the ingredients best.
* Cheeses should be aged over 3 months, and contain zero carbohydrates or sugars, regarding nutritional content.
Pre-sliced and pre-shredded cheese will likely contain illegal ingredients to prevent the cheese from sticking and prolong shelf life. It is always best to purchase blocks of cheese, then shred, grate, crumble or slice yourself.

DIRECTIONS

1. Preheat the waffle maker per the manufacturer's instructions. Then brush or spray the neutral oil.
2. Mix all ingredients, in a medium bowl (leaving the optional cheese to be folded into the batter last). Ladle the waffle batter into the waffle maker.
3. When the waffle maker light indicates the waffle is done, check to ensure the waffle is a golden color. Remove from waffle maker/iron when done, then allow to cool on parchment paper.
4. Waffles will store for up to 3 days in a refrigerator and can be frozen for later use. They can also be frozen for several months if wrapped in parchment, foil and stored in airtight bags.

Portable Baked Pasta

Approximate Yield	Prep Time 20 min	Estimated Macronutrients
6-8 servings	Total Time 50 min	12 g P • 19 g C • 7 g F

INGREDIENTS

8 oz (approximately 2-2 ½ cups) favorite SCD legal lentil or yellow pea pasta (penne, macaroni, agile, or spaghetti shaped) *
1 tablespoon olive oil
8 eggs*
½ teaspoon dried basil
½ teaspoon salt
½ teaspoon granulated garlic
Dash of black pepper
Butter or neutral oil for greasing baking trays

Tomato Meat
2 cups of cooked ground beef, turkey or leftover Sage Turkey Breakfast Sausage (see recipe page 72)
1 cup of shredded monterey jack cheese*
½ cup of diced tomatoes or leftover Loaded Spaghetti Sauce (see recipe page 247)
2 tablespoons grated parmesan cheese *

Bacon Chicken Parmesan
2 cups cooked chicken or leftover shredded Roasted Chicken (see recipe page 255)
½ cups of cooked and crumbled (no sugar or added sweeteners) bacon*
4 tablespoons grated parmesan cheese *
2 tablespoons minced dried onion or grated fresh shallot

KITCHEN EQUIPMENT

Large mixing bowl
Medium to large pot
Fine mesh colander or strainer
Knife or mincer
Medium bowl
Fork or whisk
Measuring spoons & measuring cups
Baking parchment muffin or mini loaf liners (recommended)
Spatula
Silicone or non-stick mini loaf baking tray or muffin baking tins/trays

SPECIAL INSTRUCTIONS/DIET INFORMATION

*Roasted Spaghetti Squash (see recipe page 177) can be substituted for pasta however the moisture will need to be squeezed from the squash in cheesecloth before baking. Also using the squash will change the macronutrients and texture.
*Always read labels carefully verify ingredients with manufacturers for prepackaged bacon.
* Cheeses should be aged over 3 months, and contain zero carbohydrates or sugars, regarding nutritional content. Pre-sliced and pre-shredded cheese will likely contain illegal ingredients to prevent the cheese from sticking and prolong shelf life. It is always best to purchase blocks of cheese, then shred, grate, crumble or slice yourself.

DIRECTIONS

1. Preheat oven to 350 degrees F. Place baking parchment liners in the tray or muffin tin as recommended or spray with oil well.
2. Boil the pasta according to the instructions, and strain off the water when cooked. Rinse the pasta in the colander with cool water and allow to drain.
3. Beat the eggs in a separate bowl with fork or whisk, then mix in remaining other seasoning. Set aside
4. Toss the pasta and olive oil in a large mixing bowl. If the pasta is the larger or longer variety, use a knife, or mincer to cut into smaller pieces, avoid mashing the pasta if possible.
5. Based on the chosen variation, toss the remaining filling ingredients in with the pasta. Then pour in the egg mixture and stir well.
6. Spoon the pasta batter into the lined muffin tin or mini loave tray.
7. Bake for 15-25 minutes (this is based on serving sizes). Insert a toothpick or knife into the center and if it comes out clean the baked pasta is done.
8. Allow to cool then refrigerate in airtight containers for up to 3-4 days.

Portable Shepherd Pies

Approximate Yield	**Prep Time 20 min**	**Estimated Macronutrients**
8-12 servings	Total Time 60 min	32g P • 35 g C • 13 g F

INGREDIENTS

1 ½ - 2 cups of Mashed No-Tato (see recipe page 211) *

3-4 mini loaves of SCD Sourdough Bread (see recipe page 312) cut lengthwise

1 ¼ cups of pasteurized liquid egg whites*

2 whole beaten eggs

2 tablespoons grated parmesan cheese*

Olive oil for greasing baking tray

Pinch of nutmeg

Dash of paprika and dried parsley for color

Meat filling

1 lb. of 93% or greater lean beef or bison

2 cups of frozen diced carrots and peas combined

12 white medium mushrooms washed and destemmed

1 cup water, or SCD Roasted Chicken Bone Broth (see recipe page 255) *

1 tablespoons olive oil

¼ cup minced dried onions or ½ cup of raw yellow onions finely chopped

2 tablespoons Worcestershire Sauce (see recipe page 120)

1 tablespoon tomato paste*

2 teaspoons dried parsley

1 ½ teaspoons fine sea salt

½ teaspoon dried thyme

¼ teaspoon fine ground black pepper

¼ teaspoon crushed rosemary leaves

Salt & pepper to taste

KITCHEN EQUIPMENT

Baking safe silicone 8 mini loaves baking tray or muffin tray (Note: Non-stick will work however it may be difficult to remove the pies from the tray without parchment paper baking liners)

Handheld meat chopper, mincer or heat-resistant spatula

Measuring spoons & measuring cups

Medium mixing bowl

Heat-resistant spoon or spatula

Large saucepan or skillet

Fork

Small spatula

SPECIAL INSTRUCTIONS/DIET INFORMATION

*The best version of No-Tato Mash recommended for this recipe is made with some SCD Nonfat Yogurt to add extra protein and less fat.

*Be careful to read all ingredients for pasteurized liquid egg whites. This should be a mono ingredient, and not contain any preservatives or additional ingredients. Regular separated egg whites can be used but they will be thicker and require many eggs.

* Cheeses should be aged over 3 months, and contain zero carbohydrates or sugars, regarding nutritional content. Pre-sliced and pre-shredded cheese will likely contain illegal ingredients to prevent the cheese from sticking and prolong shelf life. It is always best to purchase blocks of cheese, then shred, grate, crumble or slice yourself.

*Using chicken bone broth will alter the estimated macros of the dish.

*Canned tomatoes are typically not allowed under SCD. However, there are Italian brands of canned tomatoes and tomato pastes with no artificial flavors, preservatives or additives listed as ingredients, nor used in the manufacturing process. These brands are generally sold through Wellbees and a few other stores. Read store bought canned tomato and tomato paste labels carefully. If necessary, you can make your own tomato sauce or paste using fresh tomatoes or canned tomato juice (if salt is the only other ingredient).

DIRECTIONS

1. Preheat oven to 400 degrees F and grease the baking trays with some olive oil and set aside. If using nonstick muffin or baking trays, line them instead with baking parchment paper liners

2. In a food processor or blender, chop up the frozen peas and carrots, then add the mushrooms to create a coarse filling. It is ok if a few peas and carrots do not chop up completely. Set aside.

3. In a large pot or saucepan on medium to high heat, use the heat-resistant spatula (or meat mincer) to break up the ground beef with the water or bone broth. Once the meat is cooked, stir in all the vegetable mixture, remaining filling ingredients, spices and continue to cook to bubbling. Ensuring the meat and vegetables are well coated with seasonings. Remove from heat.

4. In the well-greased baking tray or tins, lay the slices of bread on the bottom. Then spoon the meat and vegetable filling on top.
5. Pour some of the egg whites over the meat filling in each tray, use a fork to press and stir the filling into the bread egg mixture. The goal is for the bread to be soaked, and egg whites will act as a binder for the filling.
6. In a small bowl mix the beaten eggs, grated parmesan and to No-Tato mash together.
7. Then spoon a layer of the No-Tato mash mixture onto the meat filling evenly. Sprinkle the top with a dash or paprika and dried parsley
8. Bake for 40-45 min or until the tops are golden. Remove from oven and allow to cool a bit (approximately 10 minutes). Serve either immediately while warm or allow to cool and place in refrigerator.
9. Once the portable shepherd pies are cooler and firmer, they can be wrapped in parchment and foil for later use as a portable meal. They also can be frozen however they will require at least 24 hours to defrost in a refrigerator before eating. Important to note, these pies are not shelf stable and will require refrigeration in a portable cooler for on the go eating. Reheat using a microwave or portable food warmer.

Portable Pie Variations

Hand pies are some of the most convenient, on the go foods for athletes. Especially if a pie is well balanced in protein, carbohydrates and fats. Each one of these variations has the option for either sweet or savory flavors. The recipes are focused on thepie crust. However there are many recipes in this book that can be used for pie fillings. Macronutrients are not provided for these recipes, as fillings and servings can vary.

INGREDIENTS

Traditional Hand Pie Crust
2 cups almond flour
⅓ cup coconut flour
2 teaspoons of unflavored, unsweetened gelatin
⅛ teaspoon sea salt
4 tablespoons chilled butter cut in squares
¼ cup of filtered water
Extra coconut flour for dusting
1 egg for wash

Easy Bread Based Crusts
3-4 cups of SCD bread, cut into cubes (ideally use breads with minimal nuts and/or dried fruits) or for a sweet variation Chewy Graham Crackers (see recipe page 275)
2 eggs lightly beaten
2 tablespoons of chilled butter
½ teaspoon of unflavored unsweetened gelatin

Tortilla/Wrap Crusts
6 Yellow Pea Wraps (see recipe page 306) or Asian Style Green Onion Wraps (see recipe page 308) or larger Pumpkin Street Tortillas (see recipe page 307) or Pumpkin Spice Sweet Wraps (see recipe page 95)

KITCHEN EQUIPMENT
Food processor
Large bowl
Small cup or bowl
Heat resistant pastry brush
Measuring cups & spoons
Baking parchment paper
Baking sheet or baking safe silicone or nonstick muffin tray
Fork
Spatula or large spoon
Rolling pin
Pie Crust/Empanada Presses or Molds
Optional: Empanada maker/press
Microwave

FILLING OPTIONS

Savory
Bison Sloppy Joe filling (see recipe page 242)
Ground Turkey Taco filling (see recipe page 236)
Sage and Turkey Breakfast Sausage crumbles (see recipe page 72)
Gyro "Döner" filling (see recipe page 215)
Sheet Pan "Combination" Sausage Egg Bake, only recommended for pie crust cups (see recipe page 71)
Bison Pad Kra Pao (see recipe page 228)
Korean Ground Beef (see recipe page 221)
Green Eggs & "Ham" Sheet Pan Egg Bake, only recommended for pie crust cups (see recipe page 70)

Sweet
Berry Compote (see recipe page 108)
Rustic Apple Sauce, not the pureed variation (see recipe page 301)
SCD Coconut Marshmallows (see recipe page 284)

FILLING OPTIONS (continued)

Lemon Coconut Yogurt Bars filling, only recommended for pie crust cups (see recipe page 279)
Pumpkin Pie (Low Fat) filling, only recommended for pie crust cups (see recipe page 288)
Cherry Swirl No-Cheesecake filling, only recommended for pie crust cups (see recipe page 274)

DIRECTIONS **Traditional Hand Pie Crust**

1. Preheat oven to 350 degrees F.
2. In small food processor, pulse together the flours, gelatin, and salt.
3. Add the chilled butter and blend until the butter has crumbled into the dough and not visible.
4. Transfer the dough into the large bowl and stir in the water. Shape the dough into a ball and refrigerate as needed for 10 minutes.

For Traditional Turnover Pies

5. Place a bit of coconut flour on a large piece of parchment paper. Separate the dough into separate balls on the parchment paper, providing enough space to roll each dough ball out. Lay another piece of parchment paper on top of the dough balls. Using the rolling pin on the parchment to prevent the dough from sticking, roll out the dough into thin pie crust circles.
6. When spooning the filling onto the pie crust, offset the placement of the filling to one side. Then gently fold over the pie crust and pinching down the edges with a fork.
7. Use the parchment paper to transfer the pies onto the baking sheet. Beat an egg in a small bowl and brush the pies with egg wash
8. Bake the pies for 20-30 minutes. This baking time depends on pie sizes.

For Pie Crust Cups

9. Grease the muffin tray well and separate the chilled dough into small balls.
10. Press the dough balls into the muffin trays, along the sides and bottom with a well in the middle for filling.
11. These crust cups can be baked separately, or fillings can be added, and pies baked for 20-30 minutes, depending on the size and filling.

DIRECTIONS **Easy Bread Based Crusts**

1. Preheat oven to 350 degrees F.
2. In small food processor, pulse together the bread, eggs, butter, and gelatin until a moist and pliable dough forms.
3. This dough can be rolled out or shaped as traditional turnover pies (see instructions above). Or the dough can be pressed into pie cups using a well-greased muffin tray or mini loaves pan.
4. The fillings can be added, and pies baked for 20-30 minutes, depending on the size and filling.

DIRECTIONS **Tortilla/Wrap Crusts**

1. Preheat oven to 350 degrees F. Line a baking sheet with parchment. If using an empanada press, preheat per instructions.
2. If the wraps are cold, microwave a wrap with filling for 10-30 seconds for more pliability and tackiness.
3. Place the wrap on the pie crust mold or press. Then fold over one side and press firmly along the edges to ensure they stick together.
4. Transfer the pie to parchment lined baking sheet or an empanada maker/press. Bake the pies for 10-15 minutes or use the empanada maker/press indicator light. Remove when golden.

French Toast Cakes

Approximate Yield	Prep Time 20 min	Estimated Macronutrients
12 servings	Total Time 55 min	17 g P • 39 g C • 19 g F

INGREDIENTS

½ -1 loaf (approximately 2-4 cups) of leftover Cloud bread, SCD "Sourdough", Zucchini, Walnut Cranberry, Raisin Bread, or Pumpkin bread *
¾ cup pasteurized liquid egg whites
¾ cup unsweetened nut milk*
3 tablespoons honey
1 teaspoon of vanilla extract
¼ teaspoon cinnamon

Butter or neutral oil for greasing baking trays

KITCHEN EQUIPMENT

Large mixing bowl
Measuring spoons & measuring cups
Whisk or mixer and beaters
Spatula
Silicone or non-stick mini loaf baking tray or muffin baking tins/trays
Fork
Aluminum foil

SPECIAL INSTRUCTIONS/DIET INFORMATION

*See the various bread recipes under Staples & Ready-Made Foods, and Breakfast Chapters. Recipes on pages 310, 312, 68, 64, 66, & 62

*Be careful to read all ingredients for pasteurized liquid egg whites. This should be a mono ingredient, and not contain any preservatives or additional ingredients. Regular separated egg whites can be used but the batter will be thicker and require many eggs.

*Any nut milks should only consist of nuts, water, or salt. No emulsifiers, gums, sweeteners or additives should be in the ingredient list. If you are unable to source a SCD legal nut milk you can make them easily at home (see recipe page 299).

DIRECTIONS

1. Preheat oven to 350 degrees F. Spray or brush the muffin or mini loaf baking tin/tray, greasing them well including the sides of the tin.
2. Cut the bread into cubes and lay in the muffin or mini loaf molds.
3. In a large mixing bowl, beat the eggs, and mix with the remaining ingredients.
4. Pour the batter over the cubed bread, and mash some of the cubes in the batter with a fork.
5. Bake for 35-40 minutes. Insert a toothpick or knife into the center and if it comes out clean the french toast cakes are done.

Crustless Sandwich Pies

For many endurance athletes the crustless sandwich is commonly used as a portable food option. Commercially made crustless sandwiches are usually found in the freezer section of many grocery stores and made with illegal SCD ingredients. This recipe is a spin-off of the crustless sandwich, which freezes well, made with SCD legal ingredients and delicious. Servings and macronutrients are not provided for this recipe, as fillings and serving sizes can vary.

INGREDIENTS

2-6 Cashew Buns (see recipe page 311), Cloud Bread (see recipe page 310) or "Sourdough" Buns (see recipe page 312)
2 tablespoons melted butter
1 egg white

Filling Variations

Peanut Butter & Banana Puree

Berry Compote (see recipe page 108) & Nut Butter

Melted SCD Coconut Marshmallow (see recipe page 284) & Nut Butter

Berry Compote (see recipe page 108) & SCD Nonfat Greek Yogurt (see recipe page 298)

KITCHEN EQUIPMENT

Baking parchment paper
Oven
Sandwich crust cutter & crimper
Spatula or large spoon
Bread knife
Small bowl
Pastry brush
Microwave
Optional: Rolling pin

DIRECTIONS

1. Preheat oven to 350 degrees F. Line a baking sheet with parchment paper.
2. Cut the 3–4-inch diameter sandwich buns in half with a bread knife.
3. Warm the sliced buns for 10-30 seconds in the microwave. As an option you can roll out the bread with a rolling pin if necessary.
4. Spoon or spread the filling on the top and bottom of each bun half (not the bready interior side). Sandwich the two halves together and using the sandwich crust cutter/ crimper, seal the sandwich edges together.
5. Place the sandwich on the parchment lined baking sheet, brush the top with melted butter, and then the sealed edges well with egg white.
6. Bake the sandwich pies for 15 minutes, or until bread is toasted and golden.
7. Remove from oven and allow to cool. These sandwich pies can also be individually wrapped in parchment and frozen in freezer safe zip top bags for use later.

Stroopwaffels
(Pumpkin Spice Sweet Wraps)

Approximate Yield **12-20 servings**	**Prep Time 10 min** **Total Time 40 min**	**Estimated Macronutrients** **5 g P • 19 g C • 2 g F**

INGREDIENTS

1 can of pumpkin puree (15 oz or 2 cups)
1 cup pasteurized liquid egg whites*
¼ cup of honey
3 ½ tablespoons coconut flour
2 teaspoons Pumpkin Spice Seasoning (see recipe page 144)
⅛ teaspoon sea salt
Neutral oil

KITCHEN EQUIPMENT

Pizzelle or waffle cone maker
Heat resistant fork, tongs or spatula
Spoon or spatula
Medium bowl
Measuring spoons & measuring cups
Optional:
Heat resistant brush & small bowl for oil
Oven or dehydrator
Oven safe taco shell holders

SPECIAL INSTRUCTION/DIET INFORMATION

*Be careful to read all ingredients for pasteurized liquid egg whites. This should be a mono ingredient, and not contain any preservatives or additional ingredients. Regular separated egg whites can be used but the batter will be thicker and require many eggs.

DIRECTIONS

1. Preheat Pizzelle or waffle cone maker per the manufacturer's instructions. Then brush or spray the maker with coconut oil.

2. Mix all ingredients in a medium bowl. Ladle approximately one tablespoon of batter into each pizzelle mold and press. Each waffle/wrap should take approximately 3-4 minutes and remove from the press when golden.

3. Cool on parchment. Waffles/wraps will store for up to 3 days in a refrigerator and can be frozen for later use. They can also be frozen for several months if wrapped in parchment, foil and airtight bags.

4. For crisp Stroopwaffles you can dehydrate them in the oven or dehydrator at 130-150 degrees F for 20-30 min. If using the waffles/wraps for Vanilla Bean Froyo Tacos (see recipe page 281), dehydrate them using oven safe taco holders to create a crispy taco shell.

5. Spread favorite nut butters, No Bake Snickerdoodle Cookie Dough, or Peanut Butter Cookie Gel (see recipes page 79 & 80) on the waffles/ wraps as dessert or for training fuel.

Blender Banana Waffles

Approximate Yield	Prep Time 15 min	Estimated Macronutrients
6-8 servings	Total Time 30 min	27 g P • 42 g C • 21 g F

INGREDIENTS

Wet

3 eggs

1-2 ripe bananas*

1 ½ tablespoons dripped SCD Nonfat Greek Yogurt (see recipe page 298)

1-3 teaspoons of honey (this is based on preference) *

½ teaspoon vanilla extract

Dry

¼ cup + 1 tablespoon coconut flour

1 tablespoon dried egg white powder*

1 teaspoon unflavored gelatin

½ teaspoon Chai Spice Mix (see recipe page 144) or Pumpkin Spice Seasoning (see recipe page 144)

½ teaspoon baking soda

⅛ teaspoon sea salt

1 tablespoon melted coconut oil

Coconut or neutral spray oil

KITCHEN EQUIPMENT

Waffle maker/iron

Blender or food processor

Measuring spoons & measuring cups

Fork

Spatula or large spoon

SPECIAL INSTRUCTION/DIET INFORMATION

*Note the number of bananas will impact the texture, taste and macronutrients. Using two bananas the waffles will be softer, chewier and higher carbohydrate count. Whereas using one banana, the waffles may be crunchier in texture and may travel easier as a portable food.

*If you are unable to eat or source dried egg white powder you can replace with almond flour in the batter. However it will not rise as high, the texture will be different, and there will be higher fat and less protein for the macronutrients.

*If you are using the waffles as portable fuel and without toppings, using more honey is recommended.

DIRECTIONS

1. Preheat the waffle maker per the manufacturer's instructions. Then brush or spray with neutral oil.
2. In a food processor or blender, add all the wet ingredients and pulse until smooth.
3. Add the dry ingredients to the waffle batter, and pulse until well mixed.
4. Pour the melted coconut oil into the batter and blend.
5. Pour or spoon the waffle batter onto the waffle maker. Using the spatula to scrape out any residual batter.
6. When the waffle maker light indicates the waffle or waffles are done (approximately 3-6 minutes), check to ensure the waffle is a golden color. Remove the waffle from the waffle maker/iron with a fork and allow to cool on parchment paper.
7. If you want a crispier waffle, you can reheat in a toaster or toaster oven. An air fryer at 350 degrees F for 2-4 minutes will also crisp the waffles.
8. Waffles will store for up to 3 days in a refrigerator and can be frozen for later use. They can also be frozen for several months if wrapped in parchment, foil and stored in airtight bags.

Blender Beet Waffles

Approximate Yield	**Prep Time 15 min**	**Estimated Macronutrients**
6 servings	**Total Time 30 min**	**25 g P • 33 g C • 21 g F**

INGREDIENTS

Wet

3 eggs

1 ½ cup cooked beets

1 ½ tablespoons dripped SCD Nonfat Greek Yogurt (see recipe page 298)

2 tablespoons of honey (this is based on preference) *

1 teaspoon vanilla extract

Dry

¼ cup + 1 tablespoon coconut flour

1 tablespoon dried egg white powder*

1 teaspoon unflavored gelatin

1 teaspoon Chai Spice Mix (see recipe page 144)

½ teaspoon baking soda

⅛ teaspoon sea salt

⅛ teaspoon ground ginger

1 tablespoon melted food grade cacao butter (approximately 6 wafers)

Coconut or neutral spray oil

KITCHEN EQUIPMENT

Waffle maker/iron

Blender or food processor

Measuring spoons & measuring cups

Fork

Spatula or large spoon

SPECIAL INSTRUCTION/DIET INFORMATION

*If you are unable to eat or source dried egg white powder you can replace with almond flour coconut flour in the batter. However it will not rise as high, the texture will be different, and there will be higher fat and less protein for the macronutrients.

*If you are using the waffles as portable fuel and without toppings, adding more honey is recommended.

DIRECTIONS

1. Preheat the waffle maker per the manufacturer's instructions. Then brush or spray with the neutral oil.
2. In a food processor or blender, add all the wet ingredients and pulse until very smooth. (Scrape the sides and check for any larger chunks of beets)
3. Add the dry ingredients to the waffle batter, and pulse until well mixed.
4. Pour the melted cacao butter into the batter and blend.
5. Pour or spoon the waffle batter onto the waffle maker. Using the spatula to scrape out any residual batter.
6. When the waffle maker light indicates the waffle or waffles are done (approximately 3-6 minutes), check to ensure the waffles are golden in color. Remove the waffle from the waffle maker/iron with a fork and allow to cool on parchment paper.
7. If you want a crispier waffle, you can reheat in a toaster or toaster oven. An air fryer at 350 degrees F for 2-4 minutes will also crisp the waffles.
8. Waffles will store for up to 3 days in a refrigerator and can be frozen for later use. They can also be frozen for several months if wrapped in parchment, foil and stored in airtight bags.

Blender Bread Balls

Approximate Yield	**Prep Time 15 min**	**Estimated Macronutrients**
24 servings	**Total Time 30 min**	**6 g P • 20 g C • 11 g F**

INGREDIENTS

Bread Balls
½ -1 loaf (approximately 2-4 cups) of leftover Zucchini, Raisin Bread, Protein Banana Bread or Pumpkin bread cut into cubes (see recipes on pages 68, 61, 62, 66) *
2 ½ tablespoon peanut butter (or other nut butter) *
1 tablespoon honey
Spray oil

Icing
½ cup coconut butter*
4 tablespoons unsweetened cashew milk*
1 tablespoon honey
½ teaspoon vanilla extract

KITCHEN EQUIPMENT

Blender or food processor
Measuring spoons & measuring cups
Microwave safe small bowl or small pot
Spatula or large spoon
Small baking sheet or large dish (one that will fit in a refrigerator or freezer)
Parchment paper

SPECIAL INSTRUCTION/DIET INFORMATION

*See the various bread recipes under the Breakfast Chapter. Recipes on pages 68, 61, 62, & 66
*Nut butters that are SCD legal should only include the nut and possibly a legal oil and/or salt. For example, peanut butter is generally roasted peanuts and salt. There are some brands that will sweeten with honey but there are very few commercially available. If you are unable to source raw cashew butter, see recipe page 300.
*Coconut butter has a different consistency than coconut oil or cacao butter. It will need to be coconut butter for this recipe.
*Any nut milks should only consist of nuts, water, or salt. No emulsifiers, gums, sweeteners or additives should be in the ingredient list. If you are unable to source a SCD legal nut milk you can make them easily at home (see recipe page 299).

DIRECTIONS

1. In a food processor or blender, add all the bread ball ingredients and pulse to a very smooth consistency and a sticky dough has formed.
2. With well-oiled hands scoop out the dough and roll into ½- 1-inch balls. Placing them on a parchment lined baking sheet or dish in the refrigerator or freezer to chill.
3. In a microwave safe bowl or small pot, melt the coconut butter in the microwave or on the stove top. (Note melted coconut butter will be soft and opaque, not liquid and clear like coconut oil) Once the coconut butter is melted, add the remaining icing ingredients stirring well until frosting consistency. Allow to cool a bit so the icing is not hot to the touch and pliable.
4. Using a spoon, spatula or your hands, coat the chilled bread balls in icing until completely covered. Place the coated balls back on the parchment lined tray. Repeat the process until all balls are covered with icing.
5. Place the balls in a freezer to allow the icing to harden. These blender balls will generally last 10 days in the refrigerator when stored in an airtight container. Preferably they can be frozen for several months and defrosted for use as needed.

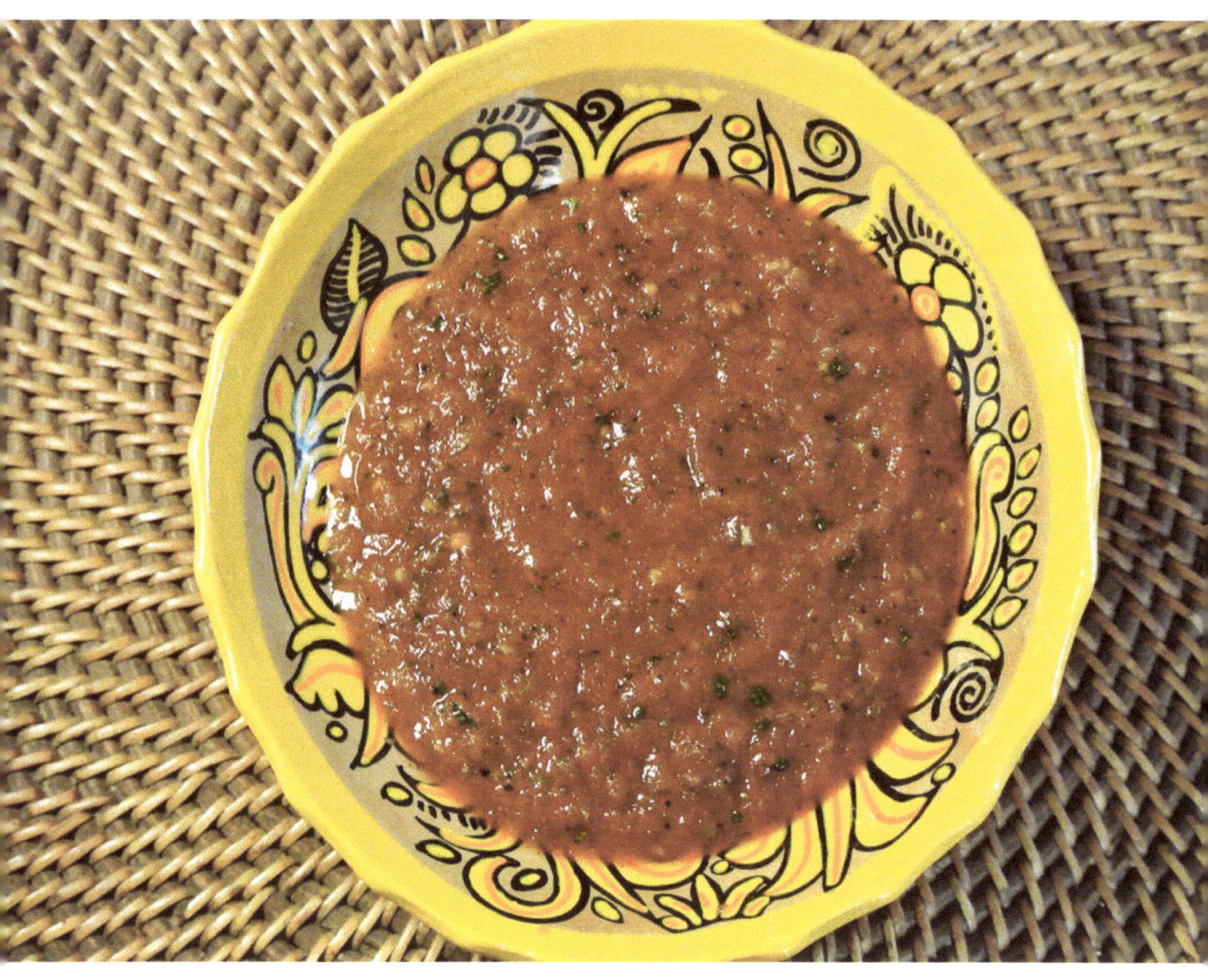

SCD Restaurant Style Salsa

Sauces & Syrups

Sauces and syrups are often overlooked, but they are the essential element that ties a dish together. For athletes, they also serve as a way to add variety to meals without significantly increasing the macronutrient or caloric count. Unfortunately, there are minimal pre-packaged sauces that sit on store shelves and follow the Specific Carbohydrate Diet guidelines.

Therefore, making your own sauces and syrups are necessary. Both are easy to make and are a measurable addition to recipes. Generally, they share the same preparation techniques but use a variety of ingredients. There are several characteristics for a good sauce such as flavor complexity, richness or depth, consistency and balanced acidity. Luckily the sauces and syrups in this cookbook are well tested and delicious.

No-"Sugar" Cookie Creamer

Approximate Yield
8-10 servings

Prep Time 15 min
Total Time 30 min

Estimated Macronutrients
1 g P • 6 g C • 4 g F

INGREDIENTS

2 tablespoons unsalted butter
½-¾ cup honey (depends on level of sweetness)
½ cup of unsweetened reduced fat coconut milk*
1 ½ tablespoons vanilla extract
1 ½ cups unsweetened cashew milk (or almond) *
⅛ teaspoon fine sea salt (omit if using salted butter)

KITCHEN EQUIPMENT

Medium pot
Heat-resistant spoon or spatula
Measuring spoons & measuring cups
Sterilized large mason jars with lids or airtight glass storage container

SPECIAL INSTRUCTIONS/DIET INFORMATION

* Coconut milk should only contain water and coconut (no additives or emulsifiers should be listed as ingredients, for example guar gum is not considered SCD legal)
*Any nut milks should only consist of nuts, water, or salt. No emulsifiers, gums, sweeteners or additives should be in the ingredient list. If you areunable to source a SCD legal nut milk you can make them easily at home (see recipe page 299).

DIRECTIONS

1. In a medium pot, add all the ingredients in order and heat on medium. Stirring occasionally.
2. Once the honey in the creamer is dissolved and simmering, remove from the heat to prevent boiling over.
3. When the pot is off the heat, allow the creamer to cool down (generally above room temperature). Transfer it into a sterilized glass container or mason jar with lid.
4. The creamer can generally be stored in a glass jar or container with airtight lid, refrigerated for up to 10 days.

Sea Salt Caramel Sauce

Approximate Yield	Prep Time 10 min	Estimated Macronutrients
10-12 servings	**Total Time 50 min**	**0 g P • 11 g C • 4 g F**

INGREDIENTS
1 cup unsweetened full fat coconut milk or cream*
½ cup of honey
1 ½ tablespoon vanilla extract
¾ teaspoon fine sea salt

KITCHEN EQUIPMENT
Medium pot or saucepan with lid
Measuring spoons & measuring cups
Heat-resistant spoon or spatula
Sterilized large mason jars with lids or appropriate glass storage container

SPECIAL INSTRUCTIONS/DIET INFORMATION
* Coconut milk should only contain water and coconut (no additives or emulsifiers should be listed as ingredients, for example guar gum is not considered SCD legal)
*Any nut milks should only consist of nuts, water, or salt. No emulsifiers, gums, sweeteners or additives should be in the ingredient list. If you are unable to source a SCD legal nut milk you can make them easily at home (see recipe page 299).

DIRECTIONS
1. In a medium pot/saucepan, add all ingredients and heat on medium. Stirring occasionally.
2. Once boiling, reduce the heat to low and let simmer, stirring until the sauce thickens. This should take approximately 30-45 minutes in total.
3. Remove the pot/saucepan off the heat and allow the sauce to cool down (generally room temperature). Transfer it into a sterilized glass container or mason jar with lid.
4. The sauce can generally be stored in a covered airtight container, refrigerated for up to one week. However the sauce will thicken when cool, and may need to be warmed or brought to room temperature for use in other recipes.

Pumpkin Spice Syrup

Approximate Yield	**Prep Time 15 min**	**Estimated Macronutrients**
10 servings	**Total Time 40 min**	**0 g P • 28 g C • 0 g F**

INGREDIENTS
½ cup canned pumpkin puree*
1 ⅓ cup of water
1 cup of honey
2 ½ teaspoons Pumpkin Spice Seasoning (see recipe page 144)
1 teaspoon vanilla extract
½ teaspoon cinnamon
Pinch of sea salt

KITCHEN EQUIPMENT
Medium pot or saucepan with lid
Measuring spoons & measuring cups
Heat-resistant spoon or spatula
Sterilized large mason jars with lids or appropriate glass storage container

SPECIAL INSTRUCTIONS/DIET INFORMATION
*Fresh pumpkin can be roasted, and the flesh finely pureed as needed for this recipe. (See page 12 for more details about canned vegetables). Always confirm ingredients and manufacturing processes.

DIRECTIONS
1. In a medium pot/saucepan, add all ingredients and heat on medium. Stirring occasionally.
2. Once boiling, reduce the heat to low and let simmer for 5-15 minutes or until the sauce thickens and volume reduced.
3. Remove the sauce from the heat and allow to cool down (generally room temperature). Transfer it into a sterilized glass container or mason jar with lid.
4. This syrup can generally be stored in an airtight container, refrigerated for up to one week.

Gingerbread Syrup

Approximate Yield	**Prep Time 15 min**	**Estimated Macronutrients**
10-18 servings	**Total Time 40 min**	**0 g P • 15 g C • 3 g F**

INGREDIENTS

1 can (13.5 oz) or 1 ¼ cup unsweetened coconut milk (reduced fat preferred) *
1 cup of honey
1 teaspoon cinnamon
1 teaspoon ground ginger
1 teaspoon vanilla extract
½ teaspoon ground cloves
⅛ teaspoon sea salt

KITCHEN EQUIPMENT

Medium pot or saucepan with lid
Measuring spoons & measuring cups
Heat-resistant spoon or spatula
Sterilized large mason jar with lid or appropriate glass storage container

SPECIAL INSTRUCTIONS/DIET INFORMATION

*Any nut milks should only consist of nuts, water, or salt. No emulsifiers, gums, sweeteners or additives should be in the ingredient list. If you are unable to source a SCD legal nut milk you can make them easily at home (see recipe page 299).

DIRECTIONS

1. In a medium pot, add all ingredients and heat on medium. Stirring occasionally.
2. Once the sauce starts to boil, reduce the heat to low and let simmer and stir for 5-15 minutes or until the sauce thickens.
3. Remove the pot off the heat and allow the sauce to cool down (generally room temperature).
4. Transfer the into a sterilized glass container or mason jar with lid. The sauce can generally be stored in the covered container, refrigerated for up to one week.

SCD Coffee Creamer Variations

<table>
<tr><td>**Approximate Yield**
10-18 servings</td><td>**Prep Time 15 min**
Total Time 40 min</td><td>Estimated macronutrients are not provided due to the different variations.</td></tr>
</table>

INGREDIENTS

Mock Maple

2 cups of unsweetened nut milk (i.e., almond, coconut or cashew) *

½ - ¾ cup honey (to taste and depends on level of sweetness)

2-3 tablespoons of date syrup (or see recipe page 107)

½ tablespoon vanilla extract

Pinch of sea salt

Vanilla Chai

2 cups of unsweetened nut milk (i.e., almond, coconut or cashew) *

½ - ¾ cup honey (to taste and depends on level of sweetness)

½ tablespoon vanilla extract

1 teaspoon Chai Spice Mix (see recipe page 144)

Pinch of sea salt

Cinnamon Streusel

2 cups of unsweetened nut milk (i.e., almond, coconut or cashew) *

½ - ¾ cup honey (to taste and depends on level of sweetness)

1 tablespoon vanilla extract

1 tablespoon of melted butter

½ teaspoon cinnamon

¼ teaspoon almond extract

Pinch of sea salt

Vanilla Bean

2 cups of unsweetened nut milk (i.e., almond, coconut or cashew) *

½ - ¾ cup honey (to taste and depends on level of sweetness)

1 vanilla bean pod seeds

1 teaspoon vanilla extract

Pinch of sea salt

Mock Peppermint Mocha

2 cups of unsweetened nut milk (i.e., almond, coconut or cashew) *

1 tablespoon finely grated food grade cacao or cocoa butter

½ - ¾ cup honey (to taste and depends on level of sweetness)

1 teaspoon mint extract

KITCHEN EQUIPMENT

Medium pot

Heat-resistant spoon or spatula

Measuring spoons & measuring cups

Sterilized large mason jars with lids or appropriate glass storage container

SPECIAL INSTRUCTIONS/DIET INFORMATION

*Any nut milks should only consist of nuts, water, or salt. No emulsifiers, gums, sweeteners or additives should be in the ingredient list. If you are unable to source a SCD legal nut milk you can make them easily at home (see recipe page 299).

DIRECTIONS

1. In a medium pot, add all ingredients in order and heat on medium. (For the Mock Peppermint Mocha, it is recommended to melt the cocoa butter in with the honey before adding cool/cold nut milk)

2. Stirring the creamer occasionally. Once simmering, remove from the heat to prevent the creamer from boiling over.

3. When the pot is off the heat, allow the creamer to cool down (generally above room temperature). Transfer it into a sterilized glass container or mason jar with lid.

4. The creamer can generally be stored in the covered container, refrigerated for up to 10 days.

Easy Crockpot Date Syrup

Approximate Yield
10-12 servings

Prep Time 15 min
Total Time 4 hours

Estimated Macronutrients
1 g P • 15 g C • 0 g F

INGREDIENTS
2 cups of dried and pitted medjool dates
2 cups of hot boiling filtered water
1 teaspoon vanilla extract
Coconut cooking oil spray

KITCHEN EQUIPMENT
Medium pot or saucepan with lid
Measuring spoons & measuring cups
Heat-resistant spoon or spatula
Immersion blender or food processor
Fine mesh metal colander
Sterilized large mason jars with lids or appropriate glass storage container

SPECIAL INSTRUCTIONS/DIET INFORMATION
*Date syrup when prepared at home, with water and dates is considered legal. However this is based on the individual's tolerance of dates and the absence of symptoms.
*Always double check the pits were fully removed from the date by cutting the date in half and feeling for any hard pit pieces with your fingers.

DIRECTIONS
1. Spray the crockpot with coconut oil and place on high to preheat.
2. Check the dates to ensure no pits or hard remnants remain in the dates.
3. Boil the water in the microwave for approximately 2 minutes. Once boiling, pour in the crockpot along with the dates and vanilla extract.
4. Cook on high for approximately 2-4 hours or until the dates are very large and soft. Using the immersion blender, puree until smooth. The dates and water can also be transferred to a food processor for blending. (If needed, use a fine mesh metal colander placed over a bowl and pour the syrup into the colander, to filter the date syrup of any larger pieces.)
5. Remove the syrup from the crockpot or bowl and transfer it into a sterilized glass container or mason jar with lid.
6. This syrup can generally be stored in the covered container, in a refrigerator for up to one week or frozen for later use.

Blueberry or Cherry Compote

Approximate Yield	Prep Time 20 min	Estimated Macronutrients
6-8 servings	Total Time 120 min	0 g P • 6 g C • 0 g F
	(To allow for refrigeration)	

INGREDIENTS
1 cup of frozen pitted cherries or blueberries
2 tablespoons water

KITCHEN EQUIPMENT
Immersion blender, food processor or blender
Measuring spoons & measuring cups
Heat-resistant spoon or spatula
Medium non-stick or ceramic pot
Glass container with airtight lid

DIRECTIONS
1. In a medium pot with lid, combine the cherries or blueberries and water. Cook the berries on medium heat, stirring to prevent them from burning on the bottom. When the berries are tender pierced with a fork, lower the heat.
2. Using a handheld immersion blender, puree the berries into a compote and be careful to not lift the blender out of the mixture to prevent splatters. If necessary, pour the compote into a food processor or blender to puree, the return it to the pot.
3. Continue cooking on low, stirring to reduce and thicken the compote. Remove from heat and place in a glass container to cool.
4. The compote can be stored in an airtight container in the refrigerator up to a week.

Blueberry Yogurt Sauce

Approximate Yield	Prep Time 15 min	Estimated Macronutrients
6-10 servings	Total Time 15 min	4 g P • 6 g C • 0 g F

INGREDIENTS
1 cup of Blueberry Compote (see recipe page 108) or defrosted frozen blueberries
1 cup of SCD Nonfat Greek Yogurt (see recipe page 298)

KITCHEN EQUIPMENT
Blender or food processor
Squeeze bottle or glass storage container with lid for pouring

SPECIAL INSTRUCTIONS/DIET INFORMATION
*This sauce compliments lemon protein pancakes, garnish for Korean tacos or added to smoothies.

DIRECTIONS
1. Place all ingredients in a food processor or blender.
2. Blend until smooth consistency and place in storage container for use in later in recipes.

Whipped Brie Cream

Approximate Yield
10-12 servings

Prep Time 20 min
Total Time 60 min
(To allow ingredients to warm)

Estimated Macronutrients
7 g P • 1 g C • 16 g F

INGREDIENTS
½ - 1 lb. of cold, aged triple cream brie*
1 cup of dripped SCD Yogurt (see recipe page 298)

KITCHEN EQUIPMENT
Food processor or handheld immersion blender
Measuring cups
Spatula or large spoon
Medium mixing bowl
Freezer safe plastic storage container with lids

SPECIAL INSTRUCTIONS/DIET INFORMATION
* Triple Cream Brie is considered an advanced cheese when following the Specific Carbohydrate Diet. Generally, cheeses should be aged over 3 months, and contain zero carbohydrates or sugars, regarding nutritional content. Pre-sliced and pre-shredded cheese will likely contain illegal ingredients to prevent the cheese from sticking and prolong shelf life. It is always best to purchase blocks or wedges of cheese, then shred, whip, grate, crumble or slice yourself.

DIRECTIONS
1. Cut the cold brie rind off all sides of the brie, and place the creamy part of the brie cheese in food processor or the mixing bowl.
2. Allow the brie to warm to room temp, then add in the dripped SCD yogurt. With the food processor or handheld blender, whip and blend the yogurt and cheese.
3. Transfer the sauce into an airtight container and refrigerate for an hour.
4. This cream sauce can generally be stored in a covered airtight container, refrigerated for up to one week. Serve with various recipes.

Mock Mac & Cheese Sauce

Approximate Yield	Prep Time 15 min	Estimated Macronutrients
4-6 servings	Total Time 30 min	7 g P • 20 g C • 6 g F

This recipe provides both dairy and dairy-free options.

INGREDIENTS
2 cups of cooked butternut squash puree or 1 (15oz) canned butternut squash*
1 cup of SCD Nonfat Greek Yogurt or ½ cup cashew cream (see recipes on page 298 & 300)
2 tablespoons butter or ghee
1 tablespoon yellow mustard*
1 teaspoon granulated onion
½ tablespoon granulated garlic
1 teaspoon fine grain sea salt
1 teaspoon paprika
1 tablespoon honey
½ teaspoon dried parsley
Pinch of ground nutmeg
Pepper to taste
*Optional unsweetened cashew milk or SCD legal bone broth (see recipes pages 255 & 299).

Optional Smoky and Spicy version:
⅛ teaspoon cayenne pepper
⅛ teaspoon chili powder
½ teaspoon smoked paprika

*Optional Cheese version:
Add the following if you
¼ cup of shredded parmesan cheese*
¼ cup of cheddar cheese*

KITCHEN EQUIPMENT
Blender or hand-held immersion blender
Medium pot
Measuring cups & measuring spoons
Heat resistant spatula or large spoon

SPECIAL INSTRUCTIONS/DIET INFORMATION
*Fresh roasted and pureed butternut squash can be substituted follow a similar recipe for Roasted Spaghetti Saquash page 177. Although there are brands of canned squash with no additives and preservatives, always verify with the manufacturer.
* If the sauce needs to be thinned, use unsweetened cashew milk or SCD legal bone broth.
* If you can tolerate cheese, add the optional cheeses to the sauce while cooking, stirring frequently until melted.
*Any nut milks should only consist of nuts, water, or salt. No emulsifiers, gums, sweeteners or additives should be in the ingredient list. If you are unable to source a SCD legal nut milk you can make them easily at home (see recipe page 299).
*There are a few commercial brands of mustard made with SCD legal ingredients. However always check ingredients carefully. Confirm with the company and determine unlisted ingredients are not being used in the manufacturing process.
* Cheeses should be aged over 3 months, and contain zero carbohydrates or sugars, regarding nutritional content. Pre-sliced and pre-shredded cheese will likely contain illegal ingredients to prevent the cheese from sticking and prolong shelf life. It is always best to purchase blocks of cheese, then shred, grate, crumble or slice yourself.

DIRECTIONS
1. In a blender or using the hand-held immersion blender, puree the buttenut squash and yogurt (or cashew cream) together until smooth.
2. In a medium pot melt the butter or ghee on medium heat. Combine all the puree and rest of the ingredients, together stirring frequently to prevent burning as the sauce thickens and simmers.
3. Serve warm with favorite SCD noodles, toss with protein and/or vegetables, or use in various recipes within this book.
4. Sauce can be frozen and stored for later use.

Creamy Greek Yogurt Taco Sauce

Approximate Yield
10-18 servings

Prep Time 15 min
Total Time 60 min
(To allow for refrigeration)

Estimated Macronutrients
1 g P • 2 g C • 3 g F

INGREDIENTS

½ cup of SCD Nonfat Greek yogurt (see recipe page 298)

⅓ cup of avocado mayonnaise (see recipe page 112) *

1 small lime juiced

½ teaspoon cumin

½ teaspoon granulated garlic

½ teaspoon salt

1 teaspoon favorite SCD legal hot sauce* (see notes)

KITCHEN EQUIPMENT

Food processor or immersion blender

Measuring spoons & measuring cups

Spatula or large spoon

Sterilized large mason jars with lids or squeeze bottle for sauce

SPECIAL INSTRUCTIONS/DIET INFORMATION

* There are limited brands of mayonnaise with legal ingredients under the Specific Carbohydrate Diet, therefore read labels carefully and verify with the manufacturer or use the recipe on page 112.

*If you do not have SCD legal hot sauce in hand, use 1 teaspoon honey, 1 teaspoon apple cider vinegar and ½ teaspoon of finely ground red pepper flakes.

DIRECTIONS

1. In food processer add all ingredients. Or if not using a food processor, in a bowl combine all ingredients and puree with an immersion blender until the sauce is well blended.
2. Transfer the sauce into a sterilized glass container or mason jar with lid and refrigerate for an hour.
3. This sauce can generally be stored in a covered airtight container, refrigerated for up to one week.

Avocado Mayonnaise

Approximate Yield **10-18 servings**	**Prep Time 20 min** **Total Time 60 min** (To allow for refrigeration)	**Estimated Macronutrients** **2 g P • 0 g C • 13 g F**

There are limited brands of avocado mayonnaise with legal ingredients under the Specific Carbohydrate Diet. Therefore reading labels and confirming ingredients with the manufacturer is essential. Many commercially made mayonnaise advertised as avocado, paleo or organic, are often sweetened with sugars, made with highly processed oils, additives and/or soy. If you are unable to source a commercially made mayonnaise with legal SCD ingredients, here is a recipe that complements many in this book.

INGREDIENTS
1 cup of avocado oil*
1 large egg room temperature
½ tablespoon white wine vinegar
½ teaspoon of salt
¼ teaspoon yellow, dijon mustard, or dry mustard powder*
⅛ teaspoon honey
Optional for garlic mayo: 2 cloves of garlic, finely grated

SPECIAL INSTRUCTIONS/DIET INFORMATION
*Avocado oil is generally mild and commonly available in stores; however sunflower oil can work as there is minimal flavor. Olive oil is not recommended as it may affect the taste of various recipes in this book.
*There are a few commercial brands of mustard made with SCD legal ingredients. However always check ingredients carefully. Confirm with the company and determine unlisted ingredients are not being used in the manufacturing process.

DIRECTIONS
1. Crack the egg into the food processor and add the salt, and mustard. Process/blend the mixture for 30 seconds. (It will appear foamy)
2. Pour in the white wine vinegar, and honey and pulse the processor for 10 seconds until well blended.
3. Blend on medium-high. then slowly start adding the oil in a very thin stream of droplets, through the lid opening of the food processor or blender. The mayonnaise will begin to thicken after half the avocado oil has been added.
4. The mayonnaise may be thinner than commercial mayonnaise, however it will become slightly denser as it chills in the refrigerator. This is the point where it can be seasoned with salt, and the optional grated garlic can be pulsed into the mixture.
5. Transfer the mayonnaise into a sterilized glass container or mason jar with lid and refrigerate for an hour.
6. The mayonnaise can generally be stored in a covered airtight container, in the refrigerator for up to one week.

White Garlic Sauce

Approximate Yield
10-18 servings

Prep Time 15 min
Total Time 60 min
(To allow for refrigeration)

Estimated Macronutrients
1 g P • 1 g C • 10 g F

INGREDIENTS

1 ¼ cup avocado mayonnaise (see recipe page 112) *
½ cup unsweetened cashew milk *
¼ cup lemon juice
12 cloves of garlic finely minced
½ teaspoon fine sea salt
½ teaspoon dried dill weed
Pinch of fine ground pepper

KITCHEN EQUIPMENT

Food processor or immersion blender
Measuring cups and measuring spoons
Spatula or large spoon
Sterilized large mason jars with lids or squeeze bottle for sauce
Optional: Sauce squeeze bottle

SPECIAL INSTRUCTIONS/DIET INFORMATION

* There are limited brands of mayonnaise with legal ingredients under the Specific Carbohydrate Diet, therefore read labels carefully and verify with the manufacturer or use the recipe on page 112.
*Note you can reduce the fat in this recipe by substituting half the mayonnaise with half SCD Nonfat Greek yogurt (see recipe page 298)
*Any nut milks should only consist of nuts, water, or salt. No emulsifiers, gums, sweeteners or additives should be in the ingredient list. If you are unable to source a SCD legal nut milk you can make them easily at home (see recipe page 299)

DIRECTIONS

1. In the food processer add all of the ingredients. Or if not using a food processor, in a bowl combine all ingredients and puree with immersion blender, until the garlic is finely minced and the sauce is well blended.
2. Pour sauce into the airtight container or squeeze bottle. Allow the sauce to marinate and chill in the refrigerator before serving. The longer the sauce marinates the stronger the garlic flavor will be
3. The sauce can generally be stored in an airtight container or squeeze bottle, refrigerated for up to one week.

Creamy Chipotle Dressing

Approximate Yield
12-24 servings

Prep Time 15 min
Total Time 60 min
(To allow for refrigeration)

Estimated Macronutrients
0 g P • 2 g C • 3 g F

INGREDIENTS

16 oz jar of whole roasted red bell peppers (drained) or 3 bell peppers (destemmed, and cut in quarters)

½ cup avocado mayonnaise (see recipe page 112) *

¼ cup apple cider vinegar

1 tablespoon honey

2 cloves of garlic minced

¼ teaspoon salt

1 teaspoon granulated onion

¼ -½ teaspoon fine chipotle chili powder

KITCHEN EQUIPMENT

Food processor or immersion blender
Measuring spoons & measuring cups
Spatula or large spoon
Sterilized large mason jars with lids or squeeze bottle for sauce
Optional: Aluminum foil or baking parchment lined baking sheet
Oven

SPECIAL INSTRUCTIONS/DIET INFORMATION

* There are limited brands of mayonnaise with legal ingredients under the Specific Carbohydrate Diet, therefore read labels carefully and verify with the manufacturer or use the recipe on page 112.

*To reduce the amount of fat in the recipe, cut the mayonnaise by ¼ and substitute with ¼ cup of SCD Nonfat Greek Yogurt. (see recipe page 298)

DIRECTIONS

1. If using roasted bell peppers preheat oven to 450 degrees F, and line baking pan with parchment paper. Place washed bell peppers on a baking sheet lined with parchment and drizzle with olive oil. Roast for 20 minutes, remove from oven and allow to cool.
2. In the food processer blend all ingredients. Or if not using a food processor, in a bowl combine all ingredients and puree with immersion blender, until the garlic is finely minced and the sauce is well blended.
3. Transfer the sauce into a sterilized glass container or mason jar with lid and refrigerate for an hour.
4. This dressing can generally be stored in a covered airtight container, in a refrigerator for up to one week.

Cilantro Jalapeno Ranch Dressing

Approximate Yield
12-24 servings

Prep Time 15 min
Total Time 60 min
(To allow for refrigeration)

Estimated Macronutrients
0 g P • 0 g C • 10 g F

INGREDIENTS

2 cups of avocado mayonnaise or (see recipe page 112) *
4 cloves of peeled garlic
2 ½ cups of fresh cilantro minced
1-2 green jalapenos deseeded and finely minced*
¼ cup of lime juice
1 ½ tablespoons SCD Ranch Dressing Mix (see recipe page 151)
Salt and pepper to taste
Optional: Unsweetened cashew milk as needed for thinning*

KITCHEN EQUIPMENT

Food processor or immersion blender
Spatula or large spoon
Measuring spoons & measuring cups
Sterilized large mason jars with lids or squeeze bottle for sauce

SPECIAL INSTRUCTIONS/DIET INFORMATION

* There are limited brands of mayonnaise with legal ingredients under the Specific Carbohydrate Diet, therefore read labels carefully and verify with the manufacturer or use the recipe on page 112.
*If mincing the jalapenos by hand be sure to wash your hands thoroughly and be careful not to touch your face or sensitive areas.
*Any nut milks should only consist of nuts, water, or salt. No emulsifiers, gums, sweeteners or additives should be in the ingredient list. If you are unable to source a SCD legal nut milk you can make them easily at home (see recipe page 299).

DIRECTIONS

1. In the food processer blend all ingredients. Or if not using a food processor, in a bowl combine all ingredients and puree with handheld immersion blender until the garlic is finely minced and the sauce is well blended.
2. Transfer the sauce into a sterilized glass container or mason jar with lid and refrigerate for an hour.
3. This dressing can generally be stored in a covered airtight container, in the refrigerator for up to one week.

Ya Ya's Greek Thousand Island Dressing

Approximate Yield	Prep Time 15 min	Estimated Macronutrients
10-12 servings	Total Time 60 min	0 g P • 2 g C • 7 g F
	(To allow for refrigeration)	

INGREDIENTS
½ cup of avocado mayonnaise (see recipe page 112) *
2 tablespoons of finely minced garlic (approximately 6-8 cloves)
2 tablespoons of favorite SCD legal ketchup or use SCD Scratch-Made Ketchup (see recipe page 117) *
2 tablespoons red wine vinegar
2 teaspoons of fresh parsley (1 teaspoon of dried parsley can be substituted)

KITCHEN EQUIPMENT
Food processor or immersion blender
Measuring spoons & measuring cups
Spatula or large spoon
Sterilized large mason jars with lids or squeeze bottle for sauce

SPECIAL INSTRUCTIONS/DIET INFORMATION
*There are limited brands of mayonnaise with legal ingredients under the Specific Carbohydrate Diet, therefore read labels carefully and verify with the manufacturer or use the recipe on page 112.
* There are a couple brands manufacturing SCD legal ketchup. You can also make your own ketchup using the recipe on page 117.

DIRECTIONS
1. In the food processer add all ingredients. Or if not using a food processor, in a bowl combine all ingredients and puree with immersion blender until the garlic is finely minced and the sauce is well blended.
2. Transfer the sauce into a sterilized glass container or mason jar with lid and refrigerate for an hour.
3. The dressing can generally be stored in a covered airtight container, refrigerated for up to one week.

SCD Scratch-Made Ketchup

Approximate Yield	**Prep Time 15 min**	**Estimated Macronutrients**
10-12 servings	**Total Time 90 min**	**1 g P • 8 g C • 0 g F**
	(To allow for refrigeration)	

INGREDIENTS

6 oz or ⅔ cup tomato paste*
¼ cup + 1 teaspoon of honey
¼ cup white vinegar
¼ cup apple cider vinegar
1 teaspoon salt
¼ teaspoon granulated garlic
⅛ teaspoon granulated onion

Optional additions for a deeper flavor:
⅛ ground cloves
⅛ teaspoon ground cinnamon
¼ teaspoon mustard powder
Dash of pepper
Pinch -⅛ teaspoon cayenne (to taste)

KITCHEN EQUIPMENT

Handheld immersion blender
Measuring spoons & measuring cups
Heat-resistant spoon or spatula
Medium pot
Sterilized large mason jars with lids or silicone ice cube trays to freeze

SPECIAL INSTRUCTIONS/DIET INFORMATION

*Canned tomatoes are typically not allowed under SCD. However, there are Italian brands of canned tomatoes and tomato pastes with no artificial flavors, sweeteners, preservatives or additives listed as ingredients or used in the manufacturing process. These brands are generally sold through Wellbees and a few other stores. Read store bought canned tomato and tomato paste labels carefully. If necessary, you can make your own tomato sauce or paste using fresh tomatoes or canned tomato juice (if salt is the only other ingredient).

DIRECTIONS

1. In a medium pot, on medium heat, add in all the ingredients and stir. Continue stirring and allow the ketchup to simmer for 20 minutes. (You will likely need to use the immersion blender or a food processor to reach ketchup consistency.)
2. Transfer the sauce into a sterilized glass container or mason jar with lid and refrigerate for an hour. Serve cool.
3. This ketchup can generally be stored in a covered airtight container, refrigerated for up to 10 days. You can also place the ketchup in silicone ice trays to freeze into cubes and use later in recipes.

Curry Ketchup Sauce

Approximate Yield	Prep Time 15 min	Estimated Macronutrients
18-24 servings	Total Time 90 min	1 g P • 5 g C • 0 g F
	(To allow for refrigeration)	

Important to note, this recipe creates a large batch of ketchup. As this is a popular low-fat sauce eaten regularly with various meat, egg and vegetable recipes.

INGREDIENTS
¾ - 1 cup of tomato paste*
1-1 ¼ cup filtered water (amount is based on desired consistency)
5 tablespoons apple cider vinegar
3 tablespoons honey
1 ½ tablespoon curry powder
1 tablespoon paprika
2 ½ teaspoons sea salt
1 teaspoon granulated garlic
1 teaspoon granulated onion
¼ teaspoon mustard powder
⅛ teaspoon ground cloves
⅛ teaspoon ground cinnamon
⅛ teaspoon pepper
Pinch -⅛ teaspoon cayenne (to taste)

KITCHEN EQUIPMENT
Handheld immersion blender
Measuring spoons & measuring cups
Heat-resistant spoon or spatula
Medium pot
Sterilized large mason jars with lids or silicone ice cube trays to freeze

SPECIAL INSTRUCTIONS/DIET INFORMATION
*Canned tomatoes are typically not allowed under SCD. However, there are Italian brands of canned tomatoes and tomato pastes with no artificial flavors, preservatives or additives listed as ingredients, nor used in the manufacturing process. These brands are generally sold through Wellbees and a few other stores. Read store bought canned tomato and tomato paste labels carefully. If necessary, you can make your own tomato sauce or paste using fresh tomatoes or canned tomato juice (if salt is the only other ingredient).

DIRECTIONS
1. In a medium pot, on medium heat, add in all ingredients and stir well. Use the immersion blender to achieve a thicker ketchup consistency. Simmer for 20 minutes and reduce the sauce.
2. Transfer the sauce into a sterilized glass container or mason jar with lid and refrigerate for an hour. Serve cool.

SCD BBQ Sauce

Approximate Yield
18-24 servings

Prep Time 15 min
Total Time 90 min
(To allow for refrigeration)

Estimated Macronutrients
0 g P • 23 g C • 0 g F

INGREDIENTS

1 ½ cups of favorite SCD legal ketchup or use homemade
Ketchup recipe (see recipe page 117)
4 cloves of garlic finely minced or grated
½ cup apple cider vinegar
¼ cup SCD Worcestershire Sauce (see recipe page 120)
¾ cup of honey
2 tablespoons yellow mustard*
1 tablespoon paprika or smoked paprika
2 teaspoons granulated onion
½ - 1 teaspoon fine ground black pepper (to taste)
Filtered water to thin the sauce as needed

KITCHEN EQUIPMENT

Handheld immersion blender
Measuring spoons & measuring cups
Heat-resistant spoon or spatula
Medium pot
Sterilized large mason jars with lids or silicone ice cube trays to freeze

SPECIAL INSTRUCTIONS/DIET INFORMATION

*There are a few commercial brands of mustard made with SCD legal ingredients. However always check ingredients carefully. Confirm with the company and determine unlisted ingredients are not being used in the manufacturing process.

DIRECTIONS

1. In a medium pot, on medium heat, add in all ingredients and stir. You will likely need to use the immersion blender to blend to BBQ sauce consistency.
2. Simmer for 20 minutes, stirring the sauce regularly. You will likely need to reduce the liquid due to the honey. However, you can also thin out the sauce as needed with water if you intend to use it as part of a marinade.
3. Transfer the sauce into a sterilized glass container or mason jar with lid and refrigerate for an hour. Serve cool.
4. This sauce can generally be stored in a covered airtight container, refrigerated for up to 10 days. You can also place in silicone ice trays to freeze into cubes and use for later in recipes.

SCD Worcestershire Sauce

Approximate Yield	Prep Time 10 min	Estimated Macronutrients
8-10 servings	**Total Time 20 min**	**1 g P • 3 g C • 0 g F**

INGREDIENTS

1/2 cup apple cider vinegar

2 tablespoons tamari or No Soy Sauce (see recipe page 121 and notes) *

1 tablespoon aged balsamic vinegar*

1 tablespoon honey

1 teaspoon ground mustard powder

¼ teaspoon granulated onion

¼ teaspoon granulated garlic

¼ teaspoon ground cinnamon

⅛ teaspoon fine ground black pepper

KITCHEN EQUIPMENT

Medium pot or saucepan with lid

Measuring spoons & measuring cups

Heat-resistant spoon or spatula

Sterilized small mason jar with lids or appropriate glass storage container with pour spout

SPECIAL INSTRUCTIONS/DIET INFORMATION

*Check the labels of the tamari, many will list rice wine vinegar and other ingredients which may be illegal when following SCD. Tamari should generally be gluten free, grain free, and sugar free. For example, tamari includes only water, organic soybeans, salt and/or organic alcohol (as part of fermentation process).

*If using No Soy Sauce (see recipe page 121) to substitute tamari, you may want to reduce or omit the amount of honey and vinegar in the recipe and just increase the amount of No Soy Sauce. This is based on personal taste and is due to the sweetness and acidity in the No Soy Sauce.

*In the book, Breaking the Vicious Cycle, explains that inexpensive vinegars may have added sugars, specifically balsamic vinegar. However balsamic vinegar aged for 15 years or more and labeled as a product of Italy (certified by the Italian controlling body for vinegar), is considered legal under SCD. Other forms of balsamic vinegar may have added sugars that are not SCD legal. Be careful to read ingredients and verify authenticity before purchasing products.

DIRECTIONS

1. In a medium pot/saucepan, add all ingredients and heat on medium. Stirring occasionally.
2. Once the sauce is at a boil, reduce the heat to low and let simmer for 2 minutes stirring occasionally.
3. Remove the pot/saucepan off the heat and allow the sauce to cool a bit. Transfer the sauce into a sterilized glass container or mason jar with lid.
4. The sauce can generally be stored in a covered, airtight container, refrigerated for up to 10 days.

No Soy Sauce

Approximate Yield	Prep Time 10 min	Estimated Macronutrients
10-12 servings	Total Time 20 min	2 g P • 8 g C • 1 g F

Important to note, when substituting No Soy Sauce for tamari, you may need to increase the salt and reduce the honey or vinegar in the recipe.

INGREDIENTS
1 cup filtered water

1 cup of cold Roasted Chicken or Beef Bone Broth (see recipes page 255 & 302) strained of fat

¼ cup aged balsamic vinegar*

4 tablespoons honey

1 ½ tablespoons apple cider vinegar

1 teaspoon salt

2 cloves of garlic grated fine or ½ teaspoon of granulated garlic

½ teaspoon ground white pepper

¼ teaspoon ginger powder

KITCHEN EQUIPMENT
Medium pot or deep saucepan with lid

Measuring spoons & measuring cups

Heat-resistant spoon or spatula

Handheld immersion blender

Sterilized large mason jars with lids or appropriate glass storage container

SPECIAL INSTRUCTIONS/DIET INFORMATION
*In the book, Breaking the Vicious Cycle, explains that inexpensive vinegars may have added sugars, specifically balsamic vinegar. However balsamic vinegar aged for 15 years or more and labeled as a product of Italy (certified by the Italian controlling body for vinegar), is considered legal under SCD. Other forms of balsamic vinegar may have added sugars that are not SCD legal. Be careful to read ingredients and verify authenticity before purchasing products.

DIRECTIONS
1. On medium heat in the pot, bring all ingredients to boil.
2. Once boiling, reduce the heat and allow the sauce to simmer until the volume is reduced by a quarter and sauce thickens. Stirring occasionally.
3. Then remove from heat and allow to cool.
4. Transfer the sauce into a sterilized glass container or mason jar with lid.
5. The sauce can generally be stored in the covered container, refrigerated for up to one week. This sauce can also be frozen into tablespoon sized or quarter cup silicon freezer trays. Freeze sauce for later use in recipes.

Teri-**YAY**-ki Sauce

(SCD Unagi Sauce)

Approximate Yield **10-12 servings**	**Prep Time 15 min** **Total Time 40 min**	**Estimated Macronutrients** **2 g P • 23 g C • 2 g F**

INGREDIENTS

1 cup of honey

½ cup of tamari or No Soy Sauce (see recipe page 121 and notes) *

3 tablespoons fish sauce* (If making unagi sauce increase amount to 4 tablespoons)

1 tablespoon + 1 teaspoon toasted sesame oil

KITCHEN EQUIPMENT

Medium pot or saucepan with lid

Measuring spoons & measuring cups

Heat-resistant spoon or spatula

Sterilized large mason jars with lids or appropriate glass storage container

SPECIAL INSTRUCTIONS/DIET INFORMATION

* Check the labels of the tamari, many will list rice wine vinegar and other ingredients which may be illegal when following SCD. Tamari should generally be gluten free, grain free, and sugar free. For example, tamari includes only water, organic soybeans, salt and/or organic alcohol (as part of fermentation process).

*If using No Soy Sauce (see recipe page 121) to substitute tamari, you may want to increase the amount of No Soy Sauce by ¼ cup, reduce the amount of honey in the recipe and add ¼ teaspoon of fine sea salt. This is based on personal taste and is due to the sweetness of the No Soy Sauce.

*Fish sauce should not have added ingredients except fish (generally anchovies) and salt.

DIRECTIONS

1. In a medium saucepan, add all ingredients and heat on medium heat. Stirring occasionally.
2. Once the sauce is boiling, reduce the heat to low and let simmer from 10-15 minutes or until the sauce thickens and volume is reduced.
3. Remove the saucepan off the heat and allow the sauce to cool down (generally room temperature).
4. Transfer the sauce into a sterilized glass container or mason jar with lid. The sauce can generally be stored in the covered, airtight container, refrigerated for up to one week.

No Oyster Sauce

Approximate Yield
10-12 servings

Prep Time 10 min
Total Time 50 min

Estimated Macronutrients
3 g P • 6 g C • 4 g F

INGREDIENTS

1 cup of cleaned and minced shitake mushrooms
½ cup + 2 tablespoons filtered water
½ cup tamari or No Soy Sauce (see recipe page 121 and notes) *
1 tablespoon cashew butter*
1 tablespoon fish sauce*
1 tablespoon honey

KITCHEN EQUIPMENT

Medium pot or deep saucepan with lid
Handheld immersion blender
Sterilized large mason jars with lids or appropriate glass storage container

SPECIAL INSTRUCTIONS/DIET INFORMATION

*Check the labels of the tamari, many will list rice wine vinegar and other ingredients which may be illegal when following SCD. Tamari should generally be gluten free, grain free, and sugar free. For example, tamari includes only water, organic soybeans, salt and/or organic alcohol (as part of fermentation process).

*If using No Soy Sauce (see recipe page 121) to substitute tamari, you may want to reduce the amount of honey and fish sauce in the recipe. This is based on personal taste and is due to the sweetness of the No Soy Sauce.

*Nut butters that are SCD legal should only include the nut and possibly a legal oil and/or salt. For example, peanut butter is generally roasted peanuts and salt. There are some brands that will sweeten with honey but there are very few commercially available.

*Fish sauce should not have added ingredients except fish (generally anchovies) and salt.

DIRECTIONS

1. On medium heat in the pot, add mushrooms and ½ cup of filtered water. Boil the mushrooms until softened. Reduce the heat.
2. Then add in the cashew butter and all other ingredients. Stirring til cashew butter has melted.
3. Using the immersion blender puree, the sauce well til smooth. Then remove from heat. (If using a food processor allow the sauce to cool a bit before blending)
4. Transfer the sauce into a sterilized glass container or mason jar with lid.
5. The sauce can generally be stored in a covered container, refrigerated for up to one week. This sauce can also be frozen into tablespoon sized or quarter cup silicon freezer trays. Freeze sauce for later use in recipes.

Honey Hoisin Sauce

Approximate Yield 10-12 servings	Prep Time 10 min Total Time 50 min	Estimated Macronutrients 3 g P • 21 g C • 3 g F

INGREDIENTS

1 tablespoon unsweetened seedless raisins (dark preferred not golden)
4 medjool dates (dried, pitted and chopped)
½ cup filtered water
¼ cup tamari or No Soy Sauce (see recipe page 121 and notes) *
1 tablespoon sesame oil
2 tablespoons white vinegar
2 tablespoons peanut butter*
2 garlic cloves minced
1 teaspoon fine red chili flakes
¼ teaspoon fine ground pepper
¼ cup of honey
Optional: ½ teaspoon of Chinese five spice (omit if sensitivity)

KITCHEN EQUIPMENT

Medium pot or deep saucepan with lid
Microwave safe glass bowl or large measuring cup
Measuring spoons
Heat-resistant spoon or spatula
Handheld immersion blender or food processor
Sterilized large mason jars with lids or appropriate glass storage container

SPECIAL INSTRUCTIONS/DIET INFORMATION

*Nut butters that are SCD legal should only include the nut and possibly a legal oil and/or salt. For example, peanut butter is generally roasted peanuts and salt. There are some brands that will sweeten with honey but there are very few commercially available.

*Check the labels of the tamari, many will list rice wine vinegar and other ingredients which may be illegal when following SCD. Tamari should generally be gluten free, grain free, and sugar free. For example, tamari includes only water, organic soybeans, salt and/or organic alcohol (as part of fermentation process).

*If using No Soy Sauce (see recipe page 121) to substitute tamari, you may want to reduce or omit the amount of honey and vinegar in the recipe. This is based on personal taste and is due to the sweetness and vinegar in the No Soy Sauce.

DIRECTIONS

1. In the microwave safe bowl or glass measuring cup, heat the water to a boil.
2. Check each of the dates for any pits or hard remnants. Add the dates, and raisins to the water. Allowing them to steep for 5-10 minutes.
3. When the dates and raisins are softened, add in the minced garlic and puree with the immersion blender or food processor. (Be careful not to puree if water is still hot, wait until its cooled.)
4. On medium heat add the puree and all other ingredients into the pot. Stirring until the peanut butter is thoroughly melted and mixed well.
5. Next raise the heat and keep stirring to reduce the sauce to desired thickness. You will likely need to bring the sauce to a low boil and continue to stir to prevent it from boiling/foaming over.
6. Once the sauce has reached the desired darker color and thickness of hoisin sauce (approximately 10-15 min), remove the pot/saucepan off the heat and allow the sauce to cool down (generally to slightly above room temperature). This may be an opportunity to use the immersion blender or food processor to puree it again til the sauce is smooth. Transfer it into a sterilized glass container or mason jar with lid.
7. The sauce can generally be stored in the covered container, refrigerated for up to one week.

Plum Sauce

Approximate Yield	Prep Time 10 min	Estimated Macronutrients
10-12 servings	Total Time 50 min	1 g P • 25 g C • 2 g F

INGREDIENTS

12 oz of dried unsweetened pitted prunes
6 medjool pitted dried dates
2 cups of filtered water (for steeping)
½ sweet yellow onion (grated)
3-4 cloves of garlic (grated)
1 tablespoon grated fresh ginger (approximately thumb-size)
½ apple cider vinegar
⅓ cup of honey
¼ cup of tamari or No Soy Sauce (see recipe page 121 and notes) *
1 tablespoon toasted sesame oil
1 ¼ teaspoons sea salt
1 ⅛ teaspoons ground Chinese five spice

KITCHEN EQUIPMENT

Medium pot or deep saucepan with lid
Heat-resistant spoon or spatula
Microwave safe glass bowl or large measuring cup
Grater or micro grater
Food processor
Handheld immersion blender
Sterilized large mason jars with lids or appropriate glass storage container

SPECIAL INSTRUCTIONS/DIET INFORMATION

*Check the labels of the tamari, many will list rice wine vinegar and other ingredients which may be illegal when following SCD. Tamari should generally be gluten free, grain free, and sugar free. For example, tamari includes only water, organic soybeans, salt and/or organic alcohol (as part of the fermentation process).

*If using No Soy Sauce (see recipe page 121) to substitute tamari, you may want to reduce the amount of honey and vinegar in the recipe. This is based on taste and is due to the sweetness and acidity of the No Soy Sauce.

DIRECTIONS

1. Always check dates and prunes for pits. Remove any pit fragments or hard remnants. This is very important because pit fragments generally don't puree and can ruin the texture of the sauce.
2. In the medium pot or deep saucepan, heat the water to a boil. Once boiling add the pitted prunes and dates. Allowing them to steep for 20- 30 minutes.
3. When the dates and prunes are softened, remove them from the water and place in the food processor. Reserve ¼ cup of the steeping water for thinning the sauce as needed. Discard the rest of the water.
4. Add in the grated garlic, ginger and yellow onion to the food processor. Then puree until everything is smooth.
5. On medium heat add the prune puree and all other ingredients into the pot; Honey, tamari (or No Soy Sauce), vinegar, oil and spices. Stirring to blend them well.
6. Next raise the heat and reduce the sauce down to the desired thickness as needed. Add some of the steeping liquid if you need to thin the sauce.
7. Once the sauce has reached the desired darker color and thickness of plum sauce (approximately 10-15 min), remove the pot/saucepan off the heat and allow the sauce to cool down (generally to slightly above room temperature). This may be an opportunity to use the immersion blender or food processor to puree it again. (The sauce should be very smooth.) Transfer it into a sterilized glass container or mason jar with lid.
8. The sauce can generally be stored in the covered container, refrigerated for up to one week. Or you can freeze the sauce in silicone freezer containers for later use.

Orange Ginger Sauce

Approximate Yield	**Prep Time 10 min**	**Estimated Macronutrients**
8-10 servings	**Total Time 50 min**	**1 g P • 34 g C • 2 g F**

INGREDIENTS

½ cup filtered water
5 pitted medjool dates (chopped/minced fine)
⅔ cup of honey
1 ½ tablespoons orange zest
⅓ cup orange juice
2 tablespoons apple cider vinegar
4 tablespoons tamari or No Soy Sauce (see recipe page 121 and notes) *
5 large cloves finely minced garlic
1 tablespoon freshly peeled and grated ginger*
1 tablespoon sesame oil
½ – 1 teaspoon finely crushed red pepper flakes (to taste)

Optional: 1 tablespoon cashew butter* to thicken

KITCHEN EQUIPMENT

Medium pot or deep saucepan with lid
Measuring spoons & measuring cups
Heat-resistant spoon or spatula
Handheld immersion blender, food processor or blender
Sterilized large mason jars with lids or appropriate glass storage container

SPECIAL INSTRUCTIONS/DIET INFORMATION

*Check the labels of the tamari, many will list rice wine vinegar and other ingredients which may be illegal when following SCD. Tamari should generally be gluten free, grain free, and sugar free. For example, tamari includes only water, organic soybeans, salt and/or organic alcohol (as part of fermentation process).

*If using No Soy Sauce (see recipe page 121) to substitute tamari, you may want to reduce or omit the amount of honey and vinegar in the recipe. This is based on personal taste and is due to the sweetness and acidity of the No Soy Sauce.

* A metal vegetable peeler is often the best way to peel ginger quickly, however, use a large piece of ginger and be careful of your fingers.

*Nut butters that are SCD legal should only include the nut and possibly a legal oil and/or salt. For example, peanut butter is generally roasted peanuts and salt. There are some brands that will sweeten with honey but there are very few commercially available.

DIRECTIONS

1. Check the dates for any pits or hard remnants. Remove and discard any before chopping or mincing.
2. In a medium pot/saucepan, add the water and dates. On medium heat cook the dates until tender. (You may need to add a bit extra water if it evaporates too quickly). When the dates have become very soft, allow them to cool a bit before using the immersion blender. Blend the dates into a puree in the pot. Or pour the water and dates into a food processor or blender to puree.
3. Next add all the remaining ingredients and heat on medium, stirring occasionally.
4. Once the sauce is at a low boil, reduce the heat to low and let simmer for 15 minutes stirring occasionally.
5. Remove the pot/saucepan off the heat and allow the sauce to cool down (generally to slightly above room temperature). This may be an opportunity to use the immersion blender and puree til the sauce is smooth. Transfer the sauce into a sterilized glass container or mason jar with lid.
6. This sauce can generally be stored in the covered container, refrigerated for up to one week.
7. If you need the sauce to be a glaze or a dipping sauce, you can later add it to a sauce pot or deep pan on medium heat, stirring and reducing it down to a glaze consistency. Then remove from heat and allow to cool and thicken.

Spicy Peanut Dressing

Approximate Yield 10-16 servings	Prep Time 15 min Total Time 40 min	Estimated Macronutrients 1 g P • 4 g C • 5 g F

INGREDIENTS

1 tablespoon avocado oil
¼ cup peanut butter*
¼ cup filtered water
2 cloves of finely minced garlic
4 tablespoons apple cider vinegar
2 tablespoons tamari or No Soy Sauce (see recipe page 121 and notes) *
2 tablespoons honey
2 tablespoons toasted sesame oil
2 tablespoons lime juice *
1 ½ teaspoon ground ginger
¼ - ½ teaspoon dried chili flakes (this is dependent on personal taste)

KITCHEN EQUIPMENT

Measuring spoons & measuring cups
Heat-resistant spoon or spatula
Large mason jars with lids or appropriate glass storage container (that can be shaken without spilling)

SPECIAL INSTRUCTIONS/DIET INFORMATION

*Nut butters that are SCD legal should only include the nut and possibly a legal oil and/or salt. For example, peanut butter is generally roasted peanuts and salt. There are some brands that will sweeten with honey but there are very few commercially available.

* Check the labels of the tamari, many will list rice wine vinegar and other ingredients which may be illegal when following SCD. Tamari should generally be gluten free, grain free, and sugar free. For example, Tamari includes only water, organic soybeans, salt and/or organic alcohol (as part of fermentation process).

*If using No Soy Sauce (see recipe page 121) to substitute tamari, you may want to reduce the amount of honey and vinegar in the recipe. This is based on personal taste and is due to the sweetness and vinegar in the No Soy Sauce.

*Fresh lime juice is best, but if using shelf stable lime juice check the labels. Verify it does not contain concentrate in the ingredients or other ingredients except water or lime juice.

DIRECTIONS

1. In a sterilized glass container or mason jar with lid add all ingredients together.
2. Close the lid tightly and give the dressing several vigorous shakes.
3. Allow the dressing to marinate in the refrigerator 1-2 hours before serving.
4. This dressing can generally be stored in the covered container, refrigerated for up to one week.

SCD Vietnamese Salad Dressing & Dipping Sauce

Approximate Yield	Prep Time 15 min	Estimated Macronutrients
10-12 servings	Total Time 60 min	3 g P • 7 g C • 5 g F
	(To allow for refrigeration)	

Recipe inspired by Prik Nam Pla.

INGREDIENTS

2 tablespoons tamari or No Soy Sauce (see recipe page 121 and notes) *
1 ½ tablespoons fish sauce*
1-2 spicy thai chili peppers (de-stemmed and chopped fine)*
5 garlic cloves minced
1 small shallot minced
¼ cup avocado oil
⅓ cup filtered water*
2 tablespoons honey*
2 tablespoons fresh lime juice
1 tablespoon fresh cilantro destemmed and minced finely
1 ½ tablespoons white vinegar

KITCHEN EQUIPMENT

Food processor or mincer
Measuring spoons & measuring cups
Sterilized large mason jar or container with lid

SPECIAL INSTRUCTIONS/DIET INFORMATION

*Check the labels of the tamari, many will list rice wine vinegar and other ingredients which may be illegal when following SCD. Tamari should generally be gluten free, grain free, and sugar free. For example, tamari includes only water, organic soybeans, salt and/or organic alcohol (as part of fermentation process).

*If using No Soy Sauce (see recipe page 121) to substitute tamari, you may want to reduce or omit the amount of honey, fish sauce and vinegar in the recipe. This is based on personal taste and is due to the sweetness and vinegar in the No Soy Sauce.

*Fish sauce should not have added ingredients except fish (generally anchovies) and salt.

*If you are unable to source thai chili peppers, substitute with a small jalapeno or serrano pepper depending on your tolerance for spice.

*The amount of honey can be increased or reduced personal preference for sweetness.

*Water can be increased or decreased depending on thickness.

DIRECTIONS

1. There are two options to prepare the sauce, for a prettier presentation you can mix all ingredients by hand. Or for a quicker option you can use the food processer, and add all ingredients, until the garlic is finely minced and the sauce is well blended.
2. Transfer the sauce into a sterilized glass container or mason jar with lid and refrigerate for an hour.
3. The sauce can generally be stored in a covered, airtight container refrigerated for up to one week.

Garlicky Sweet & Sour Sauce

Approximate Yield	Prep Time 10 min	Estimated Macronutrients
10-12 servings	**Total Time 30 min**	**0 g P • 27 g C • 1 g F**

INGREDIENTS

1 cup of crushed pineapple*
1 tablespoon minced garlic (approximately 5-6 cloves)
⅓ cup of apple cider vinegar
¾ cup of honey
5 tablespoons SCD legal ketchup*
2 tablespoons tamari or No Soy Sauce (see recipe page 121 and notes) *
1 teaspoon crushed chili flakes
1 teaspoon sesame oil

KITCHEN EQUIPMENT

Medium pot or saucepan with lid
Measuring spoons & measuring cups
Heat-resistant spoon or spatula
Handheld immersion blender
Sterilized large mason jars with lids or appropriate glass storage container

SPECIAL INSTRUCTIONS/DIET INFORMATION

*Verify the pineapple is not packed in syrup or juice concentrate with added sugar. Defrosted frozen pineapple can be substituted.

* There are a couple brands manufacturing SCD legal ketchup. You can also make your own ketchup using the recipe on page 117.

*Check the labels of the tamari, many will list rice wine vinegar and other ingredients which may be illegal when following SCD. Tamari should generally be gluten free, grain free, and sugar free. For example, tamari includes only water, organic soybeans, salt and/or organic alcohol (as part of fermentation process).

*If using No Soy Sauce (see recipe page 121) to substitute tamari, you may want to reduce or omit the amount of honey and vinegar in the recipe. This is based on personal taste and is due to the sweetness and vinegar in the No Soy Sauce.

DIRECTIONS

1. In a medium pot/saucepan, combine all ingredients together. Use the immersion blender to puree any crushed pineapple chunks, then heat on medium, stirring occasionally.
2. Once the sauce is at a low boil, reduce the heat to low and let simmer for 10-12 minutes stirring occasionally and reducing the sauce.
3. Remove the pot/saucepan off the heat and allow the sauce to cool down (to slightly above room temperature). Transfer the sauce into a sterilized glass container or mason jar with lid.
4. This sauce can generally be stored in the covered container, refrigerated for up to one week.

SCD Gochujang Paste

Approximate Yield **10-12 servings**	Prep Time **10 min** Total Time **60 min** (To allow for marinade time)	Estimated Macronutrients **3 g P • 15 g C • 5 g F**

INGREDIENTS

⅓ cup honey

¾ cup dried Korean chili coarse ground flakes*

⅓ cup tamari or No Soy Sauce

(see recipe page 121 and notes) *

7 cloves of minced garlic

⅓ cup tahini butter*

6 oz can (⅔ cup) of tomato paste + 2 tablespoons tomato paste*

2-4 tablespoons water (for thinning)

KITCHEN EQUIPMENT

Food processor or blender

Measuring spoons & measuring cups

Sterilized large mason jars with lids

Silicone food storage freezer trays/cubes with lids

SPECIAL INSTRUCTIONS/DIET INFORMATION

*Read labels carefully and confirm ingredients when sourcing (Gochugaru) Korean chili flakes.

*Check the labels of the tamari, many will list rice wine vinegar and other ingredients which may be illegal when following SCD. Tamari should generally be gluten free, grain free, and sugar free. For example, tamari includes only water, organic soybeans, salt and/or organic alcohol (as part of fermentation process).

*If using No Soy Sauce (see recipe page 121) to substitute tamari, you may want to reduce the amount of honey in the recipe. This is based on personal taste and is due to the sweetness of the No Soy Sauce.

*Canned tomatoes are typically not allowed under SCD. However, there are Italian brands of canned tomatoes and tomato pastes with no artificial flavors, preservatives or additives listed as ingredients, nor used in the manufacturing process. These brands are generally sold through Wellbees and a few other stores. Read store bought canned tomato and tomato paste labels carefully. If necessary, you can make your own tomato sauce or paste using fresh tomatoes or canned tomato juice (if salt is the only other ingredient).

*Seed butters that are SCD legal should only include the seed and possibly a legal oil and/or salt. For example, tahini is generally roasted and ground sesame seeds which may include sesame seed oil.

DIRECTIONS

1. In a food processer or blender combined all the ingredients together.
2. Transfer the paste into a sterilized glass container or mason jar with lid and refrigerate for an hour.
3. The paste can generally be stored in a covered airtight container, refrigerated for up to one week. You can also freeze the paste in silicone ice cube trays and stored in zip top freezer bags for later use in recipes.

Quick & Easy Garlic Sriracha Mayo

Approximate Yield **10-16 servings**	Prep Time **15 min** Total Time **60 min** (To allow for refrigeration)	Estimated Macronutrients **0 g P • 2 g C • 12 g F**

INGREDIENTS

1 ½ - 2 cups of roasted red peppers (jarred or fresh roasted bell peppers in olive oil) *

4-5 cloves of fresh garlic

1 – 1 ½ tablespoons apple cider vinegar (this is based on taste preference)

4 teaspoons of toasted sesame oil

1 ½ cups of avocado mayonnaise or (see recipe page 112) *

Options for adding more spice and/or color (amount to taste)

1 teaspoon of hot chili infused oil or Calabrian chili sauce/paste*

KITCHEN EQUIPMENT

Food processor or immersion blender

Spatula or large spoon

Measuring spoons & measuring cups

Sterilized large mason jars with lids or squeeze bottle for sauce

Optional: Aluminum foil or baking parchment lined baking sheet

Oven

SPECIAL INSTRUCTIONS/DIET INFORMATION

* If roasting peppers fresh you will need 3 bell peppers destemmed and cut into quarters.

* There are limited brands of mayonnaise with legal ingredients under the Specific Carbohydrate Diet, therefore read labels carefully and verify with the manufacturer or use the recipe on page 112.

*Note if using hot oil or Calabrian chili sauce/paste the ingredients should not contain any additives, and ingredients should only include chilis, oil, and/or possibly vinegar.

DIRECTIONS

1. If using fresh roasted bell peppers preheat oven to 450 degrees F, and line baking pan with parchment paper. Place washed and cut bell peppers on a baking sheet lined with parchment and drizzle with olive oil. Roast for 20 minutes, remove from oven and allow to cool.
2. In the food processer add all ingredients together. Or if not using a food processor, in a bowl combine all ingredients and puree with immersion blender until sauce is well blended.
3. Transfer the sauce into a sterilized glass container or mason jar with lid and refrigerate for an hour.
4. The sauce can generally be stored in a covered airtight container, refrigerator for up to one week.

Easy SCD Panang Curry Paste

Approximate Yield	Prep Time 10 min	Estimated Macronutrients
10-12 servings	Total Time 60 min	2 g P • 39 g C • 4 g F
	(To allow for marinade time)	

INGREDIENTS

1-2 minced thai chilis or ½-1 teaspoon of dried thai chili ground flakes and seeds (to spice tolerance)
1 minced large shallot
4 large cloves garlic minced
⅓ cup peanut butter*
¼ cup honey
1-2 tablespoons avocado or olive oil (you can also substitute with water)
4 teaspoons lime zest
2 teaspoon sea salt
1 teaspoon paprika (for coloring if using green thai chilis)
1 teaspoon ground coriander
1 teaspoon ground cumin
½ teaspoon dried lemongrass
½ teaspoon ground ginger
½ teaspoon lemon zest

KITCHEN EQUIPMENT

Food processor or blender
Spatula or large spoon
Measuring spoons & measuring cups
Sterilized large mason jars with lids

SPECIAL INSTRUCTIONS/DIET INFORMATION

*You can reduce the peanut butter and add cashew butter for a milder, less peanut flavor.
*Nut butters that are SCD legal should only include the nut and possibly a legal oil and/or salt. For example, peanut butter is generally roasted peanuts and salt. There are some brands that will sweeten with honey but there are very few commercially available.

DIRECTIONS

1. In food processer or blender add all ingredients. Pulse and blend until the paste is smooth.
2. Transfer the paste into a sterilized glass container or mason jar with lid and refrigerate for an hour.
3. This paste can generally be stored in a covered airtight container, refrigerated for up to one week. You can also freeze the paste in silicone ice cube trays for later use in recipes.

SCD Harissa Paste

Approximate Yield	Prep Time 15 min	Estimated Macronutrients
8-10 servings	Total Time 30 min	3 g P • 12 g C • 1 g F

This is a mild paste and sauce, if additional spice is necessary more cayenne pepper can easily be added.

INGREDIENTS

16 oz jar of whole roasted red bell peppers (drained) or 3 red bell peppers (destemmed, and cut in quarters)
3-4 minced garlic cloves
2 teaspoons ground coriander
2 teaspoons ground cumin
2 tablespoons fresh lemon juice
2 tablespoons olive oil + more for roasting
1 ½ teaspoon smoked paprika
¾ teaspoon cayenne pepper
½ teaspoon finely ground red pepper flakes or chipotle powder
Sea salt to taste
Optional:
1 teaspoon of toasted and ground caraway seeds
2 tablespoons tomato paste*

KITCHEN EQUIPMENT

Food processor or immersion blender
Measuring spoons & measuring cups
Spatula or large spoon
Sterilized large mason jars with lids or silicone ice cube trays to freeze
Optional: Baking sheet
Baking parchment paper
Oven

SPECIAL INSTRUCTIONS/DIET INFORMATION

*If using tomato paste, canned tomatoes are typically not allowed under SCD. However, there are Italian brands of canned tomatoes and tomato pastes with no artificial flavors, preservatives or additives listed as ingredients, nor used in the manufacturing process. These brands are generally sold through Wellbees and a few other stores. Read store bought canned tomato and tomato paste labels carefully. If necessary, you can make your own tomato sauce or paste using fresh tomatoes or canned tomato juice (if salt is the only other ingredient).

DIRECTIONS

1. If using roasted bell peppers preheat oven to 450 degrees F, and line baking pan with parchment paper. Place washed bell peppers on a baking sheet lined with parchment and drizzle with olive oil. Roast for 20 minutes, remove from oven and allow to cool.

2. In the food processer add all ingredients together and pulse until pureed. Or if not using a food processor, in a bowl combine all ingredients and puree with immersion blender until the garlic is finely minced and the paste is well blended.

3. Transfer the paste into a sterilized glass container or mason jar with lid and refrigerate for 30 minutes.

4. The paste can generally be stored in a covered airtight container, refrigerated for up to one week. You can also place in silicone ice trays to freeze into cubes and use for later.

Garlicky Jalapeno Lime Hot Sauce

Approximate Yield	Prep Time 15 min	Estimated Macronutrients
10-12 servings	Total Time 60 min	0 g P • 9 g C • 1 g F
	(To allow for refrigeration)	

INGREDIENTS

¼ cup dried minced onion or ½ a fresh onion
8 green jalapenos deseeded and coarsely chopped*
1 tablespoon olive oil
¼ cup lime juice
¾ cup filtered water
¾ cup white vinegar
5-8 cloves of garlic
1 teaspoon salt

Vinaigrette Recipe

⅓ cup of honey
¼ cup apple cider vinegar
2 teaspoons dried cilantro
1 teaspoon salt
¼ teaspoon cumin

KITCHEN EQUIPMENT

Large pot
Measuring spoons & measuring cups
Heat-resistant spoon or spatula
Food processor or handheld immersion blender
Sterilized large mason jar with lid or squeeze bottle for sauce
Optional: Electric juicer

SPECIAL INSTRUCTIONS/DIET INFORMATION

*If chopping the jalapenos by hand be sure to wash your hands thoroughly and be careful not to touch your face or sensitive areas.

DIRECTIONS

1. In a large pot on medium heat sauté and cook the jalapenos, onion and all other ingredients not part of the vinaigrette, for 8-10 minutes. Remove from heat and allow to cool for 4 minutes.
2. Transfer the jalapeno mixture to a food processer and add the remaining vinaigrette ingredients. (If using a handheld immersion blender, remove the pot form heat and add the vinaigrette ingredients directly into the pot and blend well). Transfer the sauce into a sterilized glass container or mason jar with lid and refrigerate for an hour.
3. This sauce can generally be stored in a covered airtight container, refrigerated for up to one week.
4. If you need a thinner sauce, you can use an electric juicer. When the hot sauce has cooled, use the juicer to thin the sauce further. The remaining pulp can be frozen for later use in other recipes.

Mango Habanero Hot Sauce

Approximate Yield
10-18 servings

Prep Time 15 min
Total Time 60 min
(To allow for refrigeration)

Estimated Macronutrients
1 g P • 14 g C • 0 g F

INGREDIENTS

1 ⅔ cup of filtered water
2 cups of frozen mango cubes
1 cup frozen carrots
1 habanero pepper destemmed and deseeded*
¼ cup minced dried onion or ½ of a fresh onion
2 cloves of garlic
½ cup of honey*
1 teaspoon of salt
3 tablespoons white vinegar
½ cup apple cider vinegar
¼ cup fresh lime juice
1 tablespoon tomato paste*

For a milder version add the following:
¼ cup filtered water
2 tablespoons fresh lime juice
2 tablespoons apple cider vinegar

KITCHEN EQUIPMENT

Large pot
Food processor or handheld immersion blender
Measuring spoons & measuring cups
Heat resistant tongs or spatula
Sterilized large mason jars with lids or squeeze bottle for sauce
Optional:
Electric juicer
Food grade latex gloves

SPECIAL INSTRUCTIONS/DIET INFORMATION

*If chopping the habaneros by hand be sure to wear gloves or wash your hands thoroughly. Be careful not to touch your face or sensitive areas.
*Adding honey is to taste, and more can be added after the sauce is blended well.
*Canned tomatoes are typically not allowed under SCD. However, there are Italian brands of canned tomatoes and tomato pastes with no artificial flavors, preservatives or additives listed as ingredients, nor used in the manufacturing process. These brands are generally sold through Wellbees and a few other stores. Read store bought canned tomato and tomato paste labels carefully. If necessary, you can make your own tomato sauce or paste using fresh tomatoes or canned tomato juice (if salt is the only other ingredient).

DIRECTIONS

1. In a large pot on medium heat, add all the ingredients to the pot, and cook until the carrots and mango are tender when pierced with a fork.
2. Transfer the mango and carrots to a food processer or blender and pulse until the sauce is well blended and without chunks. If using a handheld immersion blender, remove the pot form heat and blend directly in the pot
3. Transfer the sauce into a sterilized glass container or mason jar with lid and refrigerate for an hour.
4. This sauce can generally be stored in a covered airtight container, refrigerated for up to one week.
5. If you need a thinner sauce, you can use an electric juicer when the hot sauce has cooled and thin the sauce further. The remaining pulp can be frozen and/or added to other recipes.

Enchilada Sauce

Approximate Yield
10-12 servings

Prep Time 10 min
Total Time 30 min

Estimated Macronutrients
8 g P • 9 g C • 6 g F

INGREDIENTS

1-2 cups of Chicken Bone Broth (recipe on page 255 and notes below) *
6 oz can or (⅔ cups) of tomato paste*
¼ cup of chili powder
2 tablespoons apple cider vinegar
2 tablespoons avocado or olive oil
1 teaspoon granulated garlic
1 teaspoon ground cumin
1 teaspoon fine sea salt
½ teaspoon dried oregano

KITCHEN EQUIPMENT

Medium pot or deep saucepan with lid
Heat-resistant spoon or spatula
Measuring spoons & measuring cups
Handheld immersion blender
Sterilized large mason jars with lids or appropriate glass storage container
Silicone food storage freezer trays/cubes

SPECIAL INSTRUCTIONS/DIET INFORMATION

*Using 1 cup of chicken bone broth will yield a thicker enchilada sauce.
*Canned tomatoes are typically not allowed under SCD. However, there are Italian brands of canned tomatoes and tomato pastes with no artificial flavors, preservatives or additives listed as ingredients, nor used in the manufacturing process. These brands are generally sold through Wellbees and a few other stores. Read store bought canned tomato and tomato paste labels carefully. If necessary, you can make your own tomato sauce or paste using fresh tomatoes or canned tomato juice (if salt is the only other ingredient).

DIRECTIONS

1. In the pot/saucepan on medium heat, combine all ingredients for the enchilada sauce.
2. Once the sauce is at a low boil, reduce the heat to low and let simmer from 10-15 minutes stirring occasionally.
3. Remove the pot/saucepan off the heat and allow the sauce to cool down (generally to slightly above room temperature). This may be an opportunity to use the immersion blender and puree til the sauce is smooth. Transfer it into a sterilized glass container or mason jar with lid.
4. The sauce can be stored in the covered container, refrigerated for up to one week. Freeze for later use, by pouring the cooled sauce into silicone food storage freezer trays/cubes and freeze.

SCD Restaurant Style Salsa

Approximate Yield	Prep Time 15 min	Estimated Macronutrients
18 servings	**Total Time 60 min**	**1 g P • 8 g C • 0 g F**
	(To allow for refrigeration)	

There are two different variations of this recipe, one is with lemon juice and dried cilantro. The other is lime juice and fresh cilantro. Both have unique and distinct tastes. The lemon juice and dried cilantro are oftentimes more convenient to make, when fresh cilantro or limes are not available. We welcome you to try making both and see which one you enjoy most.

INGREDIENTS
1 (28 oz) can or 3-4 cups of crushed Italian tomatoes*
1-3 jalapenos (based on spice preference) *
2 limes juiced or 2 ½ tablespoons fresh squeezed lemon juice
½ white onion chopped
½ bunch of fresh cilantro (destemmed, approximately ½ cup) or ¾ tablespoon dried cilantro
4-5 green onions diced
2 teaspoons SCD Seasoning Salt (see recipe page 145)
½ teaspoon sea salt + more to taste
5- 10 cloves of garlic (this is based on personal preference and size of garlic cloves)
Optional:
1 serrano chili deseeded (save seeds based on spice preference)
Dried fine red chili flakes
2 tablespoons honey (to taste) *

KITCHEN EQUIPMENT
Food processor or blender
Measuring spoons & measuring cups
Spatula or large spoon
Sterilized large mason jars with lid

SPECIAL INSTRUCTIONS/DIET INFORMATION
*Canned tomatoes are typically not allowed under SCD. However, there are Italian brands of canned tomatoes and tomato pastes with no artificial flavors, preservatives or additives listed as ingredients, nor used in the manufacturing process. These brands are generally sold through Wellbees and a few other stores. Read store bought canned tomato and tomato paste labels carefully. If necessary, you can make your own tomato sauce or paste using fresh tomatoes or canned tomato juice (if salt is the only other ingredient).
*Jalapenos can range in heat based on their color and age. If you need more heat reserve some seeds to add to the food processor as needed.
*The honey is to help offset spice/heat and is based on your personal preference. You can add less or more as needed.

DIRECTIONS
1. In food processer or blender add all ingredients, until all vegetables are pureed and well blended.
2. Transfer the sauce into a sterilized glass container or mason jar with lid and refrigerate for an hour.
3. As the salsa marinates, test for spice and salt. Add serrano seeds, salt or red chili flakes as needed.
4. This salsa can generally be stored in a covered airtight container, refrigerated for up to one week.

Honey Mustard Vinaigrette Dressing

<table>
<tr><td>Approximate Yield
20-24 servings</td><td>Prep Time 10 min
Total Time 60 min
(To allow for refrigeration)</td><td>Estimated Macronutrients
0 g P • 4 g C • 6 g F</td></tr>
</table>

INGREDIENTS
½ to 1 cup olive oil*
¼ cup of filtered water
¼ cup apple cider vinegar
¼ cup honey
3 tablespoons Dijon or brown grain mustard*
¼ teaspoon sea salt

KITCHEN EQUIPMENT
Large mason jars with lids or appropriate glass storage container (that can be shaken without spilling)
Measuring spoons & measuring cups

SPECIAL INSTRUCTIONS/DIET INFORMATION
* You may decrease or increase the amount of olive oil to reduce the amount of fat in the recipe.
*There are a few commercial brands of mustard made with SCD legal ingredients. However always check ingredients carefully. Confirm with the company and determine unlisted ingredients are not being used in the manufacturing process.

DIRECTIONS
1. In a sterilized glass container or mason jar with lid add all ingredients together.
2. Close the lid tightly and give the dressing several good shakes.
3. Allow to marinate in the fridge 1-2 hours before serving.
4. This dressing can generally be stored in the covered container, refrigerated for up 10 days.

SCD Dressing and Marinade Variations

Servings and macronutrients are not provided for this recipe, as ingredients and serving sizes can vary.

INGREDIENTS

Teriyaki Dressing
¼ cup apple cider vinegar
½ cup olive oil or neutral oil
3 tablespoons water
2 tablespoons SCD Italian Dressing Mix (see recipe page 153)
1 tablespoon tamari or No Soy Sauce (see recipe page 121 and notes) *
1 tablespoon honey

Dijon Italian Dressing
¼ cup white wine vinegar (you can half and half with an aged balsamic vinegar)
3 tablespoons water
½ cup olive oil
1 teaspoon dijon mustard
2 tablespoons SCD Italian Dressing Mix (see recipe page 153)

Greek Dressing and Marinade
¼ cup red wine vinegar (you can half and half with an aged balsamic vinegar)
3 tablespoons water
¼ olive oil and ¼ cup vegetable oil
¼ cup crumbled cotija cheese*
2 tablespoons SCD Italian Dressing Mix (see recipe page 153)

Cherry Dressing and Marinade
¼ cup apple cider vinegar
½ cup olive oil or neutral oil
3 tablespoons water
2 tablespoons pureed Cherry Compote (see recipe page 108)
2 tablespoons SCD Italian Dressing Mix (see recipe page 153)

Lemon Dill Dressing
¼ water
3 tablespoons fresh squeezed lemon juice
½ cup oil
1 tablespoon dried dill weed
2 tablespoons SCD Italian Dressing Mix (see recipe page 153)

Cilantro Lime
¼ water
3 tablespoons fresh squeezed lime juice
½ cup oil
1 tablespoon dried cilantro
2 tablespoons SCD Italian Dressing Mix (see recipe page 153)

KITCHEN EQUIPMENT
Small glass airtight sealable jar
Measuring spoons & measuring cups

SPECIAL INSTRUCTIONS/DIET INFORMATION
*Check the labels of the tamari, many will list rice wine vinegar and other ingredients which may be illegal when following SCD. Tamari should generally be gluten free, grain free, and sugar free. For example, tamari includes only water, organic soybeans, salt and/or organic alcohol (as part of fermentation process).
*If using No Soy Sauce (see recipe page 121) to substitute tamari, you may want to reduce the amount of honey and vinegar in the recipe. This is based on personal taste and is due to the sweetness and vinegar in the No Soy Sauce.
*In the book, Breaking the Vicious Cycle, explains that inexpensive vinegars may have added sugars, specifically balsamic vinegar. However balsamic vinegar aged for 15 years or more and labeled as a product of Italy (certified by the Italian controlling body for vinegar), is considered legal under SCD. Other forms of balsamic vinegar may have added sugars that are not SCD legal. Be careful to read ingredients and verify authenticity before purchasing products.
* Cheeses should be aged over 3 months, and contain zero carbohydrates or sugars, regarding nutritional content. Pre-sliced and pre-shredded cheese will likely contain illegal ingredients to prevent the cheese from sticking and prolong shelf life. It is always best to purchase blocks of cheese, then shred, grate, crumble or slice yourself.

DIRECTIONS
1. Measure out and add each of the following seasonings into the glass jar with tight lid. Either stir or seal the jar with lid and shake to blend all ingredients well.
2. Store in the refrigerator up to a week as a dressing or use to marinade various meats.

Balsamic Honey Glaze

Approximate Yield	Prep Time 10 min	Estimated Macronutrients
12-18 servings	Total Time 55 min	0 g P • 6 g C • 0 g F

INGREDIENTS
1 cup aged balsamic vinegar*
2 tablespoons honey

KITCHEN EQUIPMENT
Medium pot or saucepan with lid
Heat-resistant spoon or spatula
Measuring spoons & measuring cups
Sterilized large mason jars with lids or appropriate glass storage container

SPECIAL INSTRUCTIONS/DIET INFORMATION
*In the book, Breaking the Vicious Cycle, explains that inexpensive vinegars may have added sugars, specifically balsamic vinegar. However balsamic vinegar aged for 15 years or more and labeled as a product of Italy (certified by the Italian controlling body for vinegar), is considered legal under SCD. Other forms of balsamic vinegar may have added sugars that are not SCD legal. Be careful to read ingredients and verify authenticity before purchasing products.
*For all vinegars avoid using the "mother" in recipes.

DIRECTIONS
1. In a medium pot/saucepan, add all ingredients and heat on medium. Stirring occasionally.
2. Once the sauce is at a low boil, reduce the heat to low and let simmer from 10-12 minutes stirring occasionally.
3. Remove the pot/saucepan off the heat, when the sauce coats the spoon and allow the sauce to cool down (to slightly above room temperature). Transfer it into a sterilized glass container or mason jar with lid.
4. This glaze can generally be stored in the covered container, in a refrigerator for up to one week.

Walnut Pesto

Approximate Yield
8 servings

Prep Time 15 min
Total Time 30 min

Estimated Macronutrients
1 g P • 4 g C • 6 g F

INGREDIENTS
4 cups of basil leaves
½ cup of shelled walnuts
8 cloves garlic finely minced
2 tablespoons lemon juice
2 tablespoons olive oil
1 teaspoon sea salt
¼ cup water*

KITCHEN EQUIPMENT
Food processor
Measuring spoons & measuring cups
Spatula or large spoon
Sterilized large mason jars with lid

SPECIAL INSTRUCTIONS/DIET INFORMATION
*Water can be increased or decreased depending on desired thickness

DIRECTIONS
1. In food processer blend all ingredients, until the walnuts and garlic are finely pureed and the pesto is well blended. Blend in the water if the pesto needs to be thinned.
2. Either toss fresh with dish, or transfer the sauce into a sterilized glass container or mason jar with lid and refrigerate.
3. The pesto can generally be stored in a covered airtight container, refrigerated for up to one week.

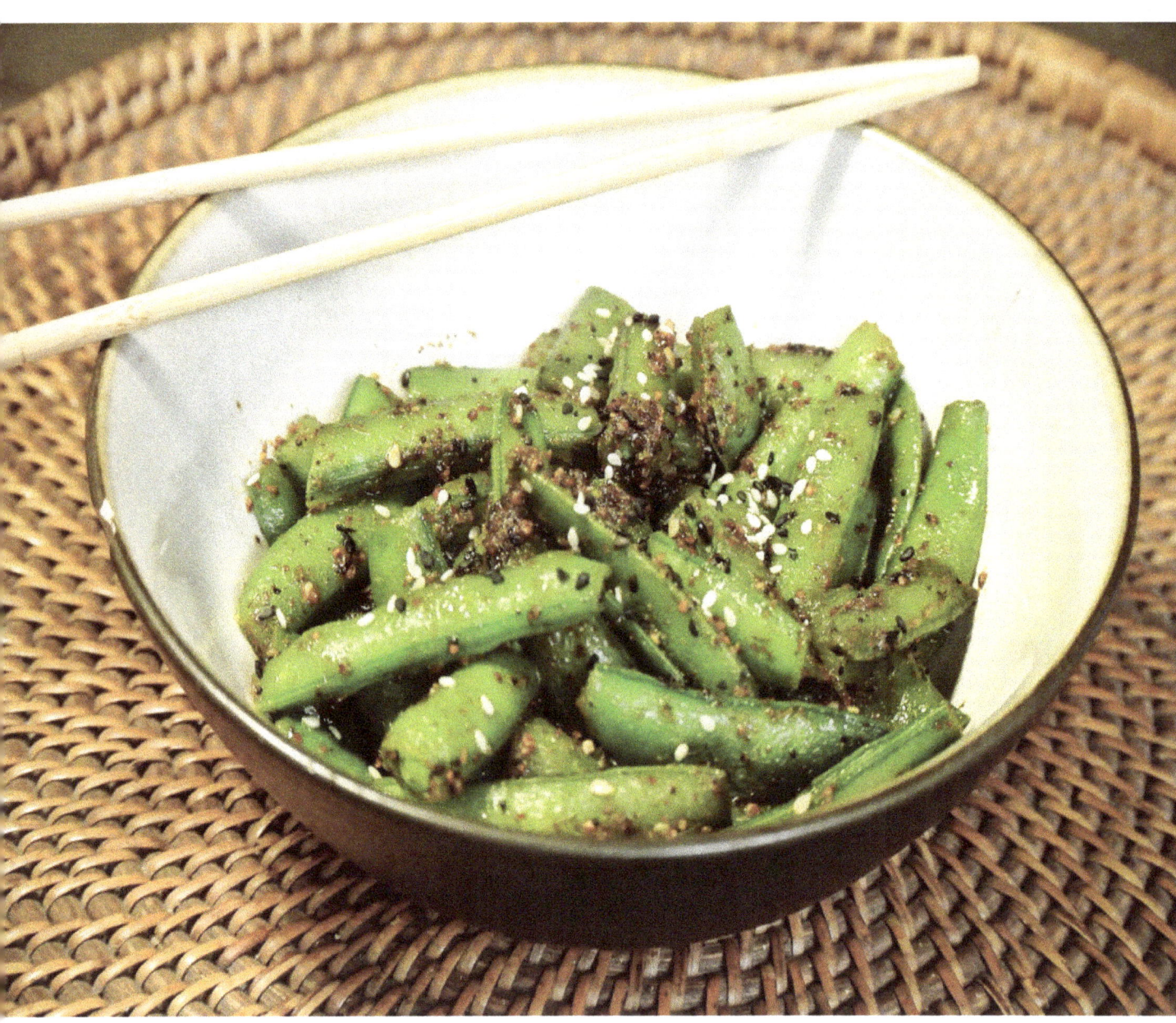

Togarashi Seasoning
on Spicy Snap Peas

Spices & Seasonings

There are many spices and seasonings on the shelves of stores, which often include undisclosed additives, anti-caking agents or ingredients you cannot pronounce. However, making your own spice or seasoning is delicious and surprisingly easy, especially when you have a well-stocked cabinet. Buying a variety of single ingredient spices and dried herbs allows you creativity in the kitchen. Many secret family recipes are derived from their homemade combinations of seasoning. For athletes, seasoning provides variety with little to no changes in calories or macronutrients. This is ideal when following a strict nutritional regimen for a sport or physique goal.

Pumpkin Spice Seasoning

Approximate Yield
10-12 servings

Total Time 10 min

Estimated Macronutrients are not available.

INGREDIENTS
2 tablespoons ground cinnamon
4 teaspoons ground ginger
2 teaspoons ground cloves
2 teaspoons ground allspice
1 teaspoon nutmeg

KITCHEN EQUIPMENT
Small glass airtight sealable jar
Measuring spoons

SPECIAL INSTRUCTIONS/DIET INFORMATION
*Since legal SCD spices should not have any concentrates, additives, anti-caking ingredients, or sugars. These spice mixes may need to be stirred or shaken regularly to prevent clumping.

DIRECTIONS
1. Measure out and add each of the following seasonings into the glass jar. Either stir the spices in the jar to mix or seal the jar with lid and shake to mix all ingredients.
2. Store along with other spices in a cool cupboard.

Chai Spice Mix

Approximate Yield
10 servings

Total Time 10 min

Estimated Macronutrients are not available.

INGREDIENTS
2 tablespoons + ¾ teaspoon ground cinnamon
1 tablespoon ground cardamom
1 tablespoon ground ginger
¾ tablespoon ground allspice
¾ tablespoon ground cloves
¾ tablespoon ground nutmeg

KITCHEN EQUIPMENT
Small glass airtight sealable jar
Measuring spoons

SPECIAL INSTRUCTIONS/DIET INFORMATION
*Since legal SCD spices should not have any concentrates, additives, anti-caking ingredients, or sugars. These spice mixes may need to be stirred or shaken regularly to prevent clumping.

DIRECTIONS
1. Measure out and add each of the following seasonings into the glass jar. Either stir the spices in the jar to mix or seal the jar with lid and shake to mix all ingredients.
2. Store along with other spices in a cool cupboard.

Italian Sage Spice Rub

Approximate Yield
12-16 servings

Total Time 10 min

Estimated Macronutrients are not
available.

INGREDIENTS
2 tablespoons salt
1 tablespoon dried thyme
1 tablespoon granulated garlic
1 teaspoon ground white pepper
3 teaspoons ground sage
2 teaspoons smoked paprika
2 teaspoons ground nutmeg
2 teaspoons basil
1 teaspoon celery seed
1 teaspoon dried rosemary
1 teaspoon oregano
½ teaspoon cayenne
¼ teaspoon ground cloves

KITCHEN EQUIPMENT
Small glass airtight sealable jar
Measuring spoons

SPECIAL INSTRUCTIONS/DIET INFORMATION
*Since legal SCD spices should not have any concentrates, additives, anti-caking ingredients, or sugars. These spice mixes may need to be stirred or shaken regularly to prevent clumping.

DIRECTIONS
1. Measure out and add each of the following seasonings into the glass jar. Either stir the spices in the jar to mix or seal the jar with lid and shake to mix all ingredients.
2. Store along with other spices in a cool cupboard.

Seasoning Salt

Approximate Yield
12-16 servings

Total Time 10 min

Estimated Macronutrients are not
available.

INGREDIENTS
¼ cup of fine sea salt
4 teaspoons fine ground black pepper
1 teaspoon granulated garlic
1 teaspoon granulated onion
1 teaspoon paprika
½ teaspoon smoked paprika
½ teaspoon cayenne pepper

KITCHEN EQUIPMENT
Small glass airtight sealable jar
Measuring spoons

SPECIAL INSTRUCTIONS/DIET INFORMATION
*Since legal SCD spices should not have any concentrates, additives, anti-caking ingredients, or sugars. These spice mixes may need to be stirred or shaken regularly to prevent clumping.

DIRECTIONS
1. Measure out and add each of the following seasonings into the glass jar. Either stir the spices in the jar to mix or seal the jar with lid and shake to mix all ingredients.
2. Store along with other spices in a cool cupboard.

Savory Greek Seasoning

Approximate Yield
10-12 servings

Total Time 10 min

Estimated Macronutrients are not available.

INGREDIENTS

3 tablespoons sea salt
3 tablespoons paprika
3 tablespoons granulated garlic
1 tablespoon + 1 teaspoon ground cumin
3 teaspoon granulated onion
1 ½ teaspoon cinnamon
1 teaspoon clove
1 teaspoon fine ground black pepper

KITCHEN EQUIPMENT

Small glass airtight sealable jar
Measuring spoons

SPECIAL INSTRUCTIONS/DIET INFORMATION

*Since legal SCD spices should not have any concentrates, additives, anti-caking ingredients, or sugars. These spice mixes may need to be stirred or shaken regularly to prevent clumping.

DIRECTIONS

1. Measure out and add each of the following seasonings into the glass jar. Either stir the spices in the jar to mix or seal the jar with lid and shake to mix all ingredients.
2. Store along with other spices in a cool cupboard.

Döner Seasoning

Approximate Yield
10-12 servings

Total Time 10 min

Estimated Macronutrients are not available.

INGREDIENTS

4 tablespoons sea salt
1 tablespoon dried oregano
1 tablespoon ground chili powder*
1 tablespoon paprika
1 tablespoon ground black pepper
1 tablespoon granulated garlic*
1 tablespoon granulated onion*
1 tablespoon dried marjoram
1 tablespoon ground cayenne
½ tablespoon ground cumin
2 teaspoons ground smoked paprika
1 teaspoon dried thyme

KITCHEN EQUIPMENT

Small glass airtight sealable jar
Measuring spoons

SPECIAL INSTRUCTIONS/DIET INFORMATION

*Since legal SCD spices should not have any concentrates, additives, anti-caking ingredients, or sugars. These spice mixes may need to be stirred or shaken regularly to prevent clumping.

DIRECTIONS

1. Measure out and add each of the following seasonings into the glass jar. Either stir the spices in the jar to mix or seal the jar with lid and shake to mix all ingredients.
2. Store along with other spices in a cool cupboard.

Taco Seasonings

**Approximate Yield
10-12 servings**

Total Time 10 min

Estimated Macronutrients are not available.

INGREDIENTS
2 tablespoons salt
2 tablespoons paprika
1 ½ tablespoons chili powder
1 tablespoon granulated garlic
1 ½ teaspoons ground cumin
1 teaspoon granulated onion powder
1 teaspoon oregano
½ teaspoon pepper
¼ teaspoon cayenne

KITCHEN EQUIPMENT
Small glass airtight sealable jar
Measuring spoons

SPECIAL INSTRUCTIONS/DIET INFORMATION
*Since legal SCD spices should not have any concentrates, additives, anti-caking ingredients, or sugars. These spice mixes may need to be stirred or shaken regularly to prevent clumping.

DIRECTIONS
1. Measure out and add each of the following seasonings into the glass jar. Either stir the spices in the jar to mix or seal the jar with lid and shake to mix all ingredients.
2. Store along with other spices in a cool cupboard.

Cilantro Onion Rub

**Approximate Yield
6 servings**

Total Time 10 min

Estimated Macronutrients are not available.

INGREDIENTS
2 tablespoons fine sea salt
1 tablespoon dried cilantro
1 tablespoon granulated onion
1 ½ teaspoon ground fine black pepper

KITCHEN EQUIPMENT
Small glass airtight sealable jar
Measuring spoons

SPECIAL INSTRUCTIONS/DIET INFORMATION
*Since legal SCD spices should not have any concentrates, additives, anti-caking ingredients, or sugars. These spice mixes may need to be stirred or shaken regularly to prevent clumping.

DIRECTIONS
1. Measure out and add each of the following seasonings into the glass jar. Either stir the spices in the jar to mix or seal the jar with lid and shake to mix all ingredients.
2. Store along with other spices in a cool cupboard.

SCD Tajin

Approximate Yield
14-16 servings

Total Time 10 min

Estimated Macronutrients are not available.

INGREDIENTS

2 limes zested
1 ½ tablespoons sea salt
1 teaspoon ground ancho chili powder
½ teaspoon ground chipotle chili powder
¼ teaspoon ground cayenne

KITCHEN EQUIPMENT

Large baking sheet
Oven or dehydrator
Baking parchment paper
Measuring spoons
Glass airtight jar or spice container
Optional: 1 gram food safe desiccant packet to prevent moisture

SPECIAL INSTRUCTIONS/DIET INFORMATION

*Since legal SCD spices should not have any concentrates, additives, anti-caking ingredients, or sugars. These spice mixes may need to be stirred or shaken regularly to prevent clumping
*Generally dehydrated lime zest can be stored in an airtight container in a dark place for up to 3-6 months depending on humidity and proper storage.

DIRECTIONS

Dehydrating lime zest in an oven

1. Preheat the oven to 200 degrees F and line a baking sheet with parchment paper.
2. Zest the lime and be sure to not include the white pith. Arrange the lime zest in a single layer on the parchment paper placed on a baking sheet
3. Bake for 2–3 hours, or until the zest is dry and starts to curl up around the edges.
4. Allow to cool and store in an airtight container for use later.

Dehydrating lime zest in a dehydrator

5. Zest the lime and be sure to not include the white pith.
6. Spread the zest in an even layer on a dehydrator tray lined with parchment paper. Place in the Dehydrator at 130 degrees F for two hours.
7. After breaking apart any clumps of zest, stir to ensure the zest is drying. Then dehydrate for an additional one to two hours at 130 degrees F.

Mixing the seasoning

8. Measure out and add each of the ingredients into the glass jar. Either stir the spices in the jar to mix or seal the jar with lid and shake to mix all ingredients.
9. Store along with other spices in a cool cupboard.

Pincho (Spanish Paprika) Spice Rub

**Approximate Yield
20-24 servings**

Total Time 10 min

Estimated Macronutrients are not available.

INGREDIENTS
½ cup smoked paprika
¼ cup of fine ground sea salt
2 tablespoons dried oregano
1 tablespoon granulated garlic*
1 tablespoon granulated onion*
1 tablespoon red pepper flakes
1 tablespoon ground cumin
1 tablespoon fine ground black pepper

KITCHEN EQUIPMENT
Small glass airtight sealable jar
Measuring spoons

SPECIAL INSTRUCTIONS/DIET INFORMATION
*Since legal SCD spices should not have any concentrates, additives, anti-caking ingredients, or sugars. These spice mixes may need to be stirred or shaken regularly to prevent clumping.

DIRECTIONS
1. Measure out and add each of the following seasonings into the glass jar. Either stir the spices in the jar to mix or seal the jar with lid and shake to mix all ingredients.
2. Store along with other spices in a cool cupboard.

Cajun Spice Seasoning

**Approximate Yield
20-24 servings**

Total Time 10 min

Estimated Macronutrients are not available.

INGREDIENTS
2 tablespoons granulated garlic
2 tablespoons paprika
2 tablespoons sea salt
1 tablespoon granulated onion
1 tablespoon dried thyme
½ tablespoon fine black ground pepper
2 teaspoons chili powder
1 teaspoon smoked paprika
½ teaspoon ground cayenne
¼ teaspoon ground cumin

KITCHEN EQUIPMENT
Small glass airtight sealable jar
Measuring spoons

SPECIAL INSTRUCTIONS/DIET INFORMATION
*Since legal SCD spices should not have any concentrates, additives, anti-caking ingredients, or sugars. These spice mixes may need to be stirred or shaken regularly to prevent clumping.

DIRECTIONS
1. Measure out and add each of the following seasonings into the glass jar. Either stir the spices in the jar to mix or seal the jar with lid and shake to mix all ingredients.
2. Store along with other spices in a cool cupboard.

Best Darn Rub (BDR) Chicken Seasoning

Approximate Yield
20-24 servings

Total Time 10 min

Estimated Macronutrients are not available.

INGREDIENTS
4 tablespoons + ¾ teaspoon fine sea salt
4 tablespoons paprika
2 tablespoons granulated garlic
1 tablespoon black pepper
½ tablespoon dried thyme
½ tablespoon ground dried mustard
½ tablespoon dried oregano
½ tablespoon dried celery seed
¾ teaspoon dried basil
¾ teaspoon dried parsley
¾ teaspoon ground white pepper
¾ teaspoon ground ginger
¾ teaspoon smoked paprika
¾ teaspoon chili powder
¼ teaspoon cayenne pepper

KITCHEN EQUIPMENT
Small glass airtight sealable jar
Measuring spoons

SPECIAL INSTRUCTIONS/DIET INFORMATION
*Since legal SCD spices should not have any concentrates, additives, anti-caking ingredients, or sugars. These spice mixes may need to be stirred or shaken regularly to prevent clumping.

DIRECTIONS
1. Measure out and add each of the following seasonings into the glass jar. Either stir the spices in the jar to mix or seal the jar with lid and shake to mix all ingredients.
2. Store along with other spices in a cool cupboard.

Greek Spice Rub

Approximate Yield
10 servings

Total Time 10 min

Estimated Macronutrients are not available.

INGREDIENTS
2 tablespoons salt
2 tablespoons granulated garlic
3 teaspoons oregano
2 teaspoons thyme
1 ½ teaspoons pepper

KITCHEN EQUIPMENT
Small glass airtight sealable jar
Measuring spoons

SPECIAL INSTRUCTIONS/DIET INFORMATION
*Since legal SCD spices should not have any concentrates, additives, anti-caking ingredients, or sugars. These spice mixes may need to be stirred or shaken regularly to prevent clumping.

DIRECTIONS
1. Measure out and add each of the following seasonings into the glass jar. Either stir the spices in the jar to mix or seal the jar with lid and shake to mix all ingredients.
2. Store along with other spices in a cool cupboard.

SCD Ranch Dressing Mix

**Approximate Yield
12-14 servings**

Total Time 10 min

Estimated Macronutrients are not
available.

INGREDIENTS

3 tablespoons dried parsley
1 tablespoon dried chives
2 teaspoons dried dill weed
2 teaspoons granulated garlic
1 ½ teaspoon sea salt
1 teaspoon granulated onion
½ teaspoon fine ground black pepper

Ranch Dressing

½ cup non-fat SCD Greek yogurt
½ cup avocado mayonnaise (see recipe page 112) *
1 ½ - 2 tablespoons SCD Ranch Dressing Mix
1 teaspoon apple cider vinegar
Splash of unsweetened cashew milk or other nut milk*
Salt & pepper to taste
Optional: ½ teaspoon of lemon juice or ½ teaspoon
Worcestershire sauce (see recipe page 120)

KITCHEN EQUIPMENT

Small glass airtight sealable jar
Measuring spoons & measuring cups
Spatula or large spoon

SPECIAL INSTRUCTIONS/DIET INFORMATION

*Since legal SCD spices should not have any concentrates, additives, anti-caking ingredients, or sugars. These spice mixes may need to be stirred or shaken regularly to prevent clumping.
* There are limited brands of mayonnaise with legal ingredients under the Specific Carbohydrate Diet, therefore read labels carefully and verify with the manufacturer or use the recipe on page 112.
*Any nut milks should only consist of nuts, water, or salt. No emulsifiers, gums, sweeteners or additives should be in the ingredient list. If you are unable to source a SCD legal nut milk you can make them easily at home (see recipe page 299).

DIRECTIONS

1. Measure out and add each of the following seasonings into the glass jar. Either stir the spices in the jar to mix or seal the jar with lid and shake to mix all ingredients.
2. Store along with other spices in a cool cupboard.
3. If you need to create the ranch dressing, mix all ingredients listed in a medium to large mason jar with lid and shake well.

Italian Herb Spice Mix

Approximate Yield
10 servings

Total Time 10 min

Estimated Macronutrients are not available.

INGREDIENTS
2 tablespoons oregano
1 ½ tablespoons basil
1 tablespoon marjoram
1 tablespoon thyme
1 tablespoon parsley

KITCHEN EQUIPMENT
Small glass airtight sealable jar
Measuring spoons

SPECIAL INSTRUCTIONS/DIET INFORMATION
*Since legal SCD spices should not have any concentrates, additives, anti-caking ingredients, or sugars. These spice mixes may need to be stirred or shaken regularly to prevent clumping.

DIRECTIONS
1. Measure out and add each of the following seasonings into the glass jar. Either stir the spices in the jar to mix or seal the jar with lid and shake to mix all ingredients.
2. Store along with other spices in a cool cupboard.

Parmesan-No Seasoning

Approximate Yield
16-18 servings

Total Time 10 min

Estimated Macronutrients are not available.

INGREDIENTS
2 tablespoons blanched almond flour
2 tablespoons fine sea salt
1 tablespoon granulated garlic
1 tablespoon granulated onion
1 tablespoon dried parsley
½ teaspoon fine ground black pepper
1 teaspoon ground mustard
⅛ teaspoon ground cumin
2 teaspoons smoked paprika
Pinch of nutmeg
*Optional for a bit of heat ¼ teaspoon of fine ground red pepper flakes

KITCHEN EQUIPMENT
Small glass airtight sealable jar
Measuring spoons

SPECIAL INSTRUCTIONS/DIET INFORMATION
*Since legal SCD spices should not have any concentrates, additives, anti-caking ingredients, or sugars. These spice mixes may need to be stirred or shaken regularly to prevent clumping.
*Reminder to always label and inform others there is almond flours in this spice mix. If necessary the almond flour can be omitted.

DIRECTIONS
1. Measure out and add each of the following seasonings into the glass jar. Either stir the spices in the jar to mix or seal the jar with lid and shake to mix all ingredients.
2. Store along with other spices in a cool cupboard.

SCD Italian Dressing Mix

Approximate Yield
10-12 servings

Total Time 10 min

Estimated Macronutrients are not available.

INGREDIENTS

2 tablespoons dried oregano
2 tablespoons + ¼ teaspoon sea salt
1 tablespoon dried parsley
1 tablespoon granulated garlic
1 tablespoon granulated onion
1 teaspoon fine ground black pepper
¼ teaspoon dried basil
¼ teaspoon celery seed

Italian Dressing
¼ cup apple cider vinegar
⅔ cup olive oil
2 tablespoons water
2 tablespoons SCD Italian Dressing Mix

KITCHEN EQUIPMENT
Small glass airtight sealable jar
Measuring spoons

SPECIAL INSTRUCTIONS/DIET INFORMATION
*Since legal SCD spices should not have any concentrates, additives, anti-caking ingredients, or sugars. These spice mixes may need to be stirred or shaken regularly to prevent clumping.

DIRECTIONS

1. Measure out and add each of the following seasonings into the glass jar. Either stir the spices in the jar to mix or seal the jar with lid and shake to mix all ingredients.
2. Store along with other spices in a cool cupboard.
3. If you need to create the Italian dressing, mix all ingredients listed in a medium to large mason jar with lid and shake well.

Asian Dry Rub

Approximate Yield
10 servings

Total Time 10 min

Estimated Macronutrients are not available.

INGREDIENTS
3 teaspoons fine sea salt
1 teaspoon dried ground ginger
½ teaspoon granulated onion powder
½ teaspoon coarse ground black pepper
½ teaspoon finely ground crushed red pepper
⅛ teaspoon granulated garlic
⅛ teaspoon Chinese five spice powder
⅛ teaspoon ground white pepper
Optional: Cayenne to taste for additional spice
If using as a sauce or marinade, add the following to coat:
2 tablespoons sesame oil
1 tablespoon honey

KITCHEN EQUIPMENT
Small glass airtight sealable jar
Measuring spoons

SPECIAL INSTRUCTIONS/DIET INFORMATION
*Since legal SCD spices should not have any concentrates, additives, anti-caking ingredients, or sugars. These spice mixes may need to be stirred or shaken regularly to prevent clumping.

DIRECTIONS
1. Measure out and add each of the following seasonings into the glass jar. Either stir the spices in the jar to mix or seal the jar with lid and shake to mix all ingredients.
2. Store along with other spices in a cool cupboard.

Togarashi Seasonings

Approximate Yield
10 servings

Total Time 10 min

Estimated Macronutrients are not available.

INGREDIENTS
2 tablespoons finely ground red chili flakes
2 teaspoons dried orange peel
1 teaspoon black sesame seeds
1 teaspoon white sesame seeds
½ teaspoon of poppy seeds
½ teaspoon of dried parsley
¼ teaspoon ground white pepper
¼ teaspoon ground ginger

KITCHEN EQUIPMENT
Small glass airtight sealable jar
Measuring spoons

SPECIAL INSTRUCTIONS/DIET INFORMATION
*Since legal SCD spices should not have any concentrates, additives, anti-caking ingredients, or sugars. These spice mixes may need to be stirred or shaken regularly to prevent clumping.

DIRECTIONS
1. Measure out and add each of the following seasonings into the glass jar. Either stir the spices in the jar to mix or seal the jar with lid and shake to mix all ingredients.
2. Store along with other spices in a cool cupboard.

Thai Spice Rub

Approximate Yield
10 servings

Prep Time 15 min
Total Time 2-4 hours
(To allow for dehydration)

Estimated Macronutrients are not available.

INGREDIENTS
4-6 Thai chilis, destemmed and chopped or ½-1 teaspoon of dried thai chilis ground into flakes (see directions below) *
2 teaspoons sea salt
1 teaspoon ground coriander
1 teaspoon ground cumin
1 teaspoon granulated onion
1 teaspoon granulated garlic
½ teaspoon dried lemongrass
½ teaspoon ground ginger

Optional:
½ teaspoon dried lemon zest*
3 teaspoons dried lime zest*

KITCHEN EQUIPMENT
Small glass airtight sealable jar
Baking sheet
Baking parchment paper
Spoon or spatula
Measuring spoons

SPECIAL INSTRUCTIONS/DIET INFORMATION
*If you are unable to source Thai chilis, Fresno or red jalapenos can be substituted.
*See SCD Tajin recipe page 148 for instructions on how to dry lime and lemon zest.
*Since legal SCD spices should not have any concentrates, additives, anti-caking ingredients, or sugars. These spice mixes may need to be stirred or shaken regularly to prevent clumping.

DIRECTIONS
Dehydrating thai chilis in an oven
1. Preheat the oven to 200 degrees F and line a baking sheet with parchment paper.
2. Arrange the chilis in a single layer on the parchment paper lining the baking sheet.
3. Bake/dehydrate the chilis for 2–4 hours, or until the chilis and the seeds are dry.
4. Allow to cool and using a high-powered blender or grinder, grind the thai chilis into flakes. Store in an airtight container for use later.

Mixing the seasoning
5. Measure out each of the ingredients and pour in the glass jar. Either stir the spices in the jar to mix, or seal the jar with lid and shake to mix all ingredients.
6. Store along with other spices in a cool cupboard.

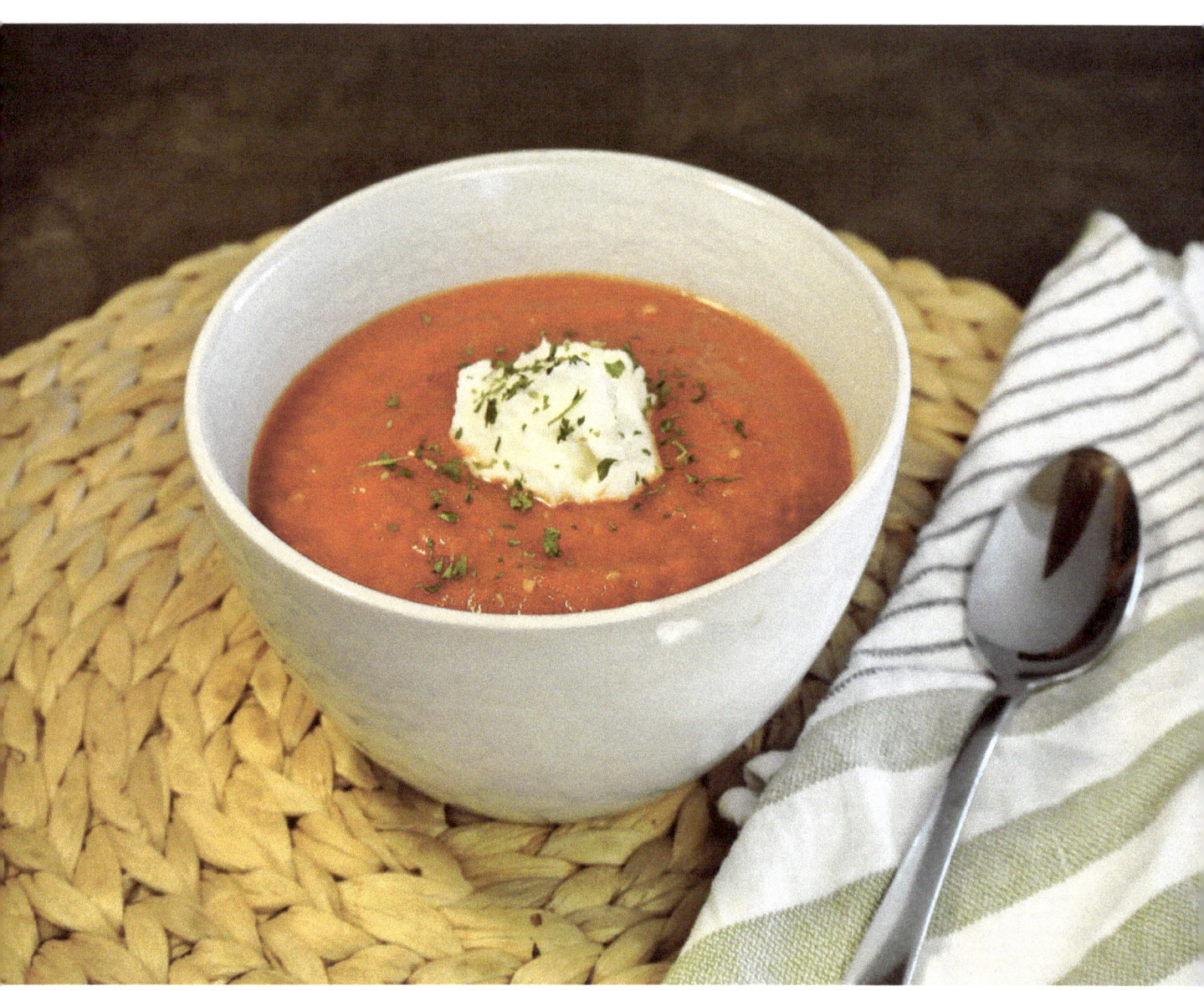

Tomato Vegetable Gazpacho
garnished with SCD Yogurt

Soups & Stews

Soups and stews are considered comfort food, but they are also a great recovery food after exercise. Soups and stews can also be very portable when stored in an insulated thermos, reheated in a portable lunch warmer, or even served cold like gazpacho. The well-cooked or pureed vegetables and soft protein sources are generally easy for digestion. Additionally the higher sodium content of a nutritious broth creates a perfect combination for a depleted athlete. After high intensity exercise, or endurance events, many athletes claim gastrointestinal distress or have minimal appetite. Therefore, a good practice is to start with foods nutritionally balanced, gentler for digestion, and will restore electrolytes like soups and stews.

Beef Pozole Rojo

Approximate Yield
10-12 servings

Prep Time 40 min
Total Time 4-10 hours
(To allow for slow cooking)

Estimated Macronutrients
32 g P • 11 g C • 7 g F

This recipe includes instructions for both stovetop and slow cooker. Cauliflower or celery root replaces the traditional ingredient of hominy which is illegal under the Specific Carbohydrate Diet.

INGREDIENTS
6-12 cups of filtered water
1 chuck roast (bone in or boneless) trimmed of excess fat (3-4 lbs.) cut into pieces fitting the Dutch oven pot or slow cooker*
1-2 tablespoons olive oil
¼ teaspoon ground black pepper
¼ teaspoon sea salt
1 white onion coarsely chopped
1 whole head of garlic (cloves peeled and hard ends cut off)
2 cups of SCD legal chicken bone broth or use Roasted Chicken Bone Broth (see recipe on page 255)
3 whole bay leaves
1 tablespoon salt
½ tablespoon black pepper
3-4 cups of cauliflower florets or celery root peeled and cut in ½ inch cubes
Salt & pepper to taste
Optional ground chipotle pepper

Red Sauce *
4 cups of filtered water
3 dried ancho chiles (stem and seeds removed)
3 dried chile guajillos (stem and seeds removed)
½ large yellow onion
4 garlic cloves peeled
1 teaspoon of salt
¾ teaspoon dried oregano
4 cups of filtered water
Drizzle of olive oil

Garnishes
Shredded cabbage
Diced white onion
Thinly sliced radishes
Lime wedges
Fresh cilantro sprigs

KITCHEN EQUIPMENT
Small to medium pot or saucepan
Blender or handheld immersion blender
Fine mesh colander/strainer
Large meat forks or tongs and knife
Parchment paper
Large dishwasher safe plate or platter (large enough to fit the roast on)
Heat resistant spoon or spatula
Large 4 Qt Dutch oven with lid (check that the roast will fit in it)
Heat resistant potholders
Stovetop
Measuring spoons
Paper towels
Ladle or large spoon
Optional: Large stove top pan and crockpot/ slow cooker
Non latex food service gloves (to wear when handling raw meat) *

SPECIAL INSTRUCTIONS
* Bone in chuck roast bone can be used later for bone broth.
*If necessary, you can substitute the Red Sauce with SCD Enchilada Sauce (see recipe page 136) with additional bone broth or water. It will not be the authentic Pozole Rojo recipe however the sauce can work in a pinch.
*Important note: Regardless of using gloves always follow best food safety practices to prevent cross contamination and food born illness when cooking with raw meat. See notes on Hygiene and General Food Safety on page 30.

DIRECTIONS

Red Sauce
1. Heat the water to boil in the small-medium pot or saucepan.
2. Remove the stem, and seeds from the dried chiles and rinse well to remove any dust or dirt.
3. Place the chiles in the boiling water with the onion garlic and spices. Cook on medium heat for about 20 minutes until the chiles are rehydrated and soft.

DIRECTIONS (continued)

4. Remove the pot from heat and allow to cool. Then transfer the contents to a blender or using the handheld immersion blender to puree the chilis into sauce.
5. Set the colander over the pot, strain the sauce through to remove excess seeds and larger pieces of chilis. Set aside the strained sauce for later.

Stovetop Only Method

1. On the stovetop, heat the olive oil on medium heat in the large dutch oven. Place parchment paper on the platter or large dish, put the roast on top of the paper and pat dry with paper towels. Salt and pepper each side of the chuck roast liberally.
2. Place the roast in the dutch oven and discard the parchment paper. Cook the roast for about 5-7 minutes and turning to brown each side. Remove the roast from the dutch oven and place on platter.
3. Add the onion and garlic to the dutch oven and sauté for 6-8 minutes or until tender. Scraping the bottom well and reduce heat to prevent burning.
4. Return the browned chuck roast to the dutch oven. Then add the bone broth, red sauce, water, bay leaves, salt and pepper.
5. Bring liquid to boil. Then cover with the lid and lower the heat to low. Simmering the soup for 2-3 hours. Note additional water may be necessary as it evaporates in the cooking process.
6. Check the beef for tenderness and then shred the beef with fork and knife. Remove the bay leaves and add in the cauliflower or cubed celery root. Continue to cook until they are tender when pierced with a fork.
7. Add salt, pepper and optional chipotle pepper as needed. Ladle into bowls and serve with garnishes.
8. This soup freezes very well once cooled and poured into freezer safe silicone cubes with lids for use later.

Stove Top & Slow Cooker Method

1. Preheat slow cooker on high.
2. On the stovetop, heat the olive oil on medium heat in large pan. Place parchment paper on the platter or large dish, put the roast on top of the paper and pat dry with paper towels. Salt and pepper each side of the chuck roast liberally.
3. Place the roast in the large pan and discard the parchment paper. Cook the roast for about 5-7 minutes and turning to brown each side. Remove the roast from the pan and place in preheated slow cooker.
4. Add the onion and garlic to the pan and sauté for 5 minutes. Scraping the bottom well and reduce heat to prevent burning. Pour the cooked garlic, remaining oil and onions over the chuck roast in the slow cooker.
5. Pour in the red sauce, bone broth, and water over the beef. Then add in the spices.
6. Cover the slow cooker with lid and change the temperature to low heat. Cooking for 7-8 hours.
7. Remove the bay leaves with fork or tongs and discard. Shred the meat with the forks or tongs. Add the cauliflower florets or celery root cubes and cook for another 30-minutes or until tender when pierced with a fork.
8. Add salt, pepper and optional chipotle pepper as needed. Ladle into bowls and serve with garnishes.
9. This soup freezes very well once cooled and poured into freezer safe silicone cubes with lids for use later.

Chicken Enchilada Soup

Approximate Yield	Prep Time 30 min	Estimated Macronutrients
10-12 servings	Total Time 60 min	23 g P • 15 g C • 3 g F

Cauliflower and bell peppers replaces the traditional corn in this recipe.

INGREDIENTS

1 ½ cups of mirepoix (½ cup diced celery, ½ cup peeled and diced carrots, ½ cup chopped onion)
2-3 tablespoons olive oil
2 (14.5 oz or approximately 2 cups) cans of diced tomatoes*
1 yellow or orange bell pepper (stem and seeds removed)
1 red bell pepper (stem and seeds removed)
Optional: 1 diced jalapeno (stem and seeds removed)
1 cup of SCD Enchilada Sauce (see recipe page 136)
2 cups SCD legal chicken bone broth or see recipe page 255
1 dried bay leaf
1 teaspoon granulated garlic or 2 cloves minced garlic
½ tablespoon Pincho Rub (see recipe page 149)
2 cups of cooked shredded chicken or use leftover Roasted Chicken (see recipe page 255)
4 cups of raw or frozen cauliflower florets
1 cup of cooked SCD Black Beans (see recipe page 199)
Salt and pepper to taste
Filtered water as needed

KITCHEN EQUIPMENT

Large pot
Measuring spoons & measuring cups
Large heat-resistant spoon or ladle
Silicone food storage freezer trays or freezer safe storage

SPECIAL INSTRUCTIONS/DIET INFORMATION

*Canned tomatoes are typically not allowed under SCD. However, there are Italian brands of canned tomatoes and tomato pastes with no artificial flavors, preservatives or additives listed as ingredients, nor used in the manufacturing process. These brands are generally sold through Wellbees and a few other stores. Read store bought canned tomato and tomato paste labels carefully. If necessary, you can make your own tomato sauce or paste using fresh tomatoes or canned tomato juice (if salt is the only other ingredient).

DIRECTIONS

1. In a large pot on medium to high heat, sauté the garlic, bell peppers, optional jalapeno, diced tomatoes mirepoix and pincho rub in olive oil. Halfway through the process add in the bone broth, enchilada sauce and remaining spices.

2. When vegetables are cooked, and the soup is simmering add in the roasted chicken, cauliflower, and black beans. Pour in the filtered water until you reach your desired consistency for the soup. Simmer until the cauliflower is tender and cooked. Taste and add salt or pepper as needed.

3. Serve warm. Cooled soup can be stored in silicone food storage freezer trays cubes or freezer safe storage, then frozen for later use.

Minestrone Soup

Approximate Yield	**Prep Time 30 min**	**Estimated Macronutrients**
12-16 servings	**Total Time 60 min**	**18 g P • 25 g C • 2 g F**

INGREDIENTS
1 cup of SCD soaked and cooked navy "white" beans or kidney beans (see recipe page 303)
1 ½ cups of mirepoix (½ cup diced celery, ½ cup peeled and diced carrots, ½ cup chopped onion)
2-3 tablespoons olive oil
1 14.5 oz can diced Italian tomatoes*
2 ½ cups of favorite SCD legal spaghetti sauce or crushed tomatoes*
4- 5 baby bella or white mushrooms
1 cup of frozen chopped spinach
2 cups SCD legal chicken bone broth or use the recipe on page 255
1 tablespoon of SCD legal tomato paste*
2-3 cloves of minced garlic
1 tablespoon of honey
1 tablespoon red wine vinegar
1 tablespoon dried oregano
1 tablespoon dried basil
2 dried bay leaves
Salt and pepper to taste

Add in 2 cups of cauliflower florets
Optional: add in 2 cups of cooked and drained favorite SCD legal pasta (lentil or yellow pea)

KITCHEN EQUIPMENT
Large pot
Measuring spoons & measuring cups
Large heat-resistant spoon or ladle
Silicone food storage freezer trays/cubes

SPECIAL INSTRUCTIONS/DIET INFORMATION
*Note there are a few commercially made SCD marinara, or spaghetti sauces made with legal ingredients. However, if you are unable to source it, use crushed tomatoes. You may need to increase the salt, add a bit of honey and red wine vinegar to taste with the crushed tomatoes.
*Canned tomatoes are typically not allowed under SCD. However, there are Italian brands of canned tomatoes and tomato pastes with no artificial flavors, preservatives or additives listed as ingredients, nor used in the manufacturing process. These brands are generally sold through Wellbees and a few other stores. Read store bought canned tomato and tomato paste labels carefully. If necessary, you can make your own tomato sauce or paste using fresh tomatoes or canned tomato juice (if salt is the only other ingredient).

DIRECTIONS
1. In a large pot on medium to high heat, sauté the chopped mushrooms, garlic, mirepoix in olive oil. Halfway through the process add in the bone broth and spices.
2. When vegetables are cooked through and the soup is simmering, add in the cauliflower, kidney beans and filtered water til the soup reaches the desired consistency. Simmer until the cauliflower is tender when pierced with a fork. Taste for salt and pepper as needed.
3. At this point you can add in your SCD legal noodles, however, keep in mind they may soak up the broth when storing leftovers. Serve warm.
4. For long term storage the soup can be stored in freezer trays/cubes and frozen for later use.

Creamy No-Tato Chicken Soup

Approximate Yield	Prep Time 30 min	Estimated Macronutrients
12-16 servings	**Total Time 60 min**	**25 g P • 8 g C • 9 g F**

INGREDIENTS

3 tablespoons olive oil
8 oz white or baby bella mushrooms (cleaned, destemmed and chopped)
1 ½ cups of mirepoix (½ cup diced celery, ½ cup peeled and diced carrots, ½ cup chopped onion)
1-2 cloves of minced garlic
2 cups SCD legal chicken bone broth or use recipe page 255
1-2 cups unsweetened cashew milk (or unsweetened coconut milk) *
2-3 cups filtered water
2 cups of shredded roasted chicken (see recipe page 255)
4 cups of cauliflower florets (fresh or frozen)
1 ½ teaspoon salt
¼ teaspoon dried thyme
¼ cup destemmed minced fresh curly leaf parsley or 1 tablespoon dried parsley
Pepper to taste

Optional thickening ingredients:
1-2 tablespoons fine ground yellow pea flour or lentil flour*
1/2 - 1 cup of cooked yellow pea mush to thicken as needed (see recipe page 304) or
¼ large tablespoons cashew cream to thicken as needed (see recipe page 300)

Garnishes

Chopped green onions
Cooked and crumbled (no sugar or added sweeteners) bacon*

KITCHEN EQUIPMENT

Large pot
Measuring spoons & measuring cups
Large heat-resistant spoon or ladle
Silicone food storage freezer trays/cubes with lids

SPECIAL INSTRUCTIONS/DIET INFORMATION

*Any nut milks should only consist of nuts, water, or salt. No emulsifiers, gums, sweeteners or additives should be in the ingredient list. If you are unable to source a SCD legal nut milk you can make them easily at home (see recipe page 299).
*If necessary, you can create a roux with butter, fine ground yellow pea flour (see recipe page 304) or SCD legal lentil flour.
*Always read labels carefully and verify ingredients with manufacturers for prepackaged bacon.

DIRECTIONS

1. In a large pot on medium to high heat, sauté the chopped mushrooms, garlic, and mirepoix in the olive oil. Halfway through the process add in the bone broth and spices.
2. When vegetables are cooked through, add cashew milk. The optional yellow pea or lentil flour, cashew cream or yellow pea mush can be used to thicken the soup to a stew as needed. Ladle some of the soup broth, into a large measuring cup or small bowl, then mix in the thickening ingredient well. Pour and stir the soup slurry back into the soup. If the soup needs to be thinned, filtered water can be added to reach desired consistency.
3. Once the soup is simmering add in the parsley, chicken and cauliflower florets. Continue to simmer until the cauliflower is tender when pierced with a fork. Taste for salt and pepper as needed.
4. Serve warm. For long term storage the soup can be frozen in silicone food storage freezer trays/cubes.

To utilize leftover soup, follow the next steps for Cheddar Biscuit Dumpling Chicken Pot Pie:

1. Preheat oven to 350 degrees F, and ladle leftover soup into a large dutch oven or cast iron pan (allowing 1- 2 inches of space for the biscuit dumplings to expand. Be careful not to ladle excess broth/liquid.
2. Mix the following ingredients in a large mixing bowl: 2 ½ cups almond flour, ¼ cup egg white powder, 1 teaspoon baking soda, ¾ teaspoon salt, ½ teaspoon granulated garlic, ¼ teaspoon ground black pepper, ½ cup of shredded cheddar cheese, 2 eggs, and 2 tablespoons melted butter.
3. Place the dough in large dollops atop the soup, and bake for 30-35 minutes or until bubbling and golden.

Cheezburger Soup

Approximate Yield	**Prep Time 30 min**	**Estimated Macronutrients**
10-12 servings	**Total Time 60 min**	**30 g P • 4 g C • 11 g F**

Note the name denotes this is a dairy free soup.

INGREDIENTS

3 tablespoons olive oil
1 (12-16 oz) package of lean ground beef or bison
1-2 cups filtered water
1 cup of diced (no sugar or added sweeteners) bacon*
1-2 cloves of minced garlic
1 ½ cups of mirepoix (½ cup diced celery, ½ cup peeled and diced carrots, ½ cup chopped onion)
½ cup diced green onion (reserve some for garnish)
2 cups SCD legal chicken bone broth or use Roasted Chicken Bone Broth (see recipe page 255)
2 tablespoons yellow mustard*
1-2 cups unsweetened cashew milk*
4 cups of cauliflower florets (fresh or frozen) or celery root (peeled and cubed)
1 ½ teaspoons salt
Pepper to taste
½ teaspoon dried parsley

Optional ingredients:
¼ cup of cooked Yellow Pea Mash or Flour (see recipe page 304) for a thickener
Turmeric as needed (for color)
Smoked paprika (for color and smokey taste)
2 tablespoons pureed cooked butternut squash or pumpkin (for color)
For garnish, diced SCD legal pickles or Quick Dill Pickles (see recipe page 182) *

Variation Notes
*Add 1 diced red bell and 8 oz white or baby bella mushrooms (cleaned, destemmed and chopped) to make it Philly Cheezsteak soup.
*Also ground beef and be substituted with shaved or diced beef.

KITCHEN EQUIPMENT
Large pot
Measuring spoons & measuring cups
Handheld meat chopper, mincer or heat-resistant spatula
Large heat-resistant spoon or ladle
Silicone food storage freezer trays/cubes

SPECIAL INSTRUCTIONS/DIET INFORMATION
*Any nut milks should only consist of nuts, water, or salt. No emulsifiers, gums, sweeteners or additives should be in the ingredient list. If you sre unable to source a SCD legal nut milk you can make them easily at home (see recipe page 299).
*There are a few commercial brands of mustard made with SCD legal ingredients. However always check ingredients carefully. Confirm with the company and determine unlisted ingredients are not being used in the manufacturing process.
* SCD legal pickles should not include any sweeteners, vague ingredients, and/or additives. The pickle ingredients used in this recipe included cucumber, water, salt, distilled white vinegar, garlic, dill weed, dill seed, mustard seed, caraway seed, calcium chloride (a natural salt), fennel seed, mace, and turmeric. If you are unable to source SCD legal pickles use the following Quick Dill Pickles, see recipe page 182.
*Always read labels carefully and verify ingredients with manufacturers for prepackaged bacon.

DIRECTIONS

1. In a large pot on medium to high heat, sauté diced bacon, ground beef and ½ cup water in olive oil. Halfway through cooking add the garlic, and mirepoix.
2. When beef is cooked, add the bone broth, cashew milk, mustard and optional butternut squash or pumpkin for color.
3. If using the yellow pea mash or flour, this should thicken the soup to a stew consistency. Add more filtered water as needed to thin or bring to desired consistency.
4. Once the soup is simmering add in the remaining spices and cauliflower florets. Allow to simmer until the cauliflower is tender when pierced with a fork. Salt and pepper to taste as needed.
5. Serve warm in bowls and garnish with some of the green onions, paprika, or pickles.
6. For long term storage freeze the soup in silicone food storage freezer trays/cubes with lids.

SCD New England Chowder

Approximate Yield	Prep Time 30 min	Estimated Macronutrients
10-12 servings	**Total Time 60 min**	**36 g P • 40 g C • 10 g F**

INGREDIENTS

3 tablespoons butter or olive oil

6 oz (no sugar or added sweeteners) bacon diced*

1 large onion finely chopped

6 small (or 4 large) celery stalks finely chopped

3 cloves of garlic minced

2 cups of clam juice, fish stock or roasted Chicken Bone Broth (see recipe page 255 and notes) *

1-2 cups of filtered water

1 teaspoon dried thyme

½ teaspoon salt

1 bay leaf

4 cups of cauliflower florets (fresh or frozen) or fresh peeled and cubed rutabaga

1 ½ cups of clams, finely chopped, approximately 3 (6.5 oz) cans or raw halibut or cod cut into bite size pieces (Deveined, shelled and cooked shrimp can be substituted as well)

1 cup of full fat SCD yogurt (see recipe page 298) *

1-2 cups of unsweetened cashew milk

1 teaspoon dried parsley or minced fresh parsley

Sea salt and pepper to taste

Garnishes

Chopped green onions or fresh chives

KITCHEN EQUIPMENT

Large pot

Handheld immersion blender

Measuring spoons & measuring cups

Large heat-resistant spoon or ladle

Silicone food storage freezer trays/cubes with lids

SPECIAL INSTRUCTIONS/DIET INFORMATION

*Note, bacon can be omitted as needed. However, if using always read labels carefully and verify ingredients with manufacturers for prepackaged bacon.

*If using chicken bone broth, cut the amount in half by 1 cup and substitute with 1 cup of water.

*If you are unable to eat dairy create a roux with cashew cream/butter and some soup broth, mixing them well in a separate bowl, then adding back into the soup.

*Any nut milks should only consist of nuts, water, or salt. No emulsifiers, gums, sweeteners or additives should be in the ingredient list. If you are unable to source a SCD legal nut milk you can make them easily at home (see recipe page 299).

DIRECTIONS

1. In a large pot on medium to high heat, add the butter or olive oil, then sauté the bacon, chopped garlic, and onion. Halfway through the process add in the chopped celery and continue to cook.

2. When the onions are translucent and bacon is crisp, add the clam juice or fish stock, salt, thyme, bay leaf and cauliflower.

3. Once the soup is simmering add in the clams or fish and water. (Note reserve some water, adding more as needed based on desired thickness.) Continue to simmer, until the seafood is cooked, and cauliflower is tender when pierced with a fork.

4. Stir in either the SCD full fat yogurt or cashew butter/cream roux, blending the soup well. Add salt and pepper to taste. Serve warm.

5. For long term storage the soup can be frozen in silicone food storage freezer trays/cubes.

Zuppa Toscano

Approximate Yield	**Prep Time 30 min**	**Estimated Macronutrients**
10-12 servings	**Total Time 60 min**	**24 g P • 8 g C • 8 g F**

INGREDIENTS

2 cups of cooked or leftover ground Sage and Turkey Sausage (see recipe page 72)
1 ½ cups of mirepoix (½ cup diced celery, ½ cup peeled and diced carrots, ½ cup chopped onion)
1-2 cloves of minced garlic
1 cup of white or baby bella mushrooms (cleaned, destemmed and chopped)
3 tablespoons olive oil
2 cups SCD legal chicken bone broth or use recipe page 255
1-2 cups unsweetened cashew milk, almond or coconut milk *
4 cups of cauliflower florets (fresh or frozen)
½ - 1 bunch of kale de-stemmed and chopped, or 3 cups of baby spinach
1 ½ teaspoons salt
¼ teaspoon dried thyme
Pepper to taste
¼ cup destemmed minced fresh curly leaf parsley or 1 tablespoon dried parsley
2-3 cups filtered water

Optional: 1 cup of cooked bacon (no sugar or added sweeteners) crumbles*
Optional thickening ingredients:
1-2 tablespoons fine ground yellow pea flour or lentil flour*

KITCHEN EQUIPMENT

Large pot
Measuring spoons & measuring cups
Large heat-resistant spoon or ladle
Silicone food storage freezer trays or cubes

SPECIAL INSTRUCTIONS/DIET INFORMATION

*Any nut milks should only consist of nuts, water, or salt. No emulsifiers, gums, sweeteners or additives should be in the ingredient list. If you are unable to source a SCD legal nut milk you can make them easily at home (see recipe page 299).
*Always read labels carefully and verify ingredients with manufacturers for prepackaged bacon.
*If necessary, you can create a roux with butter, fine ground yellow pea flour (see recipe page 304) or SCD legal lentil flour.

DIRECTIONS

1. In a large pot on medium to high heat, sauté chopped mushrooms, garlic, and mirepoix in the olive oil. Halfway through the process add in the bone broth and spices.
2. When vegetables are cooked through, add unsweetened cashew milk. Add an optional slurry or roux of lentil or yellow pea flour as needed. Or filtered water to bring it to the desired consistency.
3. Once the soup is simmering add in the parsley, cooked crumbled bacon, cooked ground turkey, kale and cauliflower florets. Allow the soup to simmer until the cauliflower is tender when pierced with a fork. Taste for salt and pepper as needed. Serve warm.
4. Leftover soup can be frozen in silicone freezer trays or cubes then in airtight container or zip top plastic freezer bags for use later.

Thai Coconut Chicken Soup

Approximate Yield	Prep Time 30 min	Estimated Macronutrients
10-12 servings	Total Time 60 min	36 g P • 9 g C • 7 g F

INGREDIENTS

2 tablespoons avocado oil
1 large shallot thinly sliced
2 cups white mushrooms (cleaned, destemmed and chopped in quarters)
1 large tomato chopped into small cubes
2 cloves of minced garlic
3 cups of SCD legal chicken bone broth or use recipe page 255
1 teaspoon dried ground lemon grass
1 teaspoon finely ground dried red chili flakes (or to taste)
Juice of 1 lime
1-2 tablespoons fish sauce (based on taste)
1 teaspoon of honey
2 cups of unsweetened coconut milk*
3-4 cups of cooked chicken or leftover Roasted Chicken (see recipe page 255)
Salt and pepper to taste
Optional: 2 tablespoons fresh Thai basil leaves julienned

Garnishes
Chopped green onions
Fresh cilantro sprigs

KITCHEN EQUIPMENT

Large pot
Measuring spoons & measuring cups
Large heat-resistant spoon or ladle
Silicone food storage freezer trays/cubes with lids

SPECIAL INSTRUCTIONS/DIET INFORMATION

*Any nut milks should only consist of nuts, water, or salt. No emulsifiers, gums, sweeteners or additives should be in the ingredient list. If you are unable to source a SCD legal nut milk you can make them easily at home (see recipe page 299).

DIRECTIONS

1. In a large pot on medium to high heat, sauté the shallot, chopped mushrooms, tomato and garlic in the olive oil. Halfway through the process add in the bone broth.
2. When vegetables are cooked through, add the fish sauce, lime juice, honey, spices coconut milk.
3. Once the soup is simmering add in the cooked chicken. Continue to simmer and taste for salt and pepper as needed. As an optional ingredient Thai basil can be added.
4. Serve the soup warm and garnish.
5. For long term storage the soup can be frozen in silicone food storage freezer trays/cubes.

Tomato Vegetable Gazpacho

<table>
<tr><td>**Approximate Yield**
8-10 servings</td><td>**Prep Time 20 min**
Total Time 60 min</td><td>**Estimated Macronutrients**
3 g P • 41 g C • 5 g F</td></tr>
</table>

As described earlier in the book, this recipe is an example of "recipe stacking". Where the goal is to build additional recipes from one and thus reduce our overall time in the kitchen. To minimize waste, this gazpacho recipe was specifically created to utilize the pulp from the Electrolyte Vegetable Juice. Also purposely designed as a large quantity for later use in the Slow Cooker Tomato Vegetable Pot Roast recipe (see recipe page 268).

INGREDIENTS

4-5 cups of leftover Electrolyte Vegetable Juice Pulp (see recipe page 84)
1-2 cups of canned finely pureed or diced tomatoes*
2 minced cloves of garlic
2 tablespoons of red wine
2 tablespoons of honey
2 tablespoons of olive oil
2 teaspoons of salt
Dash of cayenne pepper
Dash of ground white pepper to taste

Optional Garnishes
Dried or fresh parsley
Dripped SCD Yogurt (see recipe page 298)

KITCHEN EQUIPMENT

Large pot
Handheld immersion blender or food processor
Measuring spoons & measuring cups
Heat resistant spoon or spatula
Silicone freezer cubes

SPECIAL INSTRUCTIONS/DIET INFORMATION

*If you cannot source SCD legal tomato sauce, drain a large can of crushed or finely diced tomatoes over a fine mesh sieve or colander over another bowl to catch the juice. Pressing down the tomatoes to extract more juice as needed.
*Canned tomatoes are typically not allowed under SCD. However, there are Italian brands of canned tomatoes and tomato pastes with no artificial flavors, preservatives or additives listed as ingredients, nor used in the manufacturing process. These brands are generally sold through Wellbees and a few other stores. Read store bought canned tomato and tomato paste labels carefully. If necessary, you can make your own tomato sauce or paste using fresh tomatoes or canned tomato juice (if salt is the only other ingredient).

DIRECTIONS

1. In a large pot on medium heat, pour in the vegetable pulp, crushed canned tomatoes and cloves of minced garlic into the pot. Using a handheld immersion blender, puree the ingredients well. If you do not have a handheld immersion blender, puree the vegetable pulp and crushed tomatoes in a food processor. Then add the puree to the large pot.
2. Add in the remaining ingredients to the pot, stirring as the pot simmers. Taste the gazpacho and decide whether additional salt, pepper cayenne or honey may be needed.
3. Remove the pot from heat and allow to cool. Ladle the soup into bowls and refrigerate. Serve cool and add optional garnishes before serving.
4. For the leftover gazpacho, freeze in silicone freezer trays with lids for later use in the Slow Cooker Tomato Vegetable Pot Roast. (see recipe page 268)

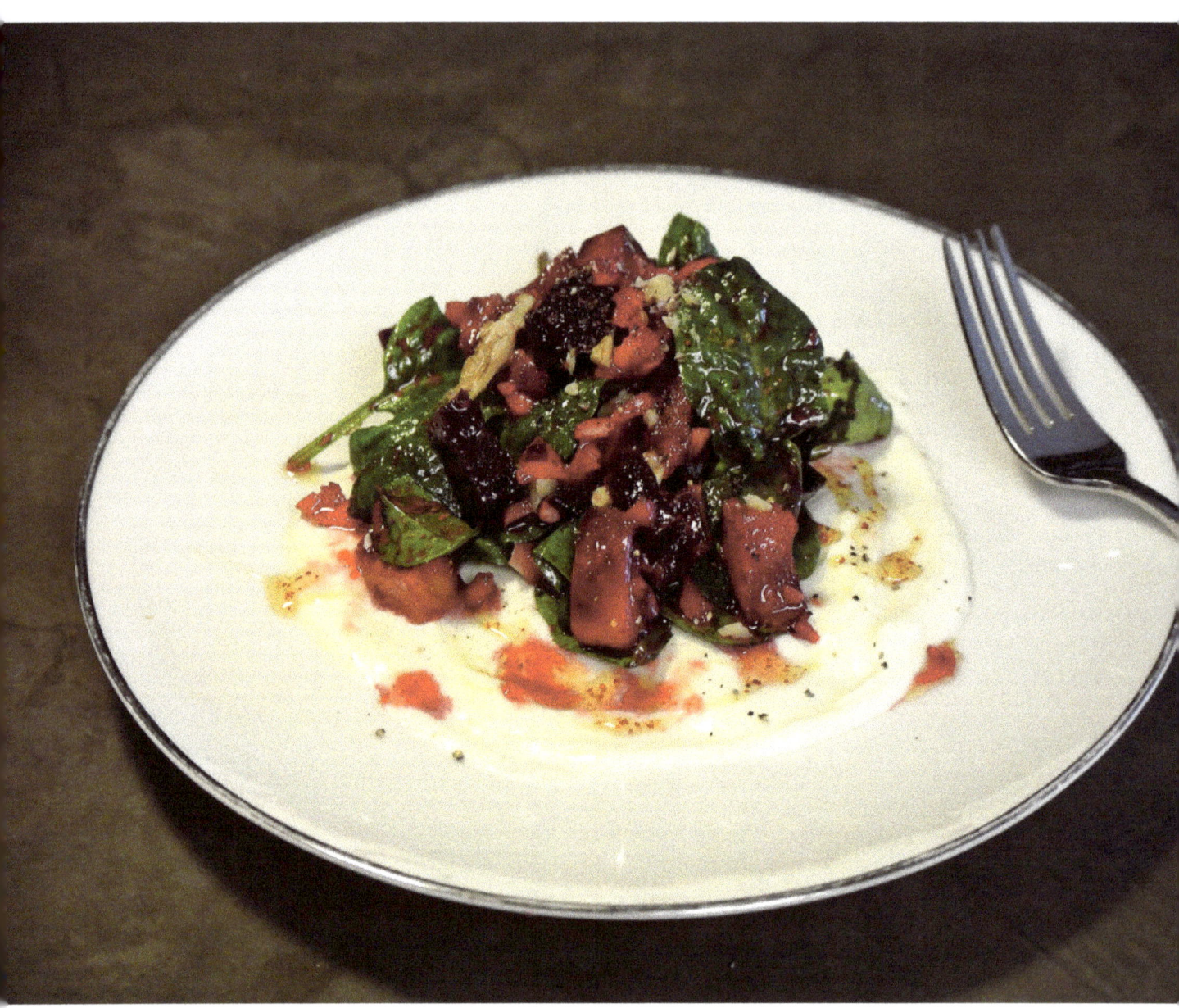

Roasted Beet and Spinach Salad
with Honey Mustard Vinaigrette Dressing
served with Whipped Brie Cream

Sides, Salads & Vegetables

These recipes are designed to provide a delicious source of fiber, nutrition and volume to any meal. Some are complete meals which contain protein, carbohydrates and fats. Unfortunately, many athletes shy away from vegetables and various sides for fear of bloating, gas or gastrointestinal distress. However, they lose out on variety, satiety and flavor. For those following the Specific Carbohydrate Diet, grains, corn, and familiar starchy tubers (like potatoes, yams, and sweet potatoes) are not allowed. Many people miss these familiar, high carbohydrate foods such as fries, popcorn, pastas, and mashed potatoes. Some even rely on those foods to fuel their athletic activities. Therefore, this collection of recipes provides appetizing alternatives and replacement options for athletes.

Smoked Curry Pea Salad

Approximate Yield	**Prep Time 20 min**	**Estimated Macronutrients**
6-8 servings	**Total Time 60 min**	**6 g P • 15 g C • 10 g F**
	(To allow for refrigeration)	

This recipe was adapted from a family recipe contributed by the author's aunt.

INGREDIENTS

1 (16oz) bag of frozen peas (defrosted in the refrigerator)
3-4 green onions chopped finely, or 1 shallot finely minced
¼ cup avocado mayonnaise (see recipe page 112) *
¼ teaspoon curry powder
½ cup of chopped Smoked Paprika Nuts (see recipe page 195) *
Salt and pepper to taste
Optional: A pinch- ⅛ teaspoon of cayenne pepper

KITCHEN EQUIPMENT

Small mixing bowl
Large mixing bowl
Measuring spoons & measuring cups
Colander/strainer
Spatula or large spoon

SPECIAL INSTRUCTIONS/DIET INFORMATION

* There are limited brands of mayonnaise with legal ingredients under the Specific Carbohydrate Diet, therefore read labels carefully and verify with the manufacturer or use the recipe on page 112.
*If you cannot tolerate nuts, then add ¼ teaspoon of smoked paprika directly to the salad and mix well.

DIRECTIONS

1. In a small mixing bowl stir the mayo, and spices together until well mixed.
2. Drain the defrosted peas of water in a colander. Then in the large mixing bowl gently combine the peas, green onion, nuts and stirring in the mayo dressing. Salt and pepper to taste.
3. Serve the salad immediately or preferably allow to chill in the refrigerator before serving.
4. For a complete meal add in chilled roasted turkey or chicken to meet your protein needs.

Quick Candied Jalapeno "Cowboy Candy"

Approximate Yield
8-10 servings

Prep Time 20 min
Total Time 2 hours
(To allow for cooling)

Estimated Macronutrients
1 g P • 5 g C • 1 g F

INGREDIENTS
4-6 large and firm jalapenos
1 finely minced garlic clove
½ cup of apple cider vinegar*
½ cup filtered water
1 ½ cup honey
1 teaspoon pickling spice
1 teaspoon salt

KITCHEN EQUIPMENT
Non latex food service gloves
Heat-resistant spoon or spatula
Measuring spoons & measuring cups
Canning or mason jar with lid
Slotted spoon

SPECIAL INSTRUCTIONS/DIET INFORMATION
*You may substitute distilled white vinegar, but this may require more honey to sweeten.

DIRECTIONS
1. Rinse the jalapenos. Wearing gloves to protect your hands from being burned by the jalapeno oils, remove the stems and then slice each jalapeno is ¼ inch rounds.
2. In a medium saucepan combine the vinegar, honey, salt, water and pickling spices. Bring to a boil, stirring occasionally until all ingredients are well mixed.
3. Add the jalapenos and garlic, returning the liquid to boil and simmer until the peppers have shrunk slightly and are glossy. This takes approximately 6 minutes.
4. Using the slotted spoon, transfer the jalapenos and garlic to the canning jar. Then bring the liquid back to boil reducing to a syrup. This should take approximately 8-10 minutes.
5. Pour the syrup over the jalapenos and garlic, pressing them down to keep them submerged. Then allow to cool before adding the lid and sealing.
6. You may need to stir or shake the container to keep the jalapenos covered with syrup. Serve when cool. Generally, the candied jalapenos will last up to 10 days refrigerated.

Quick Pickled Cabbage

Approximate Yield
6-8 servings

Prep Time 20 min
Total Time 60 min
(To allow for refrigeration)

Estimated Macronutrients
1 g P • 10 g C • 0 g F

INGREDIENTS
¼ head of thinly sliced red or purple cabbage
½ cup of apple cider vinegar*
½ cup of filtered water
1 tablespoon of honey
1 clove of minced garlic
1 teaspoon sea salt
⅛ teaspoon ground black pepper

KITCHEN EQUIPMENT
Glass mason jar container with airtight lid for storage
Small pot
Measuring spoons & measuring cups
Heat-resistant spoon or spatula

SPECIAL INSTRUCTIONS/DIET INFORMATION
*You may substitute distilled white vinegar, but this may require more honey to sweeten.

DIRECTIONS
1. Wash and cut the cabbage thinly and remove the core. Place the cabbage in the glass jar, filling to the top and then adding the minced garlic.
2. In a small pot on medium heat add water, vinegar, honey, salt and pepper. Stirring until all ingredients are mixed well. Bring to a boil, then remove from heat.
3. Pour mixture over the cabbage and garlic in the glass jar. Place lid on the container.
4. You may need to stir or shake the container to keep the cabbage covered with pickling liquid.

Quick Pickled Cucumber Salad

Approximate Yield
4-5 servings

Prep Time 20 min
Total Time 60 min
(To allow for refrigeration)

Estimated Macronutrients
1 g P • 18 g C • 0 g F

INGREDIENTS
4 medium persian cucumbers thinly sliced
⅓ cup of white distilled vinegar*
3 green onions thinly sliced
1 cup filtered water
2 tablespoons of honey
1 ½ teaspoons sea salt

KITCHEN EQUIPMENT
Glass mason jar container with airtight lid for storage
Small pot
Measuring spoons & measuring cups
Heat-resistant spoon or spatula

SPECIAL INSTRUCTIONS/DIET INFORMATION
*You may substitute white distilled with apple cider vinegar, but this will change the taste.

DIRECTIONS
1. Wash and cut the vegetables. Place the vegetables in the glass jar or container, filling to the top.
2. In a small pot on medium heat, add the water, honey, and salt. Stirring until all ingredients are mixed well, and honey and salt are dissolved. Set aside to cool.
3. Once cool, add in the vinegar, and pour the mixture over the green onions and cucumbers. Place the lid on the container and immediately refrigerate to cool.
4. You may need to stir or shake the container to keep the vegetables covered with pickling liquid. Important to note, the cumbers need to be eaten in a couple days and quick pickling is not meant for long term storage.

Korean Easy Pickled Vegetables Salad

Approximate Yield	**Prep Time 20 min**	**Estimated Macronutrients**
4-5 servings	**Total Time 60 min**	**4 g P • 33 g C • 3 g F**
	(To allow for refrigeration)	

INGREDIENTS

3 medium persian or 1 english cucumber thinly sliced
1 ¼ cup of shredded carrots
½ a red onion, finely sliced
¼ cup of white distilled vinegar*
¼ cup of filtered water
1 tablespoon of honey
¾ tablespoon sea salt

KITCHEN EQUIPMENT

Large bowl or glass container for storage with airtight lid
Measuring spoons & measuring cups
Tongs, spatula or large spoon

SPECIAL INSTRUCTIONS/DIET INFORMATION

*You may substitute white distilled vinegar with apple cider vinegar, but this will change the taste and sweeten the salad.

DIRECTIONS

1. Wash and cut the vegetables. Place the vegetables in a large bowl or glass container.
2. In a small pot on medium heat add water, vinegar, honey, and salt. Stirring until all ingredients are mixed well. Bring to a boil, then remove from heat.
3. Pour the mixture over the vegetables in the bowl or container. Place lid on the container (or plastic wrap the bowl) and immediately refrigerate to cool.
4. You may need to stir salad in the bowl or container to keep the vegetables covered with pickling liquid. This salad is meant to be eaten within 3 days of making.

Spicy Snap Peas

Approximate Yield	**Prep Time 10 min**	**Estimated Macronutrients**
4 servings	**Total Time 15-20 min**	**3 g P • 8 g C • 5 g F**

INGREDIENTS

1 teaspoon sea salt
2 tablespoons toasted sesame oil
10 oz-16 oz of raw snap peas in shells *
1 tablespoon of legal SCD togarashi seasoning or see recipe
on page 154*
Coarse flaked sea salt to taste
Red pepper flakes to taste
Optional garnish: black sesames

Ice and water for ice bath

KITCHEN EQUIPMENT

Medium to large ceramic or nonstick skillet
Measuring spoons & measuring cups
Heat resistant spatula
Bowl
Medium to large cooking pot
Slotted spoon or colander

SPECIAL INSTRUCTIONS/DIET INFORMATION

*Be careful as many commercially made togarashi seasonings have dried seaweed, sugar and/or other SCD illegal additives. Read labels carefully and always verify with the manufacturer or use the following recipe (see recipe page 154).

DIRECTIONS

1. Rinse the snap peas and cut off any fibrous or hard tips.
2. Bring a large pot of water to boil. Add a teaspoon of salt then add the snap peas.
3. Blanche the snap peas until bright green and heated through, 3 minutes (you do not want to overcook to allow the snap peas to retain some crunch). Then either drain the water with a colander or using a slotted spoon remove the snap peas. Placing the snap peas in an ice bath of water to prevent over cooking.
4. In a large non-stick skillet heating the sesame oil on medium high heat. Add in the par cooked snap peas and sauté briefly before adding in the togarashi seasoning and flaked sea salt, tossing until all the snap peas are coated with spices. Garnish with optional black sesame seeds.
5. Remove from heat and serve warm.

Asian Chicken "Noodle" Salad

Approximate Yield	**Prep Time 20 min**	**Estimated Macronutrients**
5-6 servings	**Total Time 60 min**	**32 g P • 42 g C • 10 g F**

INGREDIENTS

2 cups of spiralized cucumbers or heart of palm or SCD legal lentil or yellow pea noodles*

2 cups of chicken breast cooked and shredded (preferably roasted with the Asian Dry Rub (see recipe page 154)

4 medium persian cucumbers spiralized into noodles or thinly sliced*

¼ green cabbage finely chopped/shredded

¼ purple cabbage finely chopped/ shredded

1 ¼ cup of shredded carrots

½ finely sliced red onion

3 green onions finely sliced

½- 1 cup of Spicy Peanut Dressing (see recipe page 127)

KITCHEN EQUIPMENT

Large salad bowl
Large serving spoon or tongs

SPECIAL INSTRUCTIONS/DIET INFORMATION

*If unable to source SCD legal noodles or reducing carbohydrates and/or fats, use spiralized cucumbers to replace the noodles or heart of palm. Using a spiralizer or peeler you can shave the cucumber into thin strips to replace the noodles. Just note the cucumbers will add more moisture to the salad.

DIRECTIONS

1. If using SCD legal spaghetti or vermicelli, follow the package directions and pre-cook the noodles. Set aside and allow to cool. You also may need to toss with a neutral oil to prevent the noodles from sticking while cooling. (Heart of palm noodles or spiralized cucumbers do not require cooking so this step can be skipped.)
2. Wash and cut the vegetables, then place all in the large mixing or salad bowl.
3. Add in the chicken and noodles, then toss with the salad dressing.
4. Place lid on the mixing bowl or cover with plastic and immediately refrigerate to marinate for 20 minutes. Serve cold.

Yakisoba Style Spaghetti Squash

Approximate Yield	Prep Time 20 min	Estimated Macronutrients
8 servings	Total Time 55 min	4 g P • 29 g C • 3 g F

INGREDIENTS

3-4 cups of leftover Roasted Spaghetti Squash (see recipe page 177)
2 cups of shredded carrots
1 cup of thinly sliced shitake mushrooms*
1 cup of shredded cabbage
3 green onions finely sliced
1 tablespoon neutral oil

Sauce
1 tablespoon sesame oil
5 tablespoons tamari or No Soy Sauce (see recipe page 121 and notes) *
2 tablespoons honey*
Salt and pepper to taste
¾-1 teaspoon dried finely ground red chili flakes

KITCHEN EQUIPMENT

Measuring spoons & measuring cups
Heat-resistant tongs, spoon or spatula
Large skillet

SPECIAL INSTRUCTIONS/DIET INFORMATION

*Note mushrooms overwhelm the subtle flavors of the dish and therefore optional.
*Check the labels of the tamari, many will list rice wine vinegar and other ingredients which may be illegal when following SCD. Tamari should generally be gluten free, grain free, and sugar free. For example, tamari includes only water, organic soybeans, salt and/or organic alcohol (as part of fermentation process).
*If using No Soy Sauce (see recipe page 121) to substitute tamari, you may want to reduce the amount of honey in the recipe. This is based on personal taste and is due to the sweetness of the No Soy Sauce.
*Some may not prefer a sweeter flavor profile or more heat so omit or add more red pepper flakes and honey as needed.

DIRECTIONS

1. In a small bowl whisk the ingredients for the sauce and set aside.
2. Heating the neutral oil in a large skillet on medium heat, sauté all the vegetables except the spaghetti squash.
3. Then add in the spaghetti squash, sauce and green onions are well coated, and excess moisture is reduced. Serve warm.

Roasted Spaghetti Squash

Approximate Yield **8-10 servings**	**Prep Time 20 min** **Total Time 55 min**	**Estimated Macronutrients** **1 g P • 8 g C • 4 g F**

INGREDIENTS
1 large spaghetti squash*
1 tablespoon olive oil

KITCHEN EQUIPMENT
Baking sheet pan
Measuring spoon
Baking parchment paper or aluminum foil
Bowl or airtight storage container
Grapefruit spoon or metal spoon

SPECIAL INSTRUCTIONS/DIET INFORMATION
*A best practice is to rinse and dry the outside of the spaghetti squash of any dirt and debris before cutting.

DIRECTIONS
1. Preheat oven to 400 degrees F. Line a baking sheet with parchment or aluminum foil.
2. Slice the ends off the squash, then cut the squash widthwise into rings. Try to cut the rings about the same size, around 1-1½ inches thick. Then using a metal or grapefruit spoon to scrape out and discard the seeds.
3. Place the squash on the parchment paper lined baking sheet, and drizzle with olive oil.
4. Bake the spaghetti squash for 30-40 minutes and flip the spaghetti squash rings halfway through roasting.
5. The spaghetti squash should be slightly tender when pierced with a knife or fork. Remove the roasted squash from the oven.
6. Allow the squash to cool to warm, then use a knife to peel away the skin and a fork to separate the strands into long spaghetti noodles. Place the spaghetti squash in a bowl or airtight container.
7. Toss the spaghetti squash with a little olive oil and salt if needed, or use in various recipes throughout the book.

Air Fried Korean Brussel Sprouts

Approximate Yield	Prep Time 10 min	Estimated Macronutrients
4 servings	Total Time 25 min	5 g P • 24 g C • 4 g F

This recipe provides an alternative instruction for roasting in the oven.

INGREDIENTS
1 (12oz) package of frozen brussel sprouts or 2 cups fresh
1 tablespoon sesame oil
2-3 tablespoons honey
1 tablespoon Parmesan-No Seasoning (see recipe page 152)*
1-2 tablespoons dried mild Korean Gochugaru chili flakes or finely ground red pepper flakes
Salt and pepper to taste

KITCHEN EQUIPMENT
Baking sheet or air fryer tray

Baking parchment paper or aluminum foil
Large bowl
Measuring spoons & measuring cups
Heat resistant tongs or spatula
Air fryer or oven

SPECIAL INSTRUCTIONS/DIET INFORMATION
*Note the amount of spice used is to taste, as once the brussel sprouts are cooked you can toss them with more seasoning, salt and pepper.
*Important reminder that the Parmesan-No Seasoning contains almond flour for those with nut sensitivities or allergies. Use an alternate seasoning or rub recipe in the book as needed.

DIRECTIONS
1. If using an oven preheat to 450 degrees F. Prepare a baking sheet with parchment paper. If using an air fryer, no need to preheat.
2. Place the brussel sprouts in the large mixing bowl and toss with all ingredients.
3. If using the oven, spread out the brussel sprouts on a baking sheet lined with parchment paper and bake for 15-20 minutes or until tender when pierced with a knife. If you prefer the brussel sprouts crisp, raise the temp to broil for an additional 1 – 2 minutes and watch to prevent burning.
4. If using the air fryer spread the artichokes out in the basket evenly, and fry at 400 degrees F for 12-15 minutes depending on desired crispness.

Quick Cucumber Kimchi

Approximate Yield	Prep Time 15 min	Estimated Macronutrients
10 servings	Total Time 60 min	1 g P • 4 g C • 0 g F
	(To allow for refrigeration)	

INGREDIENTS
1 large cucumber (rinsed) peeled, sliced thinly
2 tablespoons minced green onions
1 tablespoon fine kosher salt
1-1 ½ teaspoon dried mild gochugaru Korean Gochugaru or finely ground red chili flakes (to taste based on personal preference)*
½ teaspoon honey

KITCHEN EQUIPMENT
Medium bowl or container with airtight lid
Measuring spoons & measuring cups
Spatula or large spoon
Fine mesh colander or strainer

SPECIAL INSTRUCTIONS
*If you are unable to source dried gochugaru Korean chili flakes, mild dried red pepper flakes can be substituted.

DIRECTIONS
1. Brine the cut cucumbers with salt for 5 minutes, then rinse the cucumbers with water in the colander and pat dry.
2. Stir in the remaining ingredients in with the cucumbers.
3. Cover and refrigerate for 30 minutes to an hour.

Sesame & Sea Salt Kale Chips

Approximate Yield
4-8 servings

Prep Time 10 min
Total Time 25 min

Estimated Macronutrients
1 g P • 3 g C • 4 g F

INGREDIENTS
1 bunch or 2-3 cups of curly or dino kale (washed and destemmed)
2 tablespoons sesame oil
Flaked sea salt
Optional:
Finely ground red pepper
Everything bagel seasonings

KITCHEN EQUIPMENT
Large mixing bowl
Heat resistant tongs or spatula
Baking sheet
Measuring spoons & measuring cups
Baking parchment paper
Oven

SPECIAL INSTRUCTIONS/DIET INFORMATION
*Note the amount of spice used is to taste, as once the kale is roasted you can toss with more seasoning.

DIRECTIONS
1. Preheat oven to 425 degrees F. Prepare a baking sheet with parchment paper.
2. Place the washed and destemmed kale in a large mixing bowl. Toss the kale with sesame oil, and flaked sea salt.
3. Spread the kale evenly on the parchment paper (you will likely need two baking sheets to ensure enough space between kale leaves).
4. Roast the kale for 10-12 minutes (the kale will begin to crisp up), serve hot.

Habanero Mango Coleslaw

Approximate Yield
10 servings

Prep Time 20 min
Total Time 55 min

Estimated Macronutrients
14 g P • 13 g C • 1 g F

INGREDIENTS
¼ cup avocado mayonnaise or (see recipe page 112) *
¼ teaspoon celery seed
2 tablespoons Mango Habanero Sauce (see recipe page 135)
3 cups of shredded cabbage
1 cup shredded carrots
¼ red onion chopped thinly lengthwise
Salt and pepper to taste
Honey to taste

KITCHEN EQUIPMENT
Medium to large mixing bowl
Tongs, spatula or large spoon
Measuring spoons & measuring cups

SPECIAL INSTRUCTIONS/DIET INFORMATION
* There are limited brands of mayonnaise with legal ingredients under the Specific Carbohydrate Diet, therefore read labels carefully and verify with the manufacturer or use the recipe on page 112.

DIRECTIONS
1. Mix the habanero mango sauce, celery seed and mayo together stirring well in a bowl. Taste to determine if salt, pepper and more honey is needed. Allow the sauce to marinate for 10 minutes.
2. Toss the coleslaw dressing with cabbage, shredded carrot and red onion.
3. Cover and refrigerate for 30 minutes to an hour.

Quick Pickled Radishes

Approximate Yield	Prep Time 20 min	Estimated Macronutrients
6-12 servings	Total Time 60 min	0 g P • 11 g C • 0 g F
	(To allow for refrigeration)	

INGREDIENTS

1 bunch of radishes, (approximately 6- 8 radishes) stems and tips removed, washed and thinly sliced
2 minced garlic cloves
½ teaspoon mustard seeds
½ teaspoon black peppercorns
½ cup of white distilled vinegar
¼ cup of apple cider vinegar
¾ cup filtered water
3 ½ tablespoons of honey
2 teaspoons sea salt

KITCHEN EQUIPMENT

Glass mason jar or container with airtight lid for storage
Medium pot
Measuring spoons & cups
Heat resistant spoon or spatula

SPECIAL INSTRUCTIONS/DIET INFORMATION

*You may substitute white distilled with apple cider vinegar, but this will change the taste.

DIRECTIONS

1. Wash and cut the radishes. Place the radishes, minced garlic, peppercorns and mustard seed, in the glass jar or container filling to the top.
2. In a small pot on medium heat add water, honey, and salt. Stirring until all ingredients are dissolved. Once simmering, stir in the vinegar and remove from heat.
3. Pour the mixture over the radishes, and garlic, in the glass jar or container. Place the lid on the container and immediately refrigerate to cool. You may need to vent the lid for steam to escape as you don't want the glass container to crack. However once cool immediately snap the lid tight.
4. You may need to stir or shake the container to keep the radishes covered with pickling liquid. Important to note, the radishes should be eaten within a couple days to a week as quick pickling is not meant for long term storage.

German Style Red Cabbage "Rotkohl"

Approximate Yield	**Prep Time 20 min**	**Estimated Macronutrients**
10 servings	**Total Time 60 min**	**22 g P • 22 g C • 3 g F**

INGREDIENTS

2 tablespoons butter
1 head of thinly sliced red or purple cabbage
1 medium onion minced or ½ cup of dried onion
⅓ cup unsweetened apple sauce*
2 cups of SCD legal chicken or Chicken Bone Broth (see recipe page 255)
⅓ cup of apple cider vinegar
3 ½ tablespoons of honey (or ¼ cup honey for more sweetness)
2 teaspoons sea salt
½ teaspoon ground cloves
½ teaspoon granulated garlic
¼ teaspoon ground black pepper

KITCHEN EQUIPMENT

Large non-stick pot and lid
Measuring spoons & measuring cups
Large heat-resistant spoon or spatula
Glass container with airtight lid for storage

SPECIAL INSTRUCTIONS/DIET INFORMATION

*Read labels carefully that the apple sauce does not contain non SCD preservatives or concentrates with added sugar. You can also use the recipe on page 301 and puree the apple sauce well.

DIRECTIONS

1. Place pot on medium heat, add the butter and melt it.
2. Add cabbage and onions. Followed by remaining ingredients, stirring with spoon to coat the cabbage with spices and broth.
3. Cook the cabbage approximately 45 minutes, with regular stirring to prevent any burning on the bottom of the pot. You may lower the heat as the cabbage softens.
4. Remove the pot from heat when the cabbage has reached a soft or tender texture when pierced with a fork. Salt and pepper to taste as needed.
5. Store in an airtight glass container in the refrigerator if not serving immediately.

Quick Dill Pickles

Approximate Yield 4-5 servings	Prep Time 20 min Total Time 48 hours (To allow for refrigeration)	Estimated Macronutrients 14 g P • 13 g C • 1 g F

INGREDIENTS

4-5 medium pickling cucumbers depending on size *
4-6 cloves of garlic sliced (this amount depends on personal taste)
1 ½ tablespoon dill seeds
1 handful of fresh dill
1-2 bay leaf
1 teaspoon mustard seeds
¼ teaspoon fennel seeds
¼ teaspoon caraway seed
⅛ teaspoon mace
⅛ teaspoon turmeric
Pinch of red pepper flakes
1 cup of white distilled vinegar *
3 tablespoons pickling salt (or kosher) *
4 cups filtered water (note you will have extra for a second batch)

KITCHEN EQUIPMENT

1-2 glass mason jars or glass container with airtight lid for storage
Small- medium pot
Measuring spoons & measuring cups
Heat-resistant spoon or spatula
Optional: Funnel for pouring the pickling liquid

SPECIAL INSTRUCTIONS/DIET INFORMATION

* Pickling cucumbers or often referred to as the Kirby variety, is recommended however Persian cucumbers can work as needed. Also verify there is no wax on the skin.
*Pickling salt is a finer grain and ideal for clear brines, whereas kosher is coarser and may or may not contain anti-caking agents. Note the pickling salt is pure sodium chloride and will taste saltier.
*The vinegar amount is to taste; some people may prefer a more acidic pickle flavor.

DIRECTIONS

1. Wash and cut the end tips of the cucumbers off. Or as an option, cut the cucumbers lengthwise in halves or quarter spears and set aside.
2. Place the sliced garlic in a small saucepan of water and bring to a boil. Boiling the garlic for one minute then remove quickly.
3. Place the blanched garlic, fresh dill, bay leaf, and spices in the jar (or jars).
4. Place the cucumbers in the glass jars or containers, standing the whole cucumbers or cut spears upright.
5. In a small pot on medium heat add water, vinegar, and salt then bring to a boil. Stirring until all ingredients are mixed well, and salt is dissolved.
6. Pour the hot liquid over the cucumbers until they are completely submerged. (Note you will likely have extra pickling liquid to accommodate for various jar sizes and for filling them to the top.) Then let the jars cool completely to room temperature before securing with lids and placing in refrigerator.
7. The pickles will be ready to eat after 48 hours in the refrigerator.
8. Important to note, the cucumbers need to be stored in the refrigerator and eaten within 10 days. Quick pickling is not meant for long term storage.

Dill Pickle Hummus Dip

Approximate Yield	Prep Time 20 min	Estimated Macronutrients
10 servings	**Total Time 55 min**	**14 g P • 13 g C • 1 g F**

INGREDIENTS

2 cups soaked, cooked and drained red lentils or navy "white" beans (see recipe page 303)
¼ cup of sliced SCD legal dill pickles or Quick Dill Pickles (see recipe page 182) *
3 cloves of garlic minced
2 tablespoons olive oil
2 tablespoons of SCD legal pickle juice *
2 tablespoons thick tahini butter*
½ teaspoon of salt
¼ teaspoon dried dill weed
⅛ teaspoon cumin
Sprinkle of olive oil
Dash of dried dill weed

KITCHEN EQUIPMENT

Food processor
Measuring spoons & measuring cups
Spatula or spoon
Sterilized plastic food storage container with lids or silicone cups with lids to freeze

SPECIAL INSTRUCTIONS/DIET INFORMATION

*SCD legal pickles should not include any sweeteners, vague ingredients, and/or additives. The pickle ingredients used in this recipe included cucumber, water, salt, distilled white vinegar, garlic, dill weed, dill seed, mustard seed, caraway seed, calcium chloride (a natural salt), fennel seed, mace, and turmeric. If you are unable to source SCD legal pickles use the following Quick Dill Pickles, see recipe page 182.
*Seed butters that are SCD legal should only include the seed and possibly a legal oil and/or salt. For example, tahini is generally roasted and ground sesame seeds which may include sesame seed oil.

DIRECTIONS

1. Add all ingredients to the food processor and puree to the smooth consistency of hummus.
2. Garnish with a dash of dill weed and sprinkling of olive oil.
3. Place in airtight containers or freeze as needed.

Mediterranean Hummus Dip

Approximate Yield 10-12 servings	Prep Time 15 min Total Time 30 min	Estimated Macronutrients 4 g P • 8 g C • 6 g F

INGREDIENTS

2 cups soaked, cooked and drained red lentils or navy "white" beans (see recipe page 303)
4 cloves of garlic minced
3 tablespoons olive oil
2 tablespoons thick tahini butter*
1 teaspoon of salt
Zest and juice of medium whole lemon (approximately 2 tablespoon of juice and 1 teaspoon of zest)
½ teaspoon cumin
Dash of ground paprika or smoked paprika
Sprinkle of olive oil

KITCHEN EQUIPMENT

Food processor
Measuring spoons & measuring cups
Spatula or spoon
Sterilized plastic food storage container with lids or silicone cups with lids to freeze.

SPECIAL INSTRUCTIONS/DIET INFORMATION

*Seed butters that are SCD legal should only include the seed and possibly a legal oil and/or salt. For example, tahini is generally roasted and ground sesame seeds which may include sesame seed oil.

DIRECTIONS

1. Add all ingredients to the food processor and puree to the smooth consistency of hummus.
2. Garnish with a dash of paprika and sprinkling of olive oil.
3. Place in airtight containers or freeze as needed.

Red Pepper Hummus Dip

Approximate Yield 10-12 servings	Prep Time 15 min Total Time 30 min	Estimated Macronutrients 6 g P • 10 g C • 9 g F

INGREDIENTS

2 cups soaked, cooked and drained red lentils or navy "white" beans (see recipe page 303)
4 cloves of garlic minced
3 tablespoons olive oil
1 cup (approximately 3) whole roasted mild red peppers
2 tablespoons thick tahini butter*
½ -1 teaspoon of salt
Zest and juice of ½ small lemon (approximately 1½ tablespoons of juice and 1 teaspoon of zest)
½ teaspoon cumin
¼ teaspoon paprika
⅛ teaspoon smoked paprika
Sprinkle of olive oil

KITCHEN EQUIPMENT

Food processor or blender
Measuring spoons & measuring cups
Spatula or spoon
Sterilized plastic food storage container with lids or silicone cups with lids to freeze

SPECIAL INSTRUCTIONS/DIET INFORMATION

*Seed butters that are SCD legal should only include the seed and possibly a legal oil and/or salt. For example, tahini is generally roasted and ground sesame seeds which may include sesame seed oil.

DIRECTIONS

1. Add all ingredients to the food processor and puree to the smooth consistency of hummus.
2. Garnish with a dash of paprika and sprinkling of olive oil.
3. Place in airtight containers or freeze as needed.

Greek White Bean, Cucumber and Tomato Salad

Approximate Yield	Prep Time 20 min	Estimated Macronutrients
10-12 servings	Total Time 60 min	14 g P • 12 g C • 8 g F
	(To allow for refrigeration)	

INGREDIENTS

2 cups of cooked and cooled white (navy) beans (see recipe page 303) *

5-6 medium persian cucumbers, chopped and peeled

1 cup of halved grape or small cherry tomatoes

¼ large red onion, sliced thinly

¾ cup of crumbled cotija cheese*

Optional: 2 cups of roasted sliced or shredded chicken or use leftover Roasted Chicken (see recipe page 255)

Dressing

¼ cup of red wine vinegar

3 tablespoons olive oil

1 tablespoon of Italian Herb Mix (see recipe page 153)

½ teaspoon sea salt

¼ teaspoon black pepper

Additional salt and pepper to taste as needed

KITCHEN EQUIPMENT

Small mixing bowl
Measuring spoons & measuring cups
Spatula or large spoon
Large mixing bowl

SPECIAL INSTRUCTIONS/DIET INFORMATION

*White or navy beans can be soaked and cooked using the same crockpot method as yellow peas, for more information see the recipe page 303.

*Cheeses should be aged over 3 months, and contain zero carbohydrates or sugars, regarding nutritional content. Pre-sliced and pre-shredded cheese will likely contain illegal ingredients to prevent the cheese from sticking and prolong shelf life. It is always best to purchase blocks of cheese, then shred, grate, crumble or slice yourself.

DIRECTIONS

1. In a small mixing bowl combine the dressing ingredients and stir until well blended. Set aside.
2. In a large mixing bowl combine the beans, cucumbers, cotija, onion and tomatoes. Tossing gently with the salad dressing.
3. Serve immediately or preferably allow to marinate in the refrigerator before serving.
4. For a complete meal you can add chilled roasted turkey or chicken to meet your protein needs.

Harissa Honey Carrots

Approximate Yield	Prep Time 10 min	Estimated Macronutrients
4 servings	Total Time 25 min	1 g P • 10 g C • 4 g F

INGREDIENTS

2 cups of carrots cut in crosscut slices or roll cut slices

1 tablespoon of Harissa paste/sauce (see recipe page 133)

1 tablespoon honey

Salt & pepper to taste

1 tablespoon olive oil or avocado spray oil

Optional:

Parmesan-No Seasoning can be used to taste

(see recipe page 152)*

Garnish or serve with Whipped Brie Cream

 (see recipe page 109)

KITCHEN EQUIPMENT

Large bowl

Measuring spoons & measuring cups

Baking parchment paper or silicone tray/baking liner

Baking sheet or air fryer tray

Air fryer or oven

SPECIAL INSTRUCTIONS/DIET INFORMATION

*Note the amount of spice used is to taste, as once the carrots are cooked you can toss them with more salt, pepper or seasoning.

*Important reminder that the Parmesan-No Seasoning contains almond flour for those with nut sensitivities or allergies. Use an alternate seasoning or rub recipe in the book as needed.

DIRECTIONS

1. If using an oven preheat to 450 degrees F. Prepare a baking sheet with parchment paper. If using an air fryer, no need to preheat.

2. Place the carrots in the large mixing bowl and toss with Harissa paste, honey and oil.

3. If using the oven, spread out the carrots on a baking sheet lined with parchment paper. Bake for 10-15 minutes or until tender when pierced with a fork. If you prefer the carrots caramelized, raise the temperature to broil and bake for an additional 1 – 2 minutes watching carefully to prevent burning.

4. If using the air fryer spread the carrots out in the basket lined with parchment or silicone baking liner, and fry at 400 degrees F for 10-12 minutes depending on desired crispness.

5. Remove the carrots from the oven or air fryer and toss with either salt, pepper or Parmesan-No Seasoning to taste. Serve hot. You can also serve the carrots on a bed of whipped brie cream.

Savory and Spicy Roasted Cauliflower

Approximate Yield	Prep Time 10 min	Estimated Macronutrients
4 servings	**Total Time 25 min**	**4 g P • 21 g C • 11 g F**

This recipe provides an alternative instruction for air frying.

INGREDIENTS

3-4 cups of cauliflower florets
3-4 tablespoons of unsalted butter or ghee (melted)
1 teaspoon paprika
½ teaspoon cayenne pepper
1 teaspoon dried thyme
½ -1 teaspoon sea salt*

KITCHEN EQUIPMENT

Large bowl
Heat resistant tongs or spatula
Measuring spoons & measuring cups
Air fryer or oven
Baking sheet or air fryer tray
Baking parchment paper or aluminum foil

SPECIAL INSTRUCTIONS/DIET INFORMATION

*Note the amount of spice used is to taste, as once the cauliflower is cooked you can toss them with more seasoning or salt.

DIRECTIONS

1. If using an oven preheat to 450 F degrees. Prepare a baking sheet with parchment paper. If using an air fryer, no need to preheat.
2. Place the cauliflower in the large mixing bowl and toss with melted butter and spices.
3. If using the oven, spread out the cauliflower on a baking sheet lined with parchment paper. Bake for 15 minutes or until tender when pierced with a knife. If you prefer the cauliflower crisp raise the temperature to broil and bake for an additional 1 – 2 minutes.
4. If using the air fryer spread the cauliflower florets out in the basket evenly, and fry at 400 degrees F for 10-12 minutes depending on desired crispness. Salt and pepper to taste. Serve hot.

Roasted Greek Broccoli

Approximate Yield	Prep Time 20 min	Estimated Macronutrients
10 servings	**Total Time 55 min**	**14 g P • 13 g C • 1 g F**

This recipe provides instruction for both oven and air frying.

INGREDIENTS

2 tablespoons olive oil
1 package (approximately 16 oz) of frozen broccoli or 3 cups of fresh broccoli*
½ tablespoon of Savory Greek Seasoning (see recipe page 146)
Sea salt and pepper to taste

KITCHEN EQUIPMENT

Large bowl
Heat resistant tongs or spatula
Baking parchment paper or aluminum foil
Measuring spoons
Air fryer or oven
Baking sheet or air fryer tray

SPECIAL INSTRUCTIONS/DIET INFORMATION

* Fresh broccoli will require a shorter roasting time.

DIRECTIONS

1. If using an oven preheat to 450 degrees F. Prepare a baking sheet with parchment paper. If using an air fryer, no need to preheat.
2. Place the broccoli in the large mixing bowl and toss with olive oil and the Savory Greek seasoning.
3. If using the oven, spread out the broccoli on the baking sheet and bake for 16-18 minutes. If you prefer the broccoli crisp raise the temperature to broil and bake for an additional 1 – 2 minutes. Serve hot.
4. If using the air fryer spread the broccoli out in the basket evenly, and fry at 400 F for 10-12 minutes depending on desired crispness. Serve hot.

Air fried Artichoke Hearts

Approximate Yield	Prep Time 10 min	Estimated Macronutrients
4 servings	Total Time 25 min	3 g P • 9 g C • 3 g F

This recipe provides an alternative instruction for roasting in the oven.

INGREDIENTS

1 (12oz) package of frozen artichoke hearts*
1 tablespoon olive or avocado oil
1-2 teaspoons of Greek Spice Rub (see recipe page 150) *

KITCHEN EQUIPMENT

Large bowl
Measuring spoons
Heat resistant tongs or spatula

Air fryer or oven
Baking sheet or air fryer tray/basket
Baking parchment paper or aluminum foil

SPECIAL INSTRUCTIONS/DIET INFORMATION

*Jarred marinated artichoke hearts can be substituted for frozen if the brine ingredients are verified and considered SCD legal. However, if the marinated artichokes are jarred in oil and seasoned, omit the spray olive or avocado oil from the recipe and reduce the amount of Greek Spice Rub.
*Note the amount of spice used is to taste, as once the artichokes are cooked you can toss them with more seasoning.

DIRECTIONS

1. If using an oven preheat to 450 degrees F. Prepare a baking sheet with parchment paper. If using an air fryer, no need to preheat.
2. Place the artichoke hearts in the large mixing bowl and toss with olive oil and the Greek Spice Rub.
3. If using the oven, spread out the artichokes on a baking sheet lined with parchment paper and bake for 15 minutes or until tender when pierced with a knife. If you prefer the artichokes crisp raise the temp to broil and bake for an additional 1 – 2 minutes.
4. If using the air fryer spread the artichokes out in the basket evenly, and fry at 400 degrees F for 10-12 minutes depending on desired crispness. Serve hot.

Sweet and Spicy Pistachios

Approximate Yield	Prep Time 10 min	Estimated Macronutrients
10-12 servings	Total Time 35 min	3 g P • 13 g C • 8 g F

INGREDIENTS

2 cups shelled, raw pistachios
3 tablespoons melted butter (unsalted) or ghee
2 tablespoons + ½ teaspoon honey
1 ½ teaspoons granulated garlic
1 teaspoon paprika
1 teaspoon dried thyme
½ teaspoon cayenne

KITCHEN EQUIPMENT

Microwavable glass dish with lid or pan

Fork and knife
Measuring spoons & measuring cups
Spatula or large spoon
Cheese grater
Baking sheet pan
Baking parchment paper or aluminum foil

SPECIAL INSTRUCTIONS/DIET INFORMATION

*Note the amount of salt and cayenne pepper is to taste, as once the nuts are roasted you can toss them with more seasoning.

DIRECTIONS

1. Preheat oven 350 degrees F. Line a baking sheet with parchment paper.
2. Place the nuts in a medium mixing bowl and toss with melted butter and spices until well coated.
3. Spread the nuts evenly on the parchment paper, and roast for 30 minutes, stirring every 5-10 minutes to prevent burning.
4. When done remove from the oven and allow to cool. Toss with additional sea salt to taste and for additional spice sprinkle with ground cayenne pepper.

Cauliflower Fritters

Approximate Yield	Prep Time 15 min	Estimated Macronutrients
8-12 servings	Total Time 25 min	11 g P • 4 g C • 0 g F

INGREDIENTS

1 (12 oz) package or 1 ½ cups of frozen riced cauliflower*
3 large egg whites (separated)*
¼ teaspoon ground pepper
¼ teaspoon salt
½ teaspoon baking soda
¼ teaspoon ground cumin
⅛ teaspoon allspice
¼ teaspoon granulated garlic
Avocado or olive oil cooking spray

KITCHEN EQUIPMENT

Microwavable glass container with lid
Measuring spoons & measuring cups
Heat-resistant spoon or spatula
Small bowl
Standing or handheld electric mixer
Large non-stick ceramic skillet or non-stick sauté pan
Parchment paper lined cookie sheet

SPECIAL INSTRUCTIONS/DIET INFORMATION

*Egg whites cannot be liquid pasteurized egg whites, or they will not beat into stiff peaks.
 *Fresh steamed cauliflower can be riced and used; however, the different texture of fresh cauliflower can often vary and may affect the texture of the dish.

DIRECTIONS

1. Steam the cauliflower rice per the package instructions or in a microwavable glass container with lid.
2. In a small bowl mix the spices, salt and baking soda.
3. Beat the egg whites into stiff peaks with the electric mixer.
4. Fold in gently the cauliflower and spice mixture.
5. Lightly spray the non-stick pan, then heat to moderate or high heat.
6. When the pan is hot, spoon the fritter batter in little dollops. They should start to fry and turn golden on the bottom before flipping. When cooked and golden, gently place the fritters on the parchment sheet lined cookie sheet and serve warm.

Cacio E Pepe Broccoli

Approximate Yield	Prep Time 10 min	Estimated Macronutrients
4 servings	Total Time 15 min	2 g P • 2 g C • 7 g F

INGREDIENTS
1 (16 oz) bag (approximately 3-4 cups) of frozen broccoli*
2 tablespoons butter
2 tablespoons parmesan cheese, finely grated*
¼ teaspoon sea salt
⅛ teaspoon fresh cracked ground pepper

KITCHEN EQUIPMENT
Microwavable glass dish with lid or pan
Fork and knife
Measuring spoons & measuring cups
Spatula or large spoon
Cheese grater

SPECIAL INSTRUCTIONS/DIET INFORMATION
*Fresh steamed broccoli can be used; however, the texture tends to differ. Also cutting the broccoli very small or mincing aids in digestion.
* Cheeses should be aged over 3 months, and contain zero carbohydrates or sugars, regarding nutritional content. Pre-sliced and pre-shredded cheese will likely contain illegal ingredients to prevent the cheese from sticking and prolong shelf life. It is always best to purchase blocks of cheese, then shred, grate, crumble or slice yourself.

DIRECTIONS
1. Using a microwave or cook on stovetop, steam the broccoli per package instructions.
2. Drain any excess water from the broccoli. Melt the butter and add it to the steamed broccoli. Cut the broccoli with knife and fork into small bite size pieces or mince.
3. Toss the broccoli with parmesan cheese, salt and fresh ground black pepper.
4. Serve warm as a side with another complementary dish.

Salmon and Dill Pasta Salad

Approximate Yield
6-8 servings

Prep Time 20 min
Total Time 60 min
(To allow for refrigeration)

Estimated Macronutrients
26 g P • 24 g C • 10 g F

INGREDIENTS

6-8 oz (approximately 1 ½- 2 cups) of yellow pea or lentil, cavatappi or penne noodles*
½ cup of frozen petite peas
1 – 2 (5-6 oz) cold cooked filets (de-boned, skinless, and flaked), smoked tin salmon or use leftovers from Easy Oven Lemon Baked Salmon (see recipe page 240)

Dressing

½ cup of avocado mayonnaise (see recipe page 112) *
¼ cup unsweetened cashew milk*
1 tablespoon dried chives or 2 tablespoon fresh chives
2 tablespoons white wine vinegar
1 tablespoon lemon juice
1 finely minced shallot*
2 teaspoons dijon mustard*
1 ¼ teaspoon salt
1 teaspoon dried dillweed
1 teaspoon celery seed
1 teaspoon honey
1 teaspoon granulated garlic
⅛ teaspoon black pepper

KITCHEN EQUIPMENT

Large mixing bowl
Large pot
Strainer/colander
Immersion blender or food processor

SPECIAL INSTRUCTIONS/DIET INFORMATION

*If you are unable to source a SCD legal pasta you can also use steamed and cooled cauliflower florets as a substitute for pasta
* There are limited brands of mayonnaise with legal ingredients under the Specific Carbohydrate Diet, therefore read labels carefully and verify with the manufacturer or use the recipe on page 112.
*Any nut milks should only consist of nuts, water, or salt. No emulsifiers, gums, sweeteners or additives should be in the ingredient list. If you are unable to source a SCD legal nut milk you can make them easily at home (see recipe page 299).
* Finely shredding the shallot versus mincing the shallot allows for more flavor.
*There are a few commercial brands of mustard made with SCD legal ingredients. However always check ingredients carefully. Confirm with the company and determine unlisted ingredients are not being used in the manufacturing process.

DIRECTIONS

1. In a large pot, boil water and follow the directions to cook the SCD legal noodles. Cook the noodles until al dente, strain of water using a colander and rinse the noodles under cool water. Toss the noodles with a tablespoon of neutral oil to prevent sticking as they cool down.
2. In a separate bowl mix all the ingredients for the dressing well, cover and refrigerate until use.
3. Toss the noodles, salmon, peas and dressing, together. Stirring until well coated.
4. Preferably allow the salad to chill and marinate in the refrigerator before serving.

Walnut Pesto Pasta Salad

Approximate Yield	Prep Time 20 min	Estimated Macronutrients
5-6 servings	Total Time 30 min	15 g P • 46 g C • 5 g F

INGREDIENTS

2 cups of spiralized zucchini noodles or SCD legal lentil or yellow pea noodles*

½ finely minced shallot

1 cup of halved grape or small cherry tomatoes

1 cup of frozen (defrosted) or jarred (drained of liquid) artichoke hearts*

½- 1 cups of Walnut Pesto (see recipe page 141)

Salt and pepper to taste

Optional:

2 cups of chicken breast cooked and shredded or use recipe for Roasted Chicken (see recipe page 255)

KITCHEN EQUIPMENT

Large salad bowl
Measuring cups & spoons
Large spoon

SPECIAL INSTRUCTIONS/DIET INFORMATION

* If you are unable to source legal SCD pasta, use fresh or frozen vegetable noodles such as zucchini. However cooked butter nut squash or spaghetti squash can work as well.

*Frozen artichoke hearts will need to be defrosted before use. Also, it is common to find artichoke hearts jarred in water, olive oil and/or SCD legal spices. However, for all commercially made products it is recommended ingredients and manufacturing processes are verified before use.

DIRECTIONS

1. If using SCD legal spaghetti or vermicelli, follow the package directions and pre-cook the noodles. Once drained of water you may also need to toss the noodles with olive oil to prevent them from sticking when warm.

2. If using zucchini, thinly slice into noodles using a spiralizer and set aside. The zucchini does not need to be cooked.

3. In the large mixing or salad bowl toss the noodles or zucchini, tomatoes, shallot, artichoke hearts and optional chicken with the walnut pesto. (As a recommendation if the pesto was previously refrigerated, heat the pesto in the microwave for 30 seconds before tossing the salad to allow the flavors to marinate.)

4. Serve fresh or refrigerate until ready for serving (note the noodles and pesto texture may change as they cool).

Pesto Chicken Salad

Approximate Yield	**Prep Time 20 min**	**Estimated Macronutrients**
6-8 servings	**Total Time 60 min**	**16 g P • 14 g C • 9 g F**
	(To allow for refrigeration)	

INGREDIENTS

2 cups of chicken breast cooked and shredded or use recipe

for Roasted Chicken (see recipe page 255)

1 (16oz) bag of frozen peas (defrosted in the refrigerator)

3-4 green onions chopped finely

¼ cup of Walnut Pesto (see recipe page 141)

¼ cup avocado mayonnaise (see recipe page 112) *

Salt and pepper to taste

KITCHEN EQUIPMENT

Small mixing bowl

Large mixing bowl

Measuring spoons & measuring cups

Colander/strainer

Spatula or large spoon

SPECIAL INSTRUCTIONS/DIET INFORMATION

* There are limited brands of mayonnaise with legal ingredients under the Specific Carbohydrate Diet, therefore read labels carefully and verify with the manufacturer or use the recipe on page 112.

DIRECTIONS

1. Drain the defrosted peas of water in a colander. Then in the large mixing bowl gently combine the chicken, optional pasta, peas, green onions, walnut pesto, lemon juice and mayonnaise. Salt and pepper to taste.
2. Serve the salad immediately or preferably allow to chill in the refrigerator before serving.

Roasted Beet and Spinach Salad

Approximate Yield	Prep Time 15 min	Estimated Macronutrients
4-6 servings	Total Time 60 min	5 g P • 23 g C • 15 g F

INGREDIENTS

6 large beets peeled and cut into bite size pieces (3 golden and 3 red for variety)
2 tablespoons olive oil
Dash of sea salt
Dash of ground black pepper

4 cups of rinsed and dried baby spinach
¼ large red onion sliced thinly
¼ cup of chopped walnuts

2 tablespoons – ¼ cup of Honey Mustard Vinaigrette Dressing, to taste (see recipe page 138)

Optional Garnishes:
Whipped Brie Cream (see recipe page 109)
Crumbled cotija cheese*
¼ cup of crumbled and cooked (no sugar or added sweeteners) bacon

KITCHEN EQUIPMENT

Large mixing bowl
Vegetable peeler
Measuring spoons & measuring cups
Heat resistant tongs or spatula
Large cutting knife
Baking sheets with sides
Baking parchment paper or aluminum foil
Oven
Optional: Non latex food service gloves to protect hands from stains and a plastic cutting board
(Beets will stain your hands and wooden cutting boards)

SPECIAL INSTRUCTIONS/DIET INFORMATION

*Always read labels carefully verify ingredients with manufacturers for prepackaged bacon.
* Cheeses should be aged over 3 months, and contain zero carbohydrates or sugars, regarding nutritional content. Pre-sliced and pre-shredded cheese will likely contain illegal ingredients to prevent the cheese from sticking and prolong shelf life. It is always best to purchase blocks of cheese, then shred, grate, crumble or slice yourself.

DIRECTIONS

1. Preheat oven to 400 degrees F. Prepare the baking sheets with parchment paper or aluminum foil.
2. Wash the beets and remove the stems. Peel the beets using the vegetable peeler and then cut them into bite size pieces. Note: Beets will stain your hands and cutting boards so use gloves and/or a non-wood cutting board that can be washed in the dishwasher after use.
3. In a large mixing bowl, toss the beets with olive oil, salt and pepper.
4. Place the beets evenly on the parchment paper or aluminum lined baking sheets (you will likely need two baking pans to ensure enough space between beets).
5. Roast for 35-40 minutes (the beets should be tender when pierced with a fork).
6. Remove the beets from the oven and set aside to cool while assembling the salad.
7. In the large bowl, add the rinsed and dried baby spinach, chopped red onion, walnuts and toss all with the dressing.
8. Then add in the beets and toss with the rest of the salad. Allow the salad to marinate in the refrigerator and the spinach to absorb some of the dressing before serving.
9. Note you can plate the salad on a bed of whipped brie cream or add in some crumbled cotija cheese.

Smoked Paprika Nuts

Approximate Yield	**Prep Time 10 min**	**Estimated Macronutrients**
4-6 servings	**Total Time 35 min**	**6 g P • 11 g C • 14 g F**

INGREDIENTS

3 tablespoons of melted butter (unsalted) or ghee
1 ½ teaspoons granulated garlic
1 ½ teaspoons smoked paprika
1 teaspoon of fine sea salt (more can be added to taste after roasting) *
8-10 oz of raw nuts (almonds, peanuts, shelled pistachios and cashews work best)
Optional: A pinch- ⅛ teaspoon ground cayenne pepper

KITCHEN EQUIPMENT

Medium mixing bowl
Measuring spoons
Baking sheet
Baking parchment paper
Heat-resistant spoon or spatula
Oven

SPECIAL INSTRUCTIONS/DIET INFORMATION

*Note the amount of salt and cayenne pepper is to taste, as once the nuts are roasted you can toss them with more seasoning.

DIRECTIONS

1. In an oven preheat to 300 degrees F. Line a baking sheet with parchment paper.
2. Place the nuts in a medium mixing bowl and toss with melted butter and spices until well coated.
3. Spread the nuts evenly on the parchment paper, and roast for 30 minutes, shuffle the nuts every 10 minutes to prevent burning.
4. When done remove from the oven and allow to cool. Toss with additional sea salt and ground cayenne pepper to taste.

Watermelon Cucumber Salad

Approximate Yield
10-12 servings

Prep Time 15 min
Total Time 30 min

Estimated Macronutrients
5 g P • 25 g C • 11 g F

INGREDIENTS

Salad

5 persian cucumbers (rinsed) peeled as needed
1 medium seedless watermelon, (approximately 4 -5 cups)
removing the rind and cutting into cubes or balls
¾ of a red onion thinly sliced
½ cup of shelled and salted pistachios
¾ cup of crumbled cotija cheese*
Salt and pepper to taste

Dressing

2 jalapenos (seeds removed) and minced finely
¼ cup olive oil
2 tablespoons honey
1 lime zested and juiced
1 teaspoon dried parsley
1 teaspoon dried cilantro
½ teaspoon sea salt

KITCHEN EQUIPMENT

Large bowl or container with airtight lid
Measuring spoons & measuring cups
Spatula or large spoon
Food processor

SPECIAL INSTRUCTIONS/DIET INFORMATION

*If chopping the jalapenos by hand be sure to wash your hands thoroughly and be careful not to touch your face or sensitive areas.
*Cheeses should be aged over 3 months, and contain zero carbohydrates or sugars, regarding nutritional content.
Pre-sliced and pre-shredded cheese will likely contain illegal ingredients to prevent the cheese from sticking and prolong shelf life. It is always best to purchase blocks of cheese, then shred, grate, crumble or slice yourself.

DIRECTIONS

1. In the food processor place all ingredients of the dressing and pulse until its smooth and jalapenos are chopped fine. Set aside.
2. Add the cucumbers, watermelon and the remaining salad ingredients to the container or large bowl.
3. Pour the dressing over the salad and toss well.
4. Cover and refrigerate for 30 minutes to an hour.

Southwest Bean Salad

Approximate Yield
10-12 servings

Prep Time 20 min
Total Time 60 min
(To allow for refrigeration)

Estimated Macronutrients
9 g P • 25 g C • 16 g F

INGREDIENTS
2 cups of cooked and cooled black beans or white navy
beans (see recipe page 303) *
1 orange bell pepper, stems and seeds removed and diced
1 red bell pepper, stems and seeds removed and diced
1 yellow bell pepper, stems and seeds removed and diced
1 jalapeno, stems and seeds removed and diced
1 large, sweet onion diced
1 ½ cups of crumbled cotija cheese*
¼ cup fresh chopped cilantro or ½ teaspoon dried cilantro

Optional: 2 cups of roasted sliced or shredded chicken or
use leftover Roasted Chicken (see recipe page 255)

Dressing
¼ cup of white wine
3 tablespoons olive oil
3 tablespoons fresh lime juice
3 tablespoons of warm honey
2 tablespoons of apple cider vinegar
1 tablespoon of SCD Taco Seasoning (see recipe page 147)
¼ teaspoon of smoked paprika
⅛ teaspoon ground chipotle pepper
⅛ teaspoon cumin
Salt and pepper to taste

KITCHEN EQUIPMENT
Small mixing bowl
Measuring spoons & measuring cups
Spatula or large spoon
Large mixing bowl

SPECIAL INSTRUCTIONS/DIET INFORMATION
*Black beans or white navy beans can be soaked and cooked using the same crockpot method as yellow peas, for more information see the recipe page 303 You can also use a combination of both beans in this recipe.
*Cheeses should be aged over 3 months, and contain zero carbohydrates or sugars, regarding nutritional content. Pre-sliced and pre-shredded cheese will likely contain illegal ingredients to prevent the cheese from sticking and prolong shelf life. It is always best to purchase blocks of cheese, then shred, grate, crumble or slice yourself.

DIRECTIONS
1. In a small mixing bowl combine the dressing ingredients and stir unitl well blended. Set aside.
2. In a large mixing bowl combine the beans, peppers, cotija, and onion. Tossing gently with the salad dressing.
3. Serve immediately or preferably allow to chill in the refrigerator before serving.
4. For a complete meal you can add chilled roasted turkey or chicken to meet your protein needs. Garnish with fresh chopped cilantro.

Lime Cauliflower Rice

Approximate Yield	Prep Time 5 min	Estimated Macronutrients
2-4 servings	Total Time 10 min	5 g P • 11 g C • 2 g F

INGREDIENTS
1 16 oz bag (approximately 2 cups) of frozen cauliflower rice (steamed)*
1 teaspoon dried cilantro
1 tablespoon fresh lime juice
1 teaspoon olive oil
Salt to taste

KITCHEN EQUIPMENT
Microwavable glass dish with lid or pan
Measuring spoons & measuring cups
Heat-resistant spoon or spatula

SPECIAL INSTRUCTIONS/DIET INFORMATION
*Fresh steamed cauliflower can be riced and used; however, the different texture of fresh cauliflower can often vary and may affect the texture of the dish.

DIRECTIONS
1. Using a microwave or cook on a stovetop, steaming the cauliflower rice per package instructions. Toss the cooked cauliflower rice with all other ingredients. Then salt to taste.
2. Serve warm.

Refried Beans

Approximate Yield	Prep Time 20 min	Estimated Macronutrients
10 servings	Total Time 55 min	14 g P • 13 g C • 1 g F

INGREDIENTS
2 ½ cups soaked, cooked and drained red lentils, black beans, or navy "white" beans (see recipe page 303)
2 teaspoons olive oil
1 tablespoon SCD Taco Seasoning (see recipe page 147)
¼ teaspoon sea salt
Optional:
½ cup shredded sharp cheddar cheese or Mock Cheez Sauce (see recipe page 110) *

KITCHEN EQUIPMENT
Handheld immersion blender
Measuring spoons & measuring cups
Heat-resistant spoon or spatula
Medium saucepan or pot
Plastic containers with lids or silicone cups with lids to freeze

SPECIAL INSTRUCTIONS/DIET INFORMATION
*Cheeses should be aged over 3 months, and contain zero carbohydrates or sugars, regarding nutritional content. Pre-sliced and pre-shredded cheese will likely contain illegal ingredients to prevent the cheese from sticking and prolong shelf life. It is always best to purchase blocks of cheese, then shred, grate, crumble or slice yourself.

DIRECTIONS
1. Heat the pot/saucepan on medium heat. Then add all ingredients (except cheese) and puree with the handheld immersion blender.
2. Fold in the optional cheddar cheese if using. Serve warm or allow to cool and place in airtight containers or freeze as needed.

Savory Black Beans

Approximate Yield	Prep Time 20 min	Estimated Macronutrients
8-10 servings	**Total Time 14 hours**	**2 g P • 7 g C • 3 g F**
	(To allow for soaking)	

This recipe includes both the stovetop and crockpot/ slow cooker method for cooking beans.

INGREDIENTS

Soaking Beans
1 cup of dried black beans
4 cups of filtered water

Cooking Beans
¼ cup of dried minced onion or ½ cup of chopped fresh onion
2 tablespoons olive oil
2 bay leaves
2 tablespoons of Taco Seasoning or Pincho Spice Mix (see recipes page 147 & 149) *
1 teaspoon of baking soda
3-4 cups of filtered water (or use 3 cups of water and 1 cup of bone broth)
Salt and pepper to taste

KITCHEN EQUIPMENT
Fine mesh colander
Large bowl or storage container with lid
Measuring spoons & measuring cups
Large pot with lid or large slow cooker
Heat-resistant spoon or spatula
Freezer safe plastic storage container with lids or silicone soup containers with lids to freeze

DIRECTIONS

1. Place the dried black beans in a fine mesh colander, rinse the beans and remove any potential dirt or debris.
2. Place the rinsed beans in a container with lid, and 2 cups of water.
3. Cover with lid and place in refrigerator to soak for 6 hrs. Drain the black beans in the colander again and rinse out container. Then add the beans back to the container and refresh with another 2 cups of water. Allow to soak for another 6 hours. (If necessary, you can soak the beans up to 24 hours and refresh the water as needed.)
4. When ready to cook the beans, rinse the beans again and add to large pot or crockpot with lid. Add in the 3 cups of filtered water or a mix of water and bone broth.
5. Stir in the Taco Seasonings or Pincho Spice Mix, olive oil, dried minced or fresh onion, baking soda and bay leaf.
6. For the stovetop method, bring the beans to a boil, then reduce heat, cover and simmer until tender. Cooking approximately 45- 50 minutes. (Cooking time may vary based on the length of time the beans were soaked and age of the beans.) Serve using a slotted spoon.
7. For the crock pot/ slow cooker method, set the crockpot and cook on low for 4-6 hours or high 3-4 hours. (Cooking time may vary based on the length of time the beans were soaked and age of the beans.) Serve using a slotted spoon.

Quick Pickled Red Onion

Approximate Yield	Prep Time 20 min	Estimated Macronutrients
6-8 servings	Total Time 60 min	1 g P • 11 g C • 0 g F
	(To allow to refrigeration)	

INGREDIENTS

1 large red onion
2 finely minced garlic cloves
¾ cup of apple cider vinegar*
½ cup white vinegar or red wine vinegar*
1 ¼ cup of filtered water
3 tablespoons of honey
2 tablespoons fine sea salt
Pinch of red pepper flakes
Optional: ½ teaspoon whole yellow mustard seed

KITCHEN EQUIPMENT

Glass mason jar container with airtight lid for storage
Small pot
Measuring spoons & measuring cups
Heat-resistant spoon or spatula

SPECIAL INSTRUCTIONS/DIET INFORMATION

*Always confirm vinegars do not include added illegal sugars.
*You may substitute distilled white vinegar, but this may require more honey to sweeten.

DIRECTIONS

1. Wash and cut the onion thinly. Place in the glass jar filling to the top and add the minced garlic and pepper flakes.
2. In a small pot on medium heat combine all other ingredients. Stirring until the honey and salt are dissolved. Bring to a boil, then remove from heat. Allow to cool for 5-10 min.
3. Pour mixture over the onion and garlic in the glass jar. Place lid on the container and refrigerate. Serve cold.
4. You may need to stir or shake the container to keep the onions covered with pickling liquid. Important to note, the onions should be eaten within a couple days to a week as quick pickling is not meant for long term storage.

Goi Ga (Vietnamese Chicken Salad)

Approximate Yield	Prep Time 20 min	Estimated Macronutrients
8-10 servings	Total Time 60 min	19 g P • 30 g C • 8 g F
	(To allow for marinating)	

INGREDIENTS

2-3 cups of cooked cut chicken or Roasted Chicken (see recipe page 255)

3 medium persian cucumbers thinly sliced

2 cups of shredded or thinly julienned carrots

½ finely sliced red onion

¼ cup of chopped fresh cilantro

¼ cup of chopped fresh mint

3-4 cups of finely shredded green cabbage

3-4 green onions thinly sliced

2 shallots shredded or finely sliced

1 small daikon, outside peeled and shredded or thinly julienned, matchstick sized (a peeler works well for this) or use Quick Pickled Radishes (see recipe page 180)

Dressing

2 tablespoons lime juice

1 shredded clove of garlic

2 tablespoons honey

2 tablespoons neutral oil, avocado or olive oil

2 tablespoons white vinegar

1-2 tablespoons fish sauce (this is to taste) *

1 tablespoon filtered water

Salt to taste

Optional spice: ⅛ teaspoon of dried ground thai chili peppers

Or ½ a jalapeno seeded and minced fine

Garnish

¼ cup of shelled, roasted and salted peanuts (chopped coarsely)

KITCHEN EQUIPMENT

Glass mason jar or container with leak proof lid for dressing storage

Measuring spoons & measuring cups

Spatula or large spoon

Large bowl to toss salad

SPECIAL INSTRUCTIONS/DIET INFORMATION

*You may substitute distilled white vinegar with apple cider vinegar, but this will change the taste and sweeten the salad.

*Fish sauce should not have added ingredients except fish (generally anchovies) and salt.

DIRECTIONS

1. Combine all the salad dressing ingredients together. Placing them in a mason jar or container with leak proof lid and shake. Allow the dressing to marinate while assembling the salad.
2. Wash and cut the vegetables. Place them in a large bowl with the chicken. Toss all ingredients together with the dressing. Allow the salad to marinate together for 1 hour in the fridge.
3. One tip is to keep the salad and dressing separate to toss together in small batches as needed, as the vegetables can lose their crunch once the dressing is added.
4. Serve immediately or preferably allow to chill in the refrigerator before serving.

Bison Fried Cauliflower Rice

Approximate Yield	Prep Time 15 min	Estimated Macronutrients
10 servings	Total Time 30 min	23 g P • 9 g C • 19 g F

INGREDIENTS

16 oz of ground bison (or substitute with lean ground beef)
8 oz frozen petite peas and carrots
½ cup diced (no sugar or added sweeteners) bacon*
½ cup filtered water
¼ cup dried minced onion or ½ cup of chopped fresh onion
1 tablespoon sesame oil
1 tablespoon tamari or No Soy Sauce (see recipe page 121 and notes) *
1 (16 -24 oz) approximately 3-4 cups of frozen cauliflower rice (steamed)*
3-4 thinly sliced green onions
½ cup pasteurized liquid egg whites or 3 egg whites separated*
1 whole egg
Salt and pepper to taste

KITCHEN EQUIPMENT

Large sauté pan or wok
Microwavable dish with lid
Measuring spoons & measuring cups
Handheld meat chopper, mincer or heat-resistant spatula
Heat resistant spoon or spatula

SPECIAL INSTRUCTIONS/DIET INFORMATION

*Check the labels of the tamari, many will list rice wine vinegar and other ingredients which may be illegal when following SCD. Tamari should generally be gluten free, grain free, and sugar free. For example, tamari includes only water, organic soybeans, salt and/or organic alcohol (as part of fermentation process).

*If using No Soy Sauce (see recipe page 121) to substitute tamari, this may add sweetness and acid changing the flavor profile of the dish.

*Fresh steamed cauliflower can be riced and used; however, the different texture of fresh cauliflower can often vary and may affect the texture of the dish.

*Always read labels carefully verify ingredients with manufacturers for prepackaged bacon.

*Be careful to read all ingredients for pasteurized liquid egg whites. This should be a mono ingredient, and not contain any preservatives or additional ingredients. Regular separated egg whites can be used but the batter will be thicker and require many eggs.

DIRECTIONS

1. Pour the frozen cauliflower rice in the microwavable dish with lid and steam based on package directions (generally cook for 5-6 minutes). Set aside for later.
2. In the sauté pan on medium to high heat, add the diced bacon. Cook fully and set aside in a separate bowl. Then in the same pan/skillet sauté and break up the ground bison with the filtered water. Add the dried minced onion (or fresh onion) and continue stirring until moisture is reduced, and both the onion and meat are cooked thoroughly.
3. Add in the peas and carrots, stirring as they defrost and cook. Then fold in the cauliflower rice, and cooked bacon into the pan.
4. Stir in the sesame oil, tamari or No Soy Sauce, salt and pepper, ensuring the cauliflower rice and bison are fully coated.
5. Create a large hole in the center of the pan, and then add in the egg and egg whites, scrambling the egg and folding in with the rest of the ingredients.
6. When all ingredients are cooked well, remove from heat and serve warm.

Green Bean "Fries"

Approximate Yield 2-4 servings	Prep Time 10 min Total Time 25 min	Estimated Macronutrients 2 g P • 12 g C • 0 g F

This recipe provides an alternative instruction for roasting in the oven.

INGREDIENTS

1 (12-16 oz) package of frozen French green beans or fresh trimmed and blanched green beans*
Spray olive or avocado oil
1 – 1 ½ teaspoons of Parmesan- No Seasoning (see recipe page 152) *

KITCHEN EQUIPMENT

Large bowl
Measuring spoons
Heat resistant tongs or spatula
Air fryer or oven
Parchment paper or aluminum foil
Baking sheet or air fryer tray/basket

SPECIAL INSTRUCTIONS/DIET INFORMATION

*You can substitute frozen with fresh green beans that have been trimmed and blanched, but air frying times will be reduced.
*Note the amount of spice used is to taste, once the green beans are fried you can toss them with more seasoning.
*Important reminder that the Parmesan-No Seasoning contains almond flour for those with nut sensitivities or allergies. Use an alternate seasoning or rub recipe in the book as needed.

DIRECTIONS

1. If using an oven preheat to 450 degrees F. Line a baking sheet with parchment paper. If using an air fryer, no need to preheat.
2. Place the green beans in the large mixing bowl and toss with olive oil and the Parmesan- No Seasoning Mix.
3. If using the oven, spread out the green beans on a baking sheet lined with parchment paper and bake for 15 minutes or until tender when pierced with a knife. If you prefer the green beans crisper raise the temp to broil for an additional 1 – 2 minutes.
4. If using the air fryer spread the green beans out in the basket evenly, and fry at 400 degrees F for 20-22 minutes if frozen (if not frozen 10-12 min) depending on desired crispness.
5. When crispy, you can serve or toss the green beans in a bowl with additional seasoning as needed. Serve hot.

Air Fried Butternut Squash "Tots"

Approximate Yield	Prep Time 10 min	Estimated Macronutrients
2-4 servings	Total Time 25 min	2 g P • 18 g C • 1 g F

INGREDIENTS
1 (12oz) package of frozen cubed butternut squash or 3 cups fresh butternut squash*
Spray olive or avocado oil
1 – 1 ½ teaspoons of Parmesan- No Seasoning (see recipe page 152) *

KITCHEN EQUIPMENT
Large bowl
Measuring spoons
Heat resistant tongs or spatula
Air fryer or oven
Parchment paper or aluminum foil
Baking sheet or air fryer tray/basket

SPECIAL INSTRUCTIONS/DIET INFORMATION
*You can substitute frozen with fresh butternut squash that has been peeled and sliced into cubes, but air frying times may be reduced.
*Note the amount of spice used is to taste, once the butternut squash is fried you can toss them with more seasoning.
*Important reminder that the Parmesan-No Seasoning contains almond flour for those with nut sensitivities or allergies. Use an alternate seasoning or rub recipe in the book as needed.

DIRECTIONS
1. If using an oven preheat to 450 degrees F. Line a baking sheet with parchment paper. If using an air fryer, no need to preheat.
2. Place the butternut squash in the large mixing bowl and toss with olive oil and the Parmesan- No Seasoning Mix.
3. If using the oven, spread out the butternut squash on a baking sheet lined with parchment paper and bake for 15 minutes or until tender when pierced with a knife. If you prefer the butternut squash crisper raise the temp to broil for an additional 1 – 2 minutes.
4. If using the air fryer spread the butternut squash out in the basket evenly, and fry at 400 degrees F for 20-22 minutes if frozen (if not frozen 10-15 min) depending on desired crispness.
5. When crispy and the inside tender when pierced with a fork, you can serve or toss the butternut squash in a bowl with additional seasoning as needed. Serve hot.

Roasted Beet and Butternut Squash with Crispy Kale

Approximate Yield	Prep Time 15 min	Estimated Macronutrients
4 servings	Total Time 60 min	4 g P • 26 g C • 13 g F
	(To allow for roasting time)	

INGREDIENTS

4 large beets, washed, peeled and cut into bite size pieces (2 golden and 2 red beets for variety)

1 small – medium long neck butternut squash

2-3 tablespoons olive oil

1-1 ½ tablespoons Parmesan-No Seasoning (see recipe page 152) *

1 bunch of curly or dino kale (washed and destemmed, and cut into smaller pieces)

¼ large red onion chopped in thick pieces

2 tablespoons – ¼ cup of Honey Mustard Vinaigrette Dressing, to taste (see recipe page 138)

Optional Garnishes:
Crumbled cotija cheese*
Chopped walnuts
¼ cup of crumbled and cooked (no sugar or added sweeteners) bacon *

KITCHEN EQUIPMENT

Large mixing bowl
Vegetable peeler
Large cutting knife
Measuring spoons & measuring cups
Heat resistant tongs or spatula
2-3 Baking sheets with sides or air fryer tray/basket
Parchment paper or aluminum foil
Oven
Optional: Non-latex food service gloves to protect hands from stains and a plastic cutting board
(Beets will stain your hands and wooden cutting boards)
Air fryer

SPECIAL INSTRUCTIONS/DIET INFORMATION

*Always read labels carefully verify ingredients with manufacturers for prepackaged bacon.
*Important reminder that the Parmesan-No Seasoning contains almond flour for those with nut sensitivities or allergies. Use an alternate seasoning or rub recipe in the book as needed.
*Cheeses should be aged over 3 months, and contain zero carbohydrates or sugars, regarding nutritional content. Pre-sliced and pre-shredded cheese will likely contain illegal ingredients to prevent the cheese from sticking and prolong shelf life. It is always best to purchase blocks of cheese, then shred, grate, crumble or slice yourself.

DIRECTIONS

1. Preheat the oven to 425 degrees F. Prepare the baking sheets with parchment paper or aluminum foil.
2. Wash the beets and remove the stems. Peel the beets using the vegetable peeler and then cut them into bite size pieces. Note: Beets will stain your hands and cutting boards so use gloves and/or a non-wood cutting board that can be washed in the dishwasher after use.
3. Peel the butternut squash and cut off the neck. You can then cut the neck into bite size cubes. This also makes it easier to cut the bulb of the squash in half, scrape out the seeds and then cut the rest of squash into bite size pieces.
4. In a large mixing bowl, toss the beets, onion and butternut squash with olive oil and parmesan-no seasoning. Important Note: if you like crispier butternut squash keep the squash separate when roasting. This will also allow you to broil the squash at the end or air fry them. If air frying the squash separately, then spray the butternut squash lightly with olive oil, toss with seasoning and air fry at 400 degrees F for 20-22 minutes, flipping them over halfway.
5. If using the one pan meal method: Place the beets, onion and butternut squash evenly on the parchment paper or aluminum lined baking sheet (you will likely need two baking sheets ensuring there is enough space between the vegetables).
6. Roast for 35-45 minutes (the beets and butternut squash should be tender to pierce with a fork when done).

DIRECTIONS (continued)

You can also briefly roast them on broil for 2-4 minutes. Watching carefully to allow the vegetables to brown and crisp a little. Remove from oven and set aside to cool while assembling the salad

7. Next toss the kale in the same large mixing bowl, it will likely still have plenty or oil and seasoning in it.

8. Place the kale evenly on the parchment paper (you will likely need two baking pans ensuring there is enough space between kale leaves).

9. Roast the kale for 10-12 minutes (the kale will begin to crisp up)

10. To assemble the salad, using the large bowl toss the beets, onion and butternut squash with dressing. Then add in the crispy kale.

11. Note you can serve the salad with crumbled cotija and chopped walnuts.

Roasted Bean "Popcorn"

Approximate Yield	Prep Time 10 min	Estimated Macronutrients
10-12 servings	Total Time 25 min	3 g P • 45 g C • 4 g F

This recipe is inspired by a family favorite seasoning for popcorn, however adapted as a SCD friendly snack or garnish. The recipe provides an alternative instruction for roasting in the oven.

INGREDIENTS

2 cups of soaked, cooked and drained lima beans or navy "white" beans (see recipe page 303)
3-4 tablespoons of unsalted butter or ghee (melted)
1-1 ½ teaspoons paprika*
½ teaspoon cayenne pepper
1 teaspoon dried thyme
½ -1 teaspoon sea salt*

KITCHEN EQUIPMENT

Large bowl
Heat resistant tongs or spatula
Measuring spoons & measuring cups
Air fryer or oven
Baking sheet or air fryer tray
Baking parchment paper or aluminum foil

SPECIAL INSTRUCTIONS/DIET INFORMATION

*Note the amount of spice used is to taste, as once the beans are cooked you can toss them with more seasoning or salt.

DIRECTIONS

1. If using an oven preheat to 450 F degrees. Prepare a baking sheet with parchment paper. If using an air fryer, no need to preheat.
2. Place the cooked beans in the large mixing bowl and toss with melted butter and spices.
3. If using the oven, spread out the beans on a baking sheet lined with parchment paper. Bake for 15-20 minutes. Flipping the beans every 5 to 10 minutes to ensure they crisp up evenly and do not burn.
4. If using the air fryer spread the beans out in the basket evenly, and fry at 400 degrees F for 10-12 minutes, shuffling the basket halfway ensuring even crispness and prevent burning.
5. Remove from oven or air fryer. Allowing the beans to cool a bit and harden up on the parchment before serving.

Butternut Bacon Fritters

Approximate Yield	Prep Time 15 min	Estimated Macronutrients
10 servings	**Total Time 30 min**	**10 g P • 8 g C • 3 g F**

INGREDIENTS

**1 long neck butternut squash (peeled and shredded)
approximately 2 cups of shredded butternut squash**

2 large egg whites

**¼ cup of cooked (no sugar or added sweeteners) bacon
crumbles ***

¼ cup dried egg whites

2 tablespoon coconut flour

**1 tablespoon dried herbs of choice (i.e., Italian dried herb
mix), diced green onions or dried chives**

1 teaspoon granulated garlic

½ teaspoon salt

¼ teaspoon ground pepper

Neutral oil for frying

KITCHEN EQUIPMENT

Large mixing bowl

Heat resistant spatula

Measuring spoons & measuring cups

Standing or handheld electric mixer

Large non-stick sauté pan

Baking parchment paper lined cookie sheet.

SPECIAL INSTRUCTIONS/DIET INFORMATION

Always read labels carefully verify ingredients with
manufacturers for prepackaged bacon.

DIRECTIONS

1. In a large bowl mixing bowl, stir in all the ingredients thoroughly.
2. Heat the oil in the frying pan to moderate or high heat.
3. When the pan is hot, spoon dollops of fritter batter into the pan. They should start to fry and turn golden on the bottom before flipping each over with a spatula.
4. When fully cooked and both sides are golden, place the fritters on the parchment sheet lined cookie sheet and serve warm.

Czech Style No-Tato Salad

Approximate Yield **10-12 servings**	**Prep Time 20 min** **Total Time 2 hours** (To allow for refrigeration)	**Estimated Macronutrients** **6 g P • 15 g C • 10 g F**

INGREDIENTS

1 head of cauliflower, washed and chopped into ½ inch florets
1 16oz bag of frozen peas and carrots (defrosted in the refrigerator) *
½ red onion minced
5 SCD medium dill pickles minced or Quick Dill Pickles (see recipe page 182) *
1 ¼ cup of frozen rice cauliflower (cooked, pureed and chilled) *
Optional: 4 hard boiled eggs (shelled and minced)

Dressing

1 cup of avocado mayonnaise (see recipe page 112) *
2 tablespoons white wine or white vinegar*
2 tablespoons honey
1 tablespoon yellow mustard*
1 ½ teaspoon salt*
¼ teaspoon ground black pepper*

KITCHEN EQUIPMENT

Large mixing bowl
Measuring spoons & measuring cups
Spatula or large spoon
Large pot
Fine mesh colander/strainer or slotted spoon
Immersion blender or food processor

SPECIAL INSTRUCTIONS/DIET INFORMATION

*If you cannot source frozen peas and carrots together, then you can purchase them separately. However frozen carrots are best diced in small bite size squares and not circles.
* SCD legal pickles should not include any sweeteners, vague ingredients, and/or additives. The pickle ingredients used in this recipe included cucumber, water, salt, distilled white vinegar, garlic, dill weed, dill seed, mustard seed, caraway seed, calcium chloride (a natural salt), fennel seed, mace, and turmeric. If you are unable to source SCD legal pickles use the following Quick Dill Pickles, see recipe page 182.
*Always confirm vinegars do not include added illegal sugars.
*There are a few commercial brands of mustard made with SCD legal ingredients. However always check ingredients carefully. Confirm with the company and determine unlisted ingredients are not being used in the manufacturing process.
* There are limited brands of mayonnaise with legal ingredients under the Specific Carbohydrate Diet, therefore read labels carefully and verify with the manufacturer or use the recipe on page 112.
*A tip to prevent a watery cauliflower puree, squeeze out some of the water with a tea towel or paper towels.
*You may want to add more salt and pepper to taste.

DIRECTIONS

1. In a large pot boil water, add a tablespoon of salt.
2. Add the cauliflower florets to the boiling water and cook 5-10 minutes until al dente (slightly tender with fork). Drain the water in a colander or scoop out the cauliflower with slotted spoon. Allow the cauliflower to steam and drain for 2-5 minutes in the colander. Then place in large mixing bowl and refrigerate 2 hours or until cauliflower is cool.
3. In a separate bowl mix all the ingredients together for the dressing, cover and refrigerate until use.
4. Following the instructions for steaming the frozen cauliflower rice. Once cooked, place the riced cauliflower in a food processor or use an immersion blender to puree the cauliflower rice into a mash. Allow the mashed cauliflower to cool in the refrigerator.
5. Drain the defrosted peas and carrots of water in the colander. Then in the large mixing bowl gently combine the cauliflower florets, mashed cauliflower, peas, carrots, minced onion, pickles, and hard-boiled eggs. Stir in the preferred amount of dressing, (you may have leftover dressing).
6. Serve immediately or preferably allow to chill in the refrigerator before serving.

Elevated Egg Salad

Approximate Yield	**Prep Time 20 min**	**Estimated Macronutrients**
10-12 servings	**Total Time 60 min**	**14 g P • 8 g C • 11 g F**
	(To allow refrigeration)	

INGREDIENTS

7 hard boiled eggs (shells removed)

Dressing

1-2 tablespoons avocado mayonnaise (see recipe page 112) *
1 ½ tablespoons finely minced shallot*
1 tablespoon yellow mustard*
½ tablespoon white wine vinegar*
1-2 teaspoons honey (to taste)
⅛ teaspoon sea salt
Pinch of ground black pepper*
Optional: ⅛ teaspoon ground cumin

KITCHEN EQUIPMENT

Egg slicer
Medium glass or plastic bowl with lid for storage
Measuring spoons & measuring
Spatula or large spoon
Optional: Mincer or grater

SPECIAL INSTRUCTIONS/DIET INFORMATION

* There are limited brands of mayonnaise with legal ingredients under the Specific Carbohydrate Diet, therefore read labels carefully and verify with the manufacturer or use the recipe on page 112.
*Finely grating the shallot may be a better option for a delicate texture.
*Always confirm vinegars do not include added illegal sugars.
*You may want to add more salt and pepper to taste.
*There are a few commercial brands of mustard made with SCD legal ingredients. However always check ingredients carefully. Confirm with the company and determine unlisted ingredients are not being used in the manufacturing process.

DIRECTIONS

1. Using the egg slicer, dice the hardboiled eggs and place in the bowl.
2. Add in the remaining ingredients and mix well. Salt and pepper to taste.
3. Preferably allow the flavors to marinate and chill the egg salad in the refrigerator 1-2 hours before serving.

Best Mashed No-Tatoes

Approximate Yield **6-8 servings**	**Prep Time 15 min** **Total Time 30 min**	**Estimated Macronutrients** **11 g P • 24 g C • 5 g F**

INGREDIENTS

1 (12 oz) bag or 2 cups of frozen cauliflower rice*
¾ -1 cup of mashed Easy SCD Crockpot Yellow Peas (see recipe page 304)
½ cup of SCD Non-fat Greek Yogurt (see recipe page 298)
¼ cup of unsweetened nut milk (recommended cashew or almond) *
2 tablespoons butter or ghee
Sea salt and ground black pepper to taste

Optional mix ins:
½ cup diced cooked bacon (no sugar or added sweeteners) *
½ tablespoon chives
2 tablespoons sliced green onions

KITCHEN EQUIPMENT

Handheld immersion blender
Microwavable glass dish with lid or non-stick pot (to cook the cauliflower rice)
Measuring cups & measuring spoons
Heat resistant spatula or spoon
Medium-large pot with lid
Plastic freezer storage containers with lids or silicone cups with lids

SPECIAL INSTRUCTIONS/DIET INFORMATION

*Fresh steamed cauliflower can be riced and used; however, the different texture of fresh cauliflower can often vary and may affect the texture of the dish.
*Any nut milks should only consist of nuts, water, or salt. No emulsifiers, gums, sweeteners or additives should be in the ingredient list. If you are unable to source a SCD legal nut milk you can make them easily at home (see recipe page 299).
*If there is a nut allergy or sensitivity substitute with 2 tablespoons of SCD Non-fat Greek Yogurt well blended with 2 tablespoons water.
*Always read labels carefully verify ingredients with manufacturers for prepackaged bacon.

DIRECTIONS

1. Using a microwave or stovetop, steam the cauliflower rice per package instructions.
2. If the yellow peas are frozen, you can place them in the medium to large pot with ¼ cup of water and heat on medium heat. Stirring regularly to prevent burning and defrosting the yellow pea mash. Note, you may not need as much nut milk if you find the yellow peas are too watery.
3. Once yellow peas are defrosted, add all the other ingredients and steamed cauliflower rice to pot.
4. Using the immersion blender to puree the cauliflower mix until smooth. Salt and pepper to taste. You can also add in the optional mix-ins.
5. Cook until the mashed No-Tatos start to bubble in the pot and either serve hot or remove to cool and store in a container with lid or silicone cups for freezing.

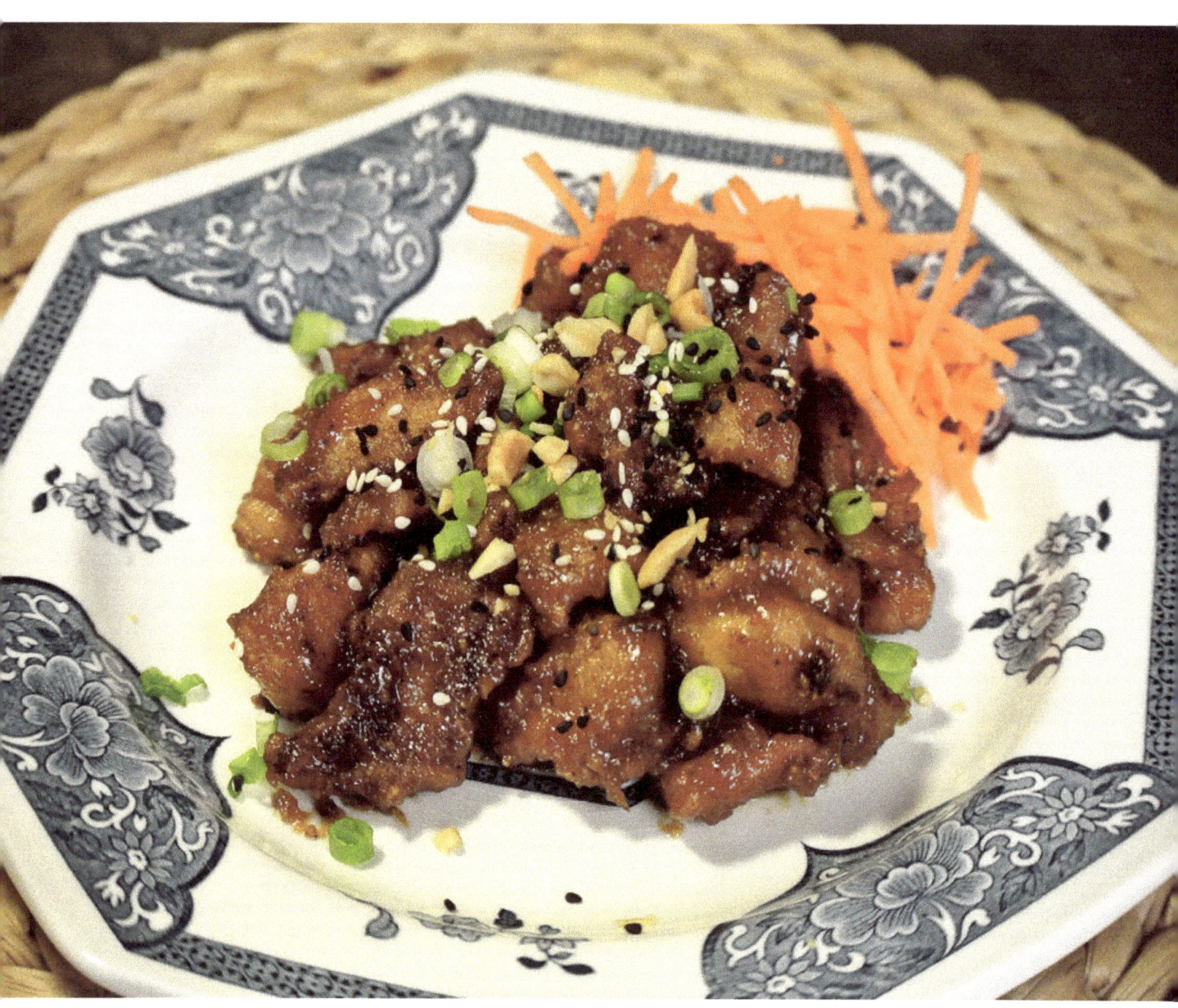

Honey Hoisin Chicken

Main Courses & Protein Sources

There is nothing better than finishing a long, strenuous day with a satisfying meal. Main courses and large meals filled with protein are essential to replenishing the body of vital nutrition. The most important aspect of a main dish or dinner is the protein source. Why? Eating protein later in the day can aid in muscle repair, help with muscle adaptation, and promotes muscle growth. Generally, a later lunch or dinner are used as "catch up" meals for macronutrient goals. Thus, the main course be nutritionally well balanced and filling. When an athlete has finished their day, a full and deliciously balanced meal will help aid in recovery.

These recipes include variety and are focused on meeting protein needs.

Chicken Paella

Approximate Yield	Prep Time 20 min	Estimated Macronutrients
6-8 servings	Total Time 60 min	34 g P • 35 g C • 10 g F

INGREDIENTS

1 24 oz bag (approximately 4 cups) of frozen cauliflower rice*

8 oz-10 oz of frozen bell peppers

8 oz-10 oz frozen petite peas

2 garlic cloves minced

¼ cup minced dried onion or ½ fresh small onion diced

⅓ cup of fresh lemon juice (to taste)

½ cup of SCD legal bone broth or use Roasted Chicken Bone Broth see recipe page 255

1 lb. of cooked and shredded boneless chicken thighs or use leftover Roasted Chicken (see recipe page 255) *

1-2 tablespoons of Cajun Seasoning (see recipe page 149)

⅓ cup cooked (no sugar or added sweeteners) bacon, crumbled *

1 large pinch of saffron

½ tablespoon turmeric

½ teaspoon finely ground red pepper flakes

½ teaspoon dried parsley

Olive oil for sauté (approximately 1 tablespoon)

KITCHEN EQUIPMENT

Large non-stick skillet with lid

Measuring spoons & measuring cups

Large heat-resistant spoon or spatula

SPECIAL INSTRUCTIONS/DIET INFORMATION

*Fresh steamed cauliflower can be riced and used; however, the different texture of fresh cauliflower can often vary and may affect the texture of the dish.

*This recipe is designed for using leftover chicken from a previous roasted chicken or air fried chicken recipes. However, if using fresh (raw) chicken breast or thighs, cut into tenders or smaller pieces and sauté separately on the stove with olive oil, and coating sparingly with Cajun seasonings.

*Always read labels carefully verify ingredients with manufacturers for prepackaged bacon.

DIRECTIONS

1. Mince the garlic cloves, and onion if using fresh. Set aside.
2. Steam the frozen rice cauliflower per package instructions or in a large microwavable casserole dish with lid. Set aside.
3. In a large measuring cup, warm up the bone broth in the microwave and add lemon juice, turmeric, and saffron. Mix well and allow to steep. Set aside.
4. In the large skillet on medium heat, add the olive oil, frozen bell peppers, minced garlic, onion, and cook til the vegetables are tender. Add in the chicken, petite frozen peas, riced cauliflower, cajun seasoning, red pepper flakes, parsley and bone broth mixture. Stirring well so all the spices and broth coat the paella.
5. Continue to sauté the ingredients, allowing the colors from the turmeric and saffron to color the cauliflower rice. Placing the lid on the pan steam the peas.
6. Once the peas are cooked, and if there is still excess liquid, increase the heat to reduce the liquid. When excess moisture is gone, reduce the heat and serve warm.

Gyro "Döner" Meat

Approximate Yield	**Prep Time 10 min**	**Estimated Macronutrients**
5-6 servings	Total Time 30 min	16 g P • 1 g C • 8 g F

INGREDIENTS

½ cup filtered water
16 oz lean shaved beef, boneless skinless chicken thighs, or ground lamb
4 tablespoons Döner Seasoning (see recipe page 146)
1 tablespoon olive oil or spray for chicken thighs

Serve with optional garnishes and/or complementary sides:

Shredded lettuce
Thinly sliced tomatoes
Thinly sliced cucumbers
Thinly sliced red onion
Crumbled cotija cheese*
Pickled Cabbage (see recipe page 172)
White Garlic Sauce (see recipe page 113)
Yellow Split Pea or Asian Style Green Onion Wraps (see recipes page 306 & 308)

KITCHEN EQUIPMENT

Large non-stick skillet or seasoned cast iron pan
Measuring spoons & measuring cups
Heat resistant tongs or spatula
Optional: Handheld meat chopper or mincer
If cooking chicken:
Air fryer or oven
Aluminum foil
Baking sheet or air fryer tray
Meat thermometer

SPECIAL INSTRUCTIONS/DIET INFORMATION

*Cheeses should be aged over 3 months, and contain zero carbohydrates or sugars, regarding nutritional content. Pre-sliced and pre-shredded cheese will likely contain illegal ingredients to prevent the cheese from sticking and prolong shelf life. It is always best to purchase blocks of cheese, then shred, grate, crumble or slice yourself.

DIRECTIONS

Shaved Beef and Lamb

1. Heat the oil in the skillet at medium to high heat, then add the ground beef or lamb, döner seasonings, and water.
2. Continue to sauté and break up the shaved beef or ground lamb until fully cooked and no pink or red is showing. Allow the meat to brown and crisp a bit, and excess water is reduced.
3. Lower the heat to warm when done and serve with accompanying sides, either plated with garnishes or in a wrap.

Chicken

1. Line a baking sheet or an air fryer tray/basket with foil. Preheat the air fryer or oven to 375 degrees F.
2. Place the chicken on the foil, and spray or drizzle with olive oil until well coated.
3. Sprinkle the döner seasoning over both sides of the chicken thighs evenly.
4. Bake or air fry the thighs for 15 minutes then flip the thighs over and continue cooking for 9-15 minutes. Using a meat thermometer to verify the internal temp of the chicken is 165 degrees F.
5. When cooked, remove the chicken from the air fryer or oven, and cut the thighs into thin strips. Serve with accompanying sides either plated or in a wrap.

Tandoori Chicken

Approximate Yield	**Prep Time 10 min**	**Estimated Macronutrients**
6 servings	**Total Time 25 min**	**24 g P • 2 g C • 10 g F**

This recipe provides instruction for both oven and air frying.

INGREDIENTS

Tandoori Rub
½ tablespoon sea salt
2 teaspoons garam masala spice
2 teaspoons paprika
1 teaspoon smoked paprika
1 teaspoon ground coriander
1 teaspoon granulated garlic
¼ teaspoon ground black pepper
¼ teaspoon ground ginger
Dash of cayenne

1-2 lbs. of boneless skinless chicken thighs or breast tenderloins
2 tablespoons lemon juice
1 tablespoon olive oil

KITCHEN EQUIPMENT

Gallon plastic zip top bag or large metal bowl
Measuring spoons
Air fryer or oven (air fryer yields the best results)
Heat resistant tongs or spatula
Baking sheet for oven method or tray/basket for air frying method
Aluminum foil
Meat thermometer

DIRECTIONS

1. Combine all the rub ingredients together and mix well. Then stir in the olive oil and lemon juice to create a paste.
2. Place the chicken thighs or breast tenderloins in a gallon plastic zip top bag or metal bowl. Then add in the rub paste, massaging it into the meat well.
3. If using an oven preheat to 375 degrees F. Prepare a baking sheet with foil. If using an air fryer no need to preheat.
4. If using the oven, spread out the thighs on a baking sheet lined with foil paper, cover with foil and bake for 30-35 minute and the internal temperature is 165 degrees F.
5. If using the air fryer set the temp to 375 degrees F, spread a piece of foil over the basket or tray, and spread the chicken evenly. You will likely need to work in small batches. Air fry for 12 minutes, flip them, and air fry for 12 minutes more.
6. When the internal temperature is 165 degrees F, remove from the air fryer and serve warm.

Panang Chicken Curry

Approximate Yield	Prep Time 10 min	Estimated Macronutrients
6-8 servings	Total Time 30 min	22 g P • 43 g C • 13 g F

INGREDIENTS

½ cup filtered water
16 oz boneless skinless chicken thighs or chicken breast cut in 1 inch diameter pieces
1 tablespoon olive or avocado oil
¼ red or white onion chopped
1 red bell pepper (stem and seeds removed) chopped julienne
2 cups of crisscross or roll cut carrots
4 cups of frozen broccoli
Optional: 1 cup of peeled and chopped cooked celery root or rutabaga (bite size pieces are ideal)

Curry Sauce

4 tablespoons favorite or SCD Panang Curry Paste or (see recipe page 132)
1 ½ teaspoon fish sauce*
1 tablespoon neutral or avocado oil
1 ½ tablespoon honey (to taste) *
1 ½ cup unsweetened coconut milk*
Juice of ½ a lime

Garnish

3 green onions
Chopped peanuts
Fresh cilantro leaves chopped

4 cups of frozen cauliflower rice

KITCHEN EQUIPMENT

Large non-stick or ceramic coated skillet
Heat resistant spatula or spoon
Measuring spoons & cups

SPECIAL INSTRUCTIONS/DIET INFORMATION

*Reduce honey to taste as needed.
*Coconut milk should only consist of coconut and water. No emulsifiers, gums, sweeteners or additives should be in the ingredient list.
*Fish sauce should not have added ingredients except fish (generally anchovies) and salt

DIRECTIONS

1. Mince and chop all the garnishes, then set aside for later.
2. Heat the oil in the skillet, add in the chicken and sear on each side, then add in the water.
3. Once the chicken is cooked remove from skillet and set aside. In the skillet add in the peppers, onion and extra cooking oil if needed. Sauté the vegetables to al dente.
4. In a microwavable container with lid, steam the frozen broccoli. You will want to steam to slightly tender (al dente) so as not to overcook the broccoli when added to the curry.
5. Return the chicken to the pan and add in the remaining ingredients for the curry sauce and optional celery root or rutabaga pieces. Allow the sauce to simmer, then add in the steamed broccoli last. Lower the heat to warm when done.
6. In a microwavable container with lid or cook the frozen cauliflower rice in bag per instructions.
7. Plate the dish with the cauliflower, the chicken curry and garnish with the peanuts, cilantro and green onions.

Teri-**Yay**-ki Chicken Thighs

| Approximate Yield
6 servings | Prep Time 10 min
Total Time 2 hours
(To allow for marinading) | Estimated Macronutrients
35 g P • 9 g C • 16 g F |

This recipe provides an alternative instruction for roasting in the oven.

INGREDIENTS
2-4 lbs. of boneless skinless chicken thighs
Fresh cracked pepper
Flaked sea salt
¼ cup of SCD Teri-Yay-ki Unagi Sauce (see recipe page 122)
Sesame seeds
Green onions

Marinade
½ cup tamari or No Soy Sauce (see recipe page 121) *
1 tablespoon of finely minced garlic
¼ teaspoon black pepper
1 tablespoon toasted sesame oil
½ cup of SCD Teri-Yay-ki Unagi Sauce (see recipe page 122)

KITCHEN EQUIPMENT
Gallon plastic zip top bag or large metal bowl
Measuring spoons & measuring cups
Heat resistant tongs or spatula
Air fryer or oven (air fryer yields the best results)
Baking parchment paper or aluminum foil
Baking sheet or air fryer tray/basket
Basting brush or small spoon

SPECIAL INSTRUCTIONS/DIET INFORMATION
*Check the labels of the tamari, many will list rice wine vinegar and other ingredients which may be illegal when following SCD. Tamari should generally be gluten free, grain free, and sugar free. For example, tamari includes only water, organic soybeans, salt and/or organic alcohol (as part of fermentation process).
*If using No Soy Sauce (see recipe page 121) to substitute tamari, you may want to reduce the amount of honey in the recipe. This is based on personal taste and is due to the sweetness of the No Soy Sauce.

DIRECTIONS
1. Combine all the marinade ingredients together and mix well.
2. Place the chicken thighs in a gallon plastic zip top bag or metal bowl. Pour half the marinade/sauce in the bag or bowl, and marinade the chicken (reserve the rest for basting)
3. If using an oven preheat to 375 degrees F. Line a baking sheet with aluminum foil. If using an air fryer, no need to preheat.
4. If using the oven, spread out the thighs on a baking sheet lined with foil. Then cover the top of the chicken thighs and baking sheet with foil and bake for 30-35 minutes. Remove the foil and baste the chicken with the remaining sauce/marinade. Bake another 10 min or until internal temp is 165 degrees F.
5. If using the air fryer set the temp to 375 degrees F. Spread a piece of foil over the basket or tray and lay the thighs evenly on it. You will likely need to work in small batches. Air fry for 12 minutes, flip them, then baste with the remaining sauce and air fry for 12 minutes more.
6. When the thighs are done and have an internal temp of 165 degrees F, remove and serve hot with flaked sea salt, fresh cracked pepper, sesame seeds and sprinkled with chopped green onions.

Vietnamese Grilled Pork with Noodle Salad

Approximate Yield 4-6 servings	**Prep Time 20 min** **Total Time 2 hours** (To allow for marinading)	**Estimated Macronutrients** 35 g P • 42 g C • 31 g F

Note the the pork can be substituted with beef or chicken as needed.

INGREDIENTS

Pork Marinade
*Note marinading overnight is recommended
2 lbs. of boneless pork shoulder (cut in ¼ of an inch thin slices) or boneless skinless chicken thighs
1 large shallot minced
1 ½ tablespoons garlic minced
⅓ cup of honey
1 tablespoon tamari or No Soy Sauce (see recipe page 121 and notes) *
1 tablespoon fish sauce*
½ tablespoon ground black pepper
3 tablespoons avocado oil

Noodles
1 cup of heart of palm noodles or cooked favorite SCD legal lentil or yellow pea spaghetti noodles
*Note you can also substitute noodles with thinly shredded cabbage

Sides and Garnishes
Fresh cilantro
Crushed roasted, salted, unshelled peanuts

Shredded romaine lettuce
Korean Easy Pickled Vegetable Salad (see recipe page 173)
SCD Vietnamese Salad Dressing or Dipping Sauce (see recipe page 128)

KITCHEN EQUIPMENT
Two baking sheets with sides or large roaster
Aluminum foil
Gallon plastic zip top bag bags or large mixing bowl
Medium pot
Various bowls for garnishes
Meat thermometer

SPECIAL INSTRUCTIONS
*Check the labels of the tamari, many will list rice wine vinegar and other ingredients which may be illegal when following SCD. Tamari should generally be gluten free, grain free, and sugar free. For example, tamari includes only water, organic soybeans, salt and/or organic alcohol (as part of fermentation process).
*If using No Soy Sauce (see recipe page 121) to substitute tamari, you may want to reduce or omit the amount of honey, fish sauce and vinegar in the recipe. This is based on personal taste and is due to the sweetness and vinegar in the No Soy Sauce.
*Fish sauce should not have added ingredients except fish (generally anchovies) and salt.

DIRECTIONS
1. In a large gallon plastic zip top bag add the sliced pork and all other marinade ingredients. Seal the bag and gently massage the meat in the bag with the marinade liquid. Refrigerate overnight.
2. After the meat is marinaded, preheat the oven to 375 degrees F. Remove the pork from refrigerator and allow to warm up a bit.
3. Line the baking sheets or large roasting pan with foil. Lay the pork strips or pieces on the foil, evenly spaced and do not overcrowd them.
4. Roast the pork in the oven for 20-40 minutes (the time is dependent on how thin the strips/pieces are cut). You will want to flip the pork pieces over a couple times to ensure they are cooking evenly. Check the internal temperature with a meat thermometer, and doneness (165 degrees F).
5. For the pork to be caramelized like BBQ, raise the oven temperature to broil, flipping the pieces to allow for even caramelization. Watch the broiler very carefully to ensure the pork does not burn entirely.
6. Remove the pork from the oven and slice into thinner bite size pieces if necessary. Plate the pork with the recommended noodles, sides and garnishes. Toss altogether with dressing as needed.

Hoisin Chicken Lettuce Cups

Approximate Yield	Prep Time 10 min	Estimated Macronutrients
6-10 servings	Total Time 40 min	24 g P • 15 g C • 11 g F

This recipe provides instruction for both oven and air frying.

INGREDIENTS

2-3 lbs of boneless skinless chicken thighs

1-1 ½ cup of Honey Hoisin Sauce (see recipe page 124)

Neutral oil spray

1 teaspoon flaked sea salt

½ teaspoon fresh cracked pepper

1 washed whole iceberg or butter leaf lettuce

Optional Garnishes

½ of shredded carrots

¼ cup sliced green onions

3 tablespoon crushed roasted and salted peanuts

½ teaspoon sesame seeds

KITCHEN EQUIPMENT

Heat-resistant fork, tongs or spatula

Measuring spoons & measuring cups

Air fryer or oven (air fryer yields the best results)

Air fryer basket/tray or baking sheet

Aluminum foil

DIRECTIONS

1. Remove and discard some of the outside leaves of lettuce. Then wash the iceberg or butter lettuce well in cold water and dry. You will want to remove and separate the lettuce leaves individually into palm sized lettuce cups. Depending on the size of the lettuce you may need to cut it in half.

2. Preheat the air fryer or oven to 375 degrees F. Line a baking sheet or the air fryer basket/tray with foil.

3. If using the oven, spray both sides of the thighs with cooking oil and sprinkle with salt and pepper. Then cover the thighs with foil and bake for 30-35 minutes, remove the foil and baste the chicken with the hoisin sauce. Bake another 10-15 min or until internal temp is 165 degrees F. You can also broil for a couple minutes to allow the sauce to caramelize, and thighs crisp up, but watch carefully to prevent burning.

4. If using the air fryer, spread the thighs evenly in the foil lined basket or tray. (You will likely need to work in small batches.) Spray the thighs with neutral oil and sprinkle with salt and black pepper. Air fry for 12 minutes, flip them, and air fry for 12 minutes more. You can then baste the thighs with hoisin sauce and air fry for 3-4 minutes. Then flip over and baste the other side with sauce, air frying for another 3- 4 minutes until the sauce is caramelized and thighs crispy.

5. You want to ensure the internal temp of the thighs are 165 degrees F, then remove from oven or air fryer.

6. When ready to serve, slice the chicken thighs into bite size pieces and place in each lettuce cup. Garnish with shredded carrots, green onion, crushed peanuts and sesame seeds.

Korean Ground Beef

Approximate Yield	Prep Time 10 min	Estimated Macronutrients
5-6 servings	Total Time 30 min	18 g P • 20 g C • 9 g F

INGREDIENTS

½ cup filtered water
16 oz lean ground beef or bison
1 tablespoon sesame oil
5 cloves of minced garlic
6 green onions chopped
¼ teaspoon finely ground red pepper flakes
¼ cup tamari or No Soy Sauce (see recipe page 121 and notes) *
¼ cup honey*
¼ teaspoon ground ginger

1 teaspoon sesame seeds for garnish

4 cups of frozen cauliflower rice (steamed)*
Serve with Korean Easy Pickled Vegetable Salad (see recipe page 173)

KITCHEN EQUIPMENT

Measuring spoons & measuring cups
Heat-resistant spoon or spatula
Large non-stick skillet
Handheld meat chopper, mincer or heat-resistant spatula

SPECIAL INSTRUCTIONS/DIET INFORMATION

*Check the labels of the tamari, many will list rice wine vinegar and other ingredients which may be illegal when following SCD. Tamari should generally be gluten free, grain free, and sugar free. For example, Tamari includes only water, organic soybeans, salt and/or organic alcohol (as part of fermentation process).

*If using No Soy Sauce (recipe page 121) to substitute tamari, increase the amount from a ¼ cup to a ½ cup of No Soy Sauce. You can also replace half of the filtered water used for cooking the beef with ¼ cup of No Soy Sauce to help flavor the meat during the cooking process. The remaining ¼ cup of No Soy can be added as directed. Due to the sweetness of the No Soy Sauce, add honey to taste.

*Fresh steamed cauliflower can be riced and used; however, the different texture of fresh cauliflower can often vary and may affect the texture of the dish.

DIRECTIONS

1. Mince the garlic, and green onions then set aside.
2. Heat the sesame oil in the skillet on medium to high heat, then add the ground beef and water.
3. Continue to sauté and break up the ground beef until well cooked. Add in the garlic, and green onions.
4. Add in the remaining ingredients and continue to sauté until all ingredients are well coated in sauce. Increase the heat to reduce the sauce and moisture from the beef. Lower the heat to warm when done.
5. In a microwavable container or steamer with lid, cook the frozen cauliflower per instructions.
6. Plate the dish with the cooked cauliflower rice, beef and garnish with sesame seeds. Serve with Korean easy pickled vegetables (see recipe page 173).

Air Fried Korean Sweet and Spicy Chicken Thighs

Approximate Yield	Prep Time 10 min	Estimated Macronutrients
6-8 servings	**Total Time 30 min**	**25 g P • 17 g C • 15 g F**

This recipe provides an alternative instruction for roasting in the oven.

INGREDIENTS

Marinade
3 tablespoons of Gochugaru Korean chili flakes
5 tablespoons Wellbees or another SCD legal ketchup (see recipe page 117) *
2 tablespoons tamari or No Soy Sauce (see recipe page 121) *
2 tablespoons crushed fine red pepper chili flakes
1 tablespoon minced garlic cloves
5 tablespoons honey
2 tablespoons sesame oil
2 tablespoons apple cider vinegar
3 tablespoons filtered water

1 -2 lbs. of boneless skinless chicken thighs
Fresh cracked pepper
Flaked sea salt

KITCHEN EQUIPMENT

Gallon plastic zip top bag or large metal bowl
Measuring spoons
Heat resistant tongs or spatula
Air fryer or oven (air fryer yields the best results)
Aluminum foil
Baking sheet or air fryer tray/basket

SPECIAL INSTRUCTIONS/DIET INFORMATION

* There are a couple brands manufacturing SCD legal ketchup. You can also make your own ketchup using the recipe on page 117.
* Check the labels of the tamari, many will list rice wine vinegar and other ingredients which may be illegal when following SCD. Tamari should generally be gluten free, grain free, and sugar free. For example, Tamari includes only water, organic soybeans, salt and/or organic alcohol (as part of fermentation process).
*If using No Soy Sauce (see recipe page 121) to substitute tamari, you may want to reduce or omit the amount of honey and vinegar in the recipe. This is based on personal taste and is due to the sweetness and vinegar in the No Soy Sauce.

DIRECTIONS

1. Combine all the marinade ingredients together except the chicken, salt and pepper.
2. Place the chicken thighs in a gallon plastic zip top bag or metal bowl. Pour half the marinade/sauce in the bag or bowl and marinade the chicken (reserve the rest for basting).
3. If using an oven preheat to 400 degrees F. Line a baking sheet with foil. If using an air fryer, no need to preheat, however line the basket or tray with foil.
4. If using the oven, spread out the thighs on a baking sheet lined with foil paper. Then cover the thighs and baking with foil and bake for 30-35 minutes. After baking, remove the foil and baste the chicken with the remaining sauce/marinade. Then bake for another 10 min or until internal temp is 165 degrees F.
5. If using the air fryer set the temp to 375 degrees F, spread a piece of foil over the basket and spread the thighs evenly. You will likely need to work in small batches. Air fry for 12 minutes, flip them, baste with the remaining sauce and air fry for 12 minutes more.
6. When the wings are done and have an internal temp of 165 degrees F remove and serve hot with flaked sea salt and fresh cracked pepper.

Zucchini Beef Japchae

Approximate Yield	**Prep Time 10 min**	**Estimated Macronutrients**
8-10 servings	**Total Time 30 min**	**20 g P • 45 g C • 10 g F**

INGREDIENTS

1 lb. of shaved beef and trimmed of excess fat
½ teaspoon finely crushed red chili peppers
½ white onion thinly sliced
6-8 oz (1 cup) shitake mushrooms, thinly sliced lengthwise
8 oz (1 cup) frozen chopped spinach
1 cup of shredded carrots
2 garlic cloves minced
3-4 long zucchinis spiralized*
3-4 sliced green onions

Sauce

8 tablespoons tamari or No Soy Sauce (see recipe page 121 and notes) *
2 tablespoons sesame oil
4 ½ teaspoons honey (add more to taste)

KITCHEN EQUIPMENT

Large wok or sauté pan
Measuring spoons & cups
Heat resistant tongs or spatula

SPECIAL INSTRUCTIONS/DIET INFORMATION

*Check the labels of the tamari, many will list rice wine vinegar and other ingredients which may be illegal when following SCD. Tamari should generally be gluten free, grain free, and sugar free. For example, Tamari includes only water, organic soybeans, salt and/or organic alcohol (as part of fermentation process).

*If using No Soy Sauce (see recipe page 121) to substitute tamari, you may want to reduce the amount of honey in the recipe. This is based on personal taste and is due to the sweetness of the No Soy Sauce.

*Note roasted spaghetti squash can be substituted for zucchini. However toss the warm squash with the sauce, beef and other vegetables. Do not overcook in wok or else it will become mushy.

DIRECTIONS

1. Mix the tamari or No Soy Sauce, 1 tablespoon sesame oil, crushed red chili peppers and honey in a small bowl or measuring cup. Set aside to marinate.
2. On moderate to high heat, sauté the green onions, garlic, and mushrooms with 1 tablespoon sesame oil (set aside in a separate bowl).
3. In the same pan, add the spinach and shredded carrots, cook until the carrots are tender and set aside.
4. Heat the ½ tablespoon sesame oil and add the spiralized zucchini, cook to slightly al dente. (Set aside in a separate bowl.)
5. Final step is to sauté the shaved beef and white onion with sesame oil and half the sauce. When cooked through add in the rest of the vegetables (except the zucchini) and the remaining sauce until liquid is reduced. Add the zucchini noodles back in, tossing all ingredients and serve warm.

Korean BBQ Chicken Tacos

Approximate Yield	Prep Time 20 min	Estimated Macronutrients
10-16 servings	Total Time 60 min	16 g P • 12 g C • 4 g F

INGREDIENTS

Chicken filling

3-4 cups of cooked boneless chicken, dark and white meat (the Roasted Chicken recipe is recommended, see recipe page 255)
2 cups of shredded carrots
2 cloves minced garlic
1 (14 oz) can or 1 cup of heart of palm, diced
¼ cup of raw cashews coarsely chopped
½ large white onion chopped
¾ cup clean and diced shitake mushrooms
¼ cup of sliced green onions
¼ cup of SCD legal chicken bone broth or use Roasted Chicken Bone Broth (see recipe page 255)
¼ cup filtered water
½ teaspoon sea salt
¼ teaspoon ground black pepper
Neutral oil

Korean BBQ Sauce

2 tablespoons – ¼ cup of SCD Gochujang Paste* (see recipe page 130)
2 tablespoons tamari or No Soy Sauce (see recipe page 121 and notes) *
3 tablespoons honey (to taste)
1 tablespoon white vinegar (to taste)
1 tablespoon sesame oil

Optional Garnishes and Taco Ingredients

Quick Pickled Cucumber Salad (see recipe page 172) or
Korean Easy Pickled Vegetable Salad (see recipe page 173)
Blueberry Yogurt Sauce (see recipe page 108)
SCD Asian Style Wraps (see recipe page 308) or washed and dried lettuce leaf wraps
Black and white sesame seeds

KITCHEN EQUIPMENT

Large ceramic or nonstick pot with lid
Bowl or large glass measuring cup
Measuring spoons & measuring cups
Heat-resistant spoon or spatula

SPECIAL INSTRUCTIONS/DIET INFORMATION

* The gochujang paste is to taste and based on your tolerance for spice. It will get spicier as it marinates with the other ingredients over time. If the paste was frozen for long term use, defrost before using in the recipe.

*Check the labels of the tamari, many will list rice wine vinegar and other ingredients which may be illegal when following SCD. Tamari should generally be gluten free, grain free, and sugar free. For example, tamari includes only water, organic soybeans, salt and/or organic alcohol (as part of fermentation process).

*If using No Soy Sauce (see recipe page 121) to substitute tamari, you may want to reduce the amount of honey and vinegar in the recipe. This is based on personal taste and is due to the sweetness and vinegar in the No Soy Sauce.

DIRECTIONS

1. In a measuring cup or bowl add the gochujang paste and tamari or No Soy Sauce. (If using the No Soy Sauce to substitute tamari, taste test the mix of gochujang and No Soy Sauce before adding the remaining ingredients. Since No Soy Sauce is both acidic and sweet)

2. Stir in the remaining ingredients for the Korean BBQ sauce and taste as you go. Set aside the Korean BBQ sauce after mixing and allow to marinate.

3. In the large pot, on medium heat, add the oil, garlic, white onion and shitake mushrooms. Sauté in the oil, cooking until the mushrooms start to soften and the onions start to become translucent.
4. Add the shredded carrots, diced heart of palm, green onion, cashews and cooked shredded chicken. Add in the filtered water, chicken bone broth salt and pepper. Keep stirring as you want to make sure all the vegetables and cashews start to soften a bit as they cook.
5. Add in the Korean BBQ sauce and keep stirring until all the chicken and vegetables are well coated with the sauce. If there is a lot of liquid just keep stirring to reduce the liquid down.
6. Taste the Korean taco filling, then add salt, pepper, SCD gochujang paste and/or honey as needed. These amounts are flexible and to your personal preference.
7. Assemble all your garnishes for your tacos and serve.

Bulgogi Beef Marinade and Glaze

Approximate Yield
6-8 servings

Prep Time 10 min
Total Time 3 hours
(To allow for marinating)

Estimated Macronutrients
25 g P • 18 g C • 19 g F

INGREDIENTS

1 lb. of sliced tri tip, sliced flank steak or shaved beef (trimmed of excess fat)
¼ white or yellow onion sliced lengthwise
3-4 sliced green onions for garnish

Marinade

5 tablespoons of tamari or No Soy Sauce (see recipe page 121 and notes) *
2 tablespoons minced garlic
2 tablespoons sesame oil
½ teaspoon ground black pepper

Reserve Glaze

3 tablespoons tamari* or No Soy Sauce (see recipe page 121 and notes) *
3 tablespoons honey
1 tablespoon sesame oil

KITCHEN EQUIPMENT

Large gallon size plastic zip top bag or large metal bowl
Heat-resistant or metal spatula
Large measuring cup or small bowl

SPECIAL INSTRUCTIONS / DIET INFORMATION

*Check the labels of the tamari, many will list rice wine vinegar and other ingredients which may be illegal when following SCD. Tamari should generally be gluten free, grain free, and sugar free. For example, tamari includes only water, organic soybeans, salt and/or organic alcohol (as part of fermentation process).

*If using No Soy Sauce (see recipe page 121) to substitute tamari, increase the amount used and base the addition of honey to taste or omit, due to the sweetness of the No Soy Sauce.

DIRECTIONS

1. Peel and finely mince the garlic cloves, placing them in the measuring cup or small bowl. Then measure out the marinade ingredients and add to the bowl mixing all the ingredients well.
2. Place the beef in the large bowl or plastic zip top bag, pour the marinade over the meat and seal or cover bowl with plastic wrap. Refrigerate for 1-3 hours.
3. Remove from refrigerator an hour before cooking. Heat a wok or skillet to moderate or high heat (dependent on thickness of beef slices) and sauté the beef with the onion. Scraping and stirring the meat to keep from burning.
4. Halfway through the process add the reserved glaze and continue stirring the beef and onions. When the meat is cooked thoroughly, remove from heat and garnish with green onions before serving.

Singapore Style Spaghetti Squash

Approximate Yield	Prep Time 20 min	Estimated Macronutrients
6-8 servings	Total Time 60 min	39 g P • 29 g C • 12 g F

INGREDIENTS
1 large spaghetti squash
1 tablespoon olive oil
1 tablespoon toasted sesame oil
1 lb. of lean ground chicken or lean ground pork (however chicken is recommended)
¼- ½ cup filtered water
2 cups of deveined, cooked medium shrimp (defrosted if frozen)
2 cups of frozen bell peppers (red, yellow and green)
1 cup of thinly sliced shitake mushrooms
½ large yellow onion
2-3 green onions cut in 2-inch slices
3 cloves of minced garlic

Sauce
3-4 tablespoons Honey Hoisin Sauce (see recipe page 124)
1 tablespoon mild curry powder
½ teaspoon salt
⅛ teaspoon ground white power
⅛ teaspoon Chinese five spice
Salt and pepper to taste
Finely ground red chili flakes to taste

Garnish
½ cup cooked minced (no sugar or added sweeteners) bacon
*
Fried shallots
Minced fresh cilantro

Optional: You can use zucchini zoodles, or SCD legal yellow pea vermicelli noodle instead of spaghetti squash if necessary. However, the flavor and textures will differ.

KITCHEN EQUIPMENT
Large nonstick skillet or sauté pan
Handheld meat chopper, mincer or heat-resistant spatula
Measuring spoons & measuring cups
Heat resistant spoon or spatula
Cookie sheet pan lined with baking parchment paper
Grapefruit spoon or metal spoon

SPECIAL INSTRUCTIONS/DIET INFORMATION
*Always read labels carefully verify ingredients with manufacturers for prepackaged bacon

DIRECTIONS
1. In a small bowl whisk the ingredients for the sauce and set aside.
2. Preheat oven to 400 degrees F. Slice the ends off the squash, then cut widthwise into rings, cutting the rings about the same size, around 1-1½ inches thick. Then using a metal or grapefruit spoon to scrape out and discard the seeds.
3. Place the squash on the parchment paper lined baking sheet, and drizzle with olive oil.
4. Bake the spaghetti squash for 30-40 minutes, while cooking the meat and vegetables. However, flip the spaghetti squash rings halfway through the roasting.
5. While the spaghetti squash is roasting, in the large skillet heat the sesame oil on medium heat and add the ground chicken and water. Using the meat mincer or spatula to break up the meat into small bits. Allow to simmer and water reduce.
6. Once the chicken is cooked, use the new spoon or spatula and add the vegetables to the pan. Stirring until the vegetables are al dente. Adding in the cooked shrimp and sauce last.
7. The spaghetti squash should be roasted and removed from the oven. Allow to cool slightly, then use a knife to peel away the skin and a fork to separate the strands into long spaghetti noodles.
8. Toss the spaghetti squash with both sauce, vegetables, meat and garnishes. Or serve the vegetables, meat, sauce and garnishes over a bed of spaghetti noodles. Important to note, you do not want to cook the squash with the sauce, as it will release water and lose its firm texture.

Bison "Pad Kra Pao"

Approximate Yield	Prep Time 10 min	Estimated Macronutrients
6 servings	**Total Time 30 min**	**22 g P • 20 g C • 12 g F**

INGREDIENTS

20 oz bison or lean ground beef
½ cup filtered water
1 tablespoon sesame oil
1 handful of thai basil leaves, destemmed
8 cloves of minced garlic
1 whole shallot minced
3 green onions chopped
4 tablespoons tamari or No Soy Sauce (see recipe page 121 and notes) *
1-3 tablespoons honey*
1 tablespoon finely ground red pepper flakes
1 tablespoon fish sauce*
Salt and pepper to taste
Optional garnish: 1 large fried egg

4 cups of frozen cauliflower rice (steamed)*

KITCHEN EQUIPMENT

Large non-stick skillet
Handheld meat chopper, mincer or heat-resistant spatula
Heat resistant large spoon or spatula
Measuring spoons & measuring cups

SPECIAL INSTRUCTIONS/DIET INFORMATION

*Check the labels of the tamari, many will list rice wine vinegar and other ingredients which may be illegal when following SCD. Tamari should generally be gluten free, grain free, and sugar free. For example, tamari includes only water, organic soybeans, salt and/or organic alcohol (as part of fermentation process).

*If using No Soy Sauce (see recipe page 121) to substitute tamari, you may want to reduce or omit the amount of honey, fish sauce and vinegar in the recipe. This is based on personal taste and is due to the sweetness and vinegar in the No Soy Sauce.

*Fish sauce should not have added ingredients except fish (generally anchovies) and salt.

*Fresh steamed cauliflower can be riced and used; however, the different texture of fresh cauliflower can often vary and may affect the texture of the dish.

DIRECTIONS

1. Wash and destem the thai basil leaves. Mince the garlic, green onions and shallots, then set aside.
2. Heat the sesame oil on medium heat in the skillet, then add the ground bison (or beef) and water.
3. Sauté and break up the bison (or beef) until well cooked. Add in the garlic, shallot, green onions, and thai basil leaves.
4. Add in the remaining ingredients and continue to sauté until all ingredients are well coated in sauce. Increase the heat to reduce the sauce. Lower the heat to warm when done.
5. In a microwavable container or pot on the stovetop, cook the frozen cauliflower per instructions.
6. If serving immediately and using the optional fried egg for garnish; In a separate small frying pan, heat with oil, crack an egg and fry until egg has reached desired doneness.
7. Plate the dish with the cauliflower ricevand bison (or beef) and top with the fried egg.

Quick Moo Shu Pork (or Chicken)

Approximate Yield	Prep Time 20 min	Estimated Macronutrients
8-10 servings	Total Time 60 min	27 g P • 28 g C • 12 g F

INGREDIENTS

1 lb. of lean ground pork or ground chicken*
1 teaspoon sesame oil
¼- ½ cup filtered water*
3 cups shredded cabbage (it can be purple, green or a mix of both)
2 cups shredded carrots
5-6 shiitake mushrooms, washed and julienned or wood ear mushrooms rehydrated and chopped in thin strips
6 green onions, cut thinly
½ large yellow onion or 1 whole small yellow onion chopped thinly
3 cloves minced garlic
3 eggs (beaten)

Optional:
1 cup of julienned celery (cut diagonally) for added texture

Sauce

3-5 tablespoons Honey Hoisin Sauce (see recipe page 124)
2 tablespoons tamari or No Soy Sauce (see recipe page 121 and notes) *
⅛ teaspoon white pepper
Salt and pepper to taste

Condiments, Complementary or Alternative Sides

Plum Sauce (see recipe page 125)
Asian Style Green Onion Wraps (see recipe page 308) or butter leaf lettuce cups
Steamed cauliflower or heart of palm rice

KITCHEN EQUIPMENT

Large and deep non-stick skillet or sauté pan
Heat resistant meat masher/mincing tool
2 small to medium bowls
Egg pan and spatula if cooking the egg separately

SPECIAL INSTRUCTIONS/DIET INFORMATION

*In traditional Moo Shu Pork thin slices of pork are used however, to minimize fat and for convenience this recipe calls for lean ground pork or chicken.
*The amount of water used is dependent of the fat percentage of the meat, the leaner the meat the more water may be needed.
*Check the labels of the tamari, many will list rice wine vinegar and other ingredients which may be illegal when following SCD. Tamari should generally be gluten free, grain free, and sugar free. For example, tamari includes only water, organic soybeans, salt and/or organic alcohol (as part of fermentation process).
*If using No Soy Sauce (see recipe page 121) to substitute tamari, you may want to reduce the amount of honey in the recipe. This is based on personal taste and is due to the sweetness of the No Soy Sauce.

DIRECTIONS

1. In a small bowl whisk all the ingredients for the sauce and set aside.
2. Beat the eggs with a fork in a separate bowl and set aside.
3. In the large skillet on medium- high heat, add the sesame oil, the ground pork and water, breaking up the meat into small bits.
4. Once the pork is cooked add the garlic, mushrooms, (optional celery) and yellow onions, stirring until the vegetables are cooked (the mushrooms are softer, and the onion lost some opaqueness).
5. Then add the sauce, cabbage, carrots, and green onions. Note you don't want these vegetables to become too overcooked if you like a bit fresher and crunchier texture.

DIRECTIONS (continued)

There are two ways to add the eggs:

- The "Quick Way": Which is to push the meat and veggies to one side of the pan and add the eggs, scrambling them, then folding them back into the meat and vegetables.
- The "Separate Way": This method is best for someone who has an egg allergy and cannot eat eggs but other people sharing the dish can eat eggs. Using a well-oiled, heated, non-stick egg pan, pour the eggs into a thin layer and rotate the pan as you would a crepe or omelet. Flip the eggs over with a spatula and remove from heat. Then cut into thin strips to serve as garnish for the top of the moo shu pork.

6. After cooking and adding in the eggs, you can taste if additional salt and pepper is needed. Note, the moo shu filling is not overly flavorful to prevent overwhelming the tastebuds when the plum sauce is added.

7. Then remove the moo shu filling from heat and be ready to serve. Assemble the moo shu wraps, by spooning a thin layer of plum sauce, and adding the moo shu pork on top. Since the wraps are small you may need to fold and eat like a taco instead of the wraps being traditionally folded like a crepe.

8. You can also eat the moo shu pork with butter leaf lettuce leaves, over steamed cauliflower rice, or heart of palm rice topped with plum sauce.

Beef Bahn Mi Bowl

Approximate Yield	Prep Time 15 min	Estimated Macronutrients
1-3 servings	Total Time 30 min	33 g P • 25 g C • 17 g F

INGREDIENTS

Beef

8 oz of leftover cooked Best Darn Tri Tip (sliced thin) or shaved Bulgogi Beef (see recipes page 238 & 226)
¼ cup Mango Habanero Sauce (see recipe page 135)
2 tablespoon lime juice
Salt and pepper to taste

Plating and Garnishes

1 cup of frozen cauliflower rice (steamed)*
Sliced jalapenos (deseeded and sliced thin) approximately 3-5 slices
¼ - ½ cup shredded matchstick carrots
¼ - ½ cup sliced cucumbers
¼ - ½ Pickled Red Onion (see recipe page 200)
Fresh cilantro
Cilantro Ranch Jalapeno Dressing (see recipe page 115)

KITCHEN EQUIPMENT

Sauté pan or medium skillet
Heat resistant spatula
Measuring spoons & measuring cups
Microwavable glass dish with lid

SPECIAL INSTRUCTIONS/DIET INFORMATION

*Fresh steamed cauliflower can be riced and used; however, the different texture of fresh cauliflower can often vary and may affect the texture of the dish.

DIRECTIONS

1. Cut and measure recommended garnishes and set aside.
2. In the sauté pan or skillet on medium heat, add the beef and all other sauce ingredients. Stirring and coating the beef with sauce and carmelizing it. Remove from heat and set aside.
3. Steam the cauliflower rice per package instructions in the microwavable glass dish.
4. Assemble the bowl with cauliflower rice, topped with beef and garnish with the recommended garnishes.

Orange Ginger Chicken

Approximate Yield	Prep Time 20 min	Estimated Macronutrients
3-4 servings	Total Time 45 min	54 g P • 31 g C • 6 g F

This recipe provides instructions for both wok frying and air frying.

INGREDIENTS

1 ½ - 2 lb. of skinless and boneless chicken breast tenderloins cut into 1-inch pieces
2 tablespoons almond flour *
2 tablespoons cooked Yellow Split Pea Flour (see recipe page 304) *
⅓ cup + 1 tablespoon neutral vegetable oil
⅛ teaspoon sea salt
1 cup of Orange Ginger Sauce (see recipe page 126)
Optional: Spray cooking oil (for air fryer method)

Garnishes & Complementary Sides
2-3 sliced green onions
Steamed cauliflower rice or Bison Fried Rice (see recipe page 202)
¼ teaspoon sesame seeds

KITCHEN EQUIPMENT

1 Large gallon size plastic zip top bag or large bowl
Measuring spoons & measuring cups
Cast iron or large skillet
Metal spatula
Large metal wok
Air Fryer with tray/basket
Paper towels or baking parchment on a plate
Tongs
Meat thermometer
Small pot

SPECIAL INSTRUCTIONS/DIET INFORMATION
*SCD legal lentil flour or coconut flour can be substituted however the texture and taste may change.

DIRECTIONS

1. In a large gallon plastic zip top bag or large bowl dredge the cut chicken tenderloins, with almond flour, pea flour and salt. Ensuring all chicken pieces are evenly coated.
2. Tip: You do not need to pat the chicken dry beforehand as the moisture from the chicken allows the pea flour to stick.

Wok Fried Method

3. In the cast iron or large skillet heat the oil on medium high. (You want the oil to bubble if testing with the end of a wooden spoon)
4. Place the pieces of chicken in the oil and be sure not to crowd them. You will likely need to fry the chicken in small batches based on the size of your skillet/cast iron pan.
5. Fry the chicken on one side for 3-5 minutes (this depends on the size of the chicken pieces) You will want the edges of the chicken to be slightly golden and crispy. Then turn the pieces over and continue to fry until all sides are a light golden color.
6. Remove from the skillet and lay on the plate covered in paper towels or parchment. If you need to confirm the chicken is cooked through, use a meat thermometer and check if the internal temp is 165 F.
7. Continue this process until all chicken is fried.
8. Heat the wok and a tablespoon of neutral oil on medium to high heat. Tip: If you sprinkle a couple drops of water and it bubbles and steams then you know the wok and oil are hot enough.
9. Add in the Orange Ginger Sauce, allow it to simmer and steam. Essentially you are trying to reduce the sauce down a bit, then add in the fried chicken. Using the metal spatula continuously stir and toss the chicken in the wok til the pieces are well coated in sauce and the sauce is reduced. The chicken will appear glossy and sticky.

DIRECTIONS (continued)

Air Fryer Method

10. If using the air fryer set the temp to 375 degrees F, spread a piece of foil over the basket and spread out the dredged chicken thigh pieces evenly. You will likely need to work in small batches so as not to crowd the pieces and allow them to crisp.

11. Lightly spray the pieces with neutral oil. Air fry for 6-9 minutes (depending on the size and thickness of pieces), flip them, continue to air fry for 4-6 minutes. When the internal temp of the chicken is 165 degrees F remove and start another batch. When all chicken pieces are air fried you can place them back on the fryer tray or in the oven on low heat to stay warm.

12. On the stove top in a small pot, heat the Orange Ginger Sauce to a simmer and allow to reduce to a thicker consistency.

13. In a large bowl toss air fried chicken with some of the warm Orange Ginger Sauce, but do not overcoat as the chicken may not stay crispy.

14. For ALL methods, top the chicken with the recommended garnishes. Serve with cauliflower rice, bison fried rice (see recipe page 202) or alongside favorite vegetables.

Habanero Mango Lime Cod

Approximate Yield	Prep Time 15 min	Estimated Macronutrients
6-10 servings	Total Time 30 min	30 g P • 14 g C • 4 g F

INGREDIENTS

2-4 fresh cod fillets (about 5-6 oz each)

⅓ cups of the Mango Habanero Sauce (see recipe page 135)

1 tablespoon minced garlic

1 lime (½ lime reserved for lime juice and ½ the lime sliced into thin rounds)

½ teaspoon salt

¼ teaspoon ground black pepper

1 teaspoon dried cilantro

1 tablespoon olive oil

Dash of paprika

Flaked sea salt and fresh ground pepper to taste

Olive oil for greasing baking dish/roaster

KITCHEN EQUIPMENT

Large glass rectangular baking dish or large roasting pan

Heat-resistant fork, tongs or spatula

Meat basting brush or spoon

Meat thermometer

Measuring spoons & measuring cups

Small bowl

DIRECTIONS

1. Preheat oven to 400 degrees F. Coat the bottom of the baking dish/roaster with olive oil.
2. Mix all the sauce, olive oil, minced garlic, lime juice and spices (except the sea salt and cracked pepper) in the small bowl or measuring cup.
3. Lay the cod filets in the baking dish/roaster (skin side down if there is skin) Coat the filets with the marinade and lay a lime slice on top of each filet.
4. Cover the entire baking dish/roaster with foil and place in oven. Roast for 12-15 minutes. Remove the foil and roast for another 2-5 minutes. Continue baking til the internal temp is 145 degrees F. Remove from oven and serve hot.

Cod Ceviche

Approximate Yield	**Prep Time 15 min**	**Estimated Macronutrients**
1-3 servings	**Total Time 30 min**	**20 g P • 20 g C • 12 g F**

This is a ceviche made with cooked, not raw cod.

INGREDIENTS

3- 6 oz of leftover Habanero Mango Lime Cod (see recipe page 234)
¼ cup red onion diced
¼ cup cucumber diced
1 avocado, skin and seed removed then diced
½ tomato diced
3 tablespoons lime juice
1 teaspoon dried cilantro or 2 tablespoons fresh cilantro
Salt and pepper to taste
Optional:
½ jalapeno (deseeded and diced)
1 tablespoon SCD Salsa Restaurant Style (see recipe page 137)

KITCHEN EQUIPMENT
Medium bowl or container with airtight lid
Measuring spoons & cups
Large spoon or spatula

DIRECTIONS

1. In a medium mixing bowl, stir together all the vegetables, lime juice. salsa, and other ingredients except the cod.
2. Remove the skin and/or bones from the leftover cooked Habanero Mango Lime Cod. Chop the filet into small pieces and add to the mixing bowl with other ingredients. Toss lightly and coat well with sauce.
3. Cover and refrigerate for 30 minutes to marinate.

Ground Turkey Tacos

Approximate Yield	Prep Time 10 min	Estimated Macronutrients
10-12 servings	**Total Time 30 min**	**16 g P • 2 g C • 5 g F**

INGREDIENTS

2 tablespoons olive oil

20 oz ground turkey (or chicken)

4 tablespoons dehydrated minced onion flakes or ½ a cup fresh minced onion

1 cup bone broth or filtered water

2- 3 tablespoons Taco Seasonings (see recipe page 147)

1 teaspoon paprika (for color)

Cayenne or ground chipotle pepper to taste

Sea salt and pepper to taste

Garnishes and Complementary Sides

Pumpkin Street Tortillas (see recipe page 307)

Lime Cauliflower Rice (see recipe page 198)

Shredded lettuce

Shredded monterey jack and cheddar cheese*

Fresh chopped cilantro

SCD Restaurant Style Salsa (see recipe page 137)

Dripped SCD Yogurt (see recipe page 298)

KITCHEN EQUIPMENT

Large non-stick skillet

Handheld meat chopper, mincer or heat-resistant spatula

Large heat-resistant spoon or spatula*

Measuring spoons & cups

SPECIAL INSTRUCTIONS/DIET INFORMATION

* Once the meat is broken up and cooked, it's a best practice to change out the spatula used in raw preparation for a new one to prevent cross contamination.

* Cheeses should be aged over 3 months, and contain zero carbohydrates or sugars, regarding nutritional content. Pre-sliced and pre-shredded cheese will likely contain illegal ingredients to prevent the cheese from sticking and prolong shelf life. It is always best to purchase blocks of cheese, then shred, grate, crumble or slice yourself.

DIRECTIONS

1. Heat the olive oil in the skillet on medium heat, then add the ground turkey or chicken, and water (or bone broth). Using the meat mincer or spatula, breaking up the meat into small bits.
2. Continue to sauté and break up the turkey. While the water is still in the skillet add in the onion, and seasonings stirring to ensure the meat is well coated. Once the meat is cooked, taste to see if more salt, pepper, or spice is needed.
3. Lower the heat on the stovetop to warm when done.
4. Remove from heat and serve or use the taco meat in other recipes or meals.

Sweet & Spicy Cowboy Chicken

Approximate Yield	**Prep Time 10 min**	**Estimated Macronutrients**
4-6 servings	**Total Time 45 min**	23 g P • 13 g C • 5 g F

This recipe provides instruction for both oven and air fryer.

INGREDIENTS
1 teaspoon Cilantro Onion Rub (see recipe page 147) *
1 lime, juiced
1 lb. of boneless and skinless chicken thighs
½ cup of Cowboy Candy (see recipe page 171) *
Avocado oil spray

KITCHEN EQUIPMENT
Measuring spoons
Heat resistant fork, tongs or spatula
Aluminum foil or baking parchment paper
Air fryer or oven
Baking sheet or air fryer tray/basket

SPECIAL INSTRUCTIONS/DIET INFORMATION
*Note the amount of spice used is to taste, as once the chicken thighs are cooked you can always sprinkle them with more seasoning.

DIRECTIONS
1. Preheat both oven or air fryer to 400 degrees F. Prepare a baking sheet or air fryer tray with parchment paper or aluminum foil.
2. If using the oven, spread out the chicken thighs on a baking sheet lined with parchment paper or foil. Spray the chicken with avocado oil, coat with lime juice and sprinkle with cilantro onion rub.
3. Bake the chicken for 30 minutes, then brush with the leftover cowboy candy sauce and place the jalapenos on top of each thigh. Finish baking the chicken another 10-15 min until internal temperature is 165 degrees F. Serve hot.
4. If using the air fryer, line the tray with foil, and spread the chicken thighs out. Coat them with avocado spray, lime juice and cilantro onion rub. Air fry them at 400 degrees F for 10-12 minutes depending on desired crispness. Turn the chicken over halfway through and bake another 9 minutes. Brush the chicken with the leftover cowboy candy sauce and top with jalapenos then finish frying for another 5-10 min (or until internal temperature of the thighs are 165 degrees F). Serve hot.

Best Darn Tri Tip Marinade

Approximate Yield	Prep Time 20 min	Estimated Macronutrients
6-10 servings	Total Time 3 hours	35 g P • 2 g C • 24 g F
	(To allow for marinating)	

This recipe provides instruction for both outdoor grill and oven.

INGREDIENTS
2- 3 lbs. of tri tip, trimmed of excess fat

Marinade

½ cup of tamari or No Soy Sauce (see recipe page 121 and notes) *
¼ cup of olive oil
12 cloves of garlic finely minced
1 tablespoon of finely ground black pepper

KITCHEN EQUIPMENT
Large gallon size plastic zip top bag or large metal bowl
Large measuring cup or small bowl
Heat resistant tongs or spatula
Measuring spoons & measuring cups
Meat thermometer
BBQ or Oven
Oven method: Large roasting pan and large stovetop pan

SPECIAL INSTRUCTIONS / DIET INFORMATION
*Check the labels of the tamari, many will list rice wine vinegar and other ingredients which may be illegal when following SCD. Tamari should generally be gluten free, grain free, and sugar free. For example, tamari includes only water, organic soybeans, salt and/or organic alcohol (as part of fermentation process).
*If using No Soy Sauce to substitute tamari, the flavor profile will be sweeter and more acidic.

DIRECTIONS
1. Peel and finely mince the garlic cloves. Add the cloves to measuring cup or small bowl. Measure out each of the remaining marinade ingredients and add to the bowl/cup. Stir and mix all ingredients well.
2. Place beef in large bowl or plastic zip top bag, pour the marinade over the meat and seal or cover bowl with plastic wrap. Refrigerate for 1-3 hours.
3. Remove the marinated tri-tip from refrigerator an hour before cooking.
4. BBQing over a charcoal or propane grill is the preferred method of cooking. Preheat the grill before adding the meat. Turn and flip the tri tip regularly to prevent burning. (Note the honey and balsamic vinegar in the No Soy Sauce may cause more charring on the outside than tamari.)
5. Approximately 20 -35 minutes to cook based on meat size and preferred level of doneness. Utilize a meat thermometer and check the meat's internal temperature until it reaches 135-145 degrees F (medium rare- medium) Remove from the oven and tent with foil allowing it to rest before slicing against the grain and serving.
6. If you do not have a BBQ grill, then an oven can be utilized. Preheat the oven to 350 degrees F. Heat large skillet/ pan on the stovetop with high heat, then add the tri tip, searing and browning the outside. Once browned, place in the roasting pan.
7. Roast in the oven for about 10 minutes per pound (approximately 20-30 minutes). Utilize a meat thermometer and check the meat's internal temperature until it reaches 135-145 degrees F (medium rare- medium) and/or desired doneness. Remove from the oven and tent with foil allowing it to rest before slicing against the grain and serving.

California Cheesesteak Bowl

Approximate Yield	Prep Time 15 min	Estimated Macronutrients
2-4 servings	Total Time 30 min	35 g P • 30 g C • 28 g F

This recipe provides instruction for both oven and air frying.

INGREDIENTS

Steak

8 oz-12 oz of cooked, sliced thin leftover Best Darn Tri Tip

(see recipe page 238)

2 cups of frozen bell pepper medley

2 cups of cremini or baby bella mushrooms

1 cup sliced onions

1 tablespoon olive oil

Salt and pepper to taste

Serve with

1 bag (16 oz) of frozen butternut squash or 2 ½- 3 cups of fresh butternut squash, peeled and cut into small cubes

1 cup shredded pepper jack or monterey jack cheese*

¼ - ½ cup Creamy Chipotle Dressing (see recip

KITCHEN EQUIPMENT

Large pan/skillet

Air fryer or oven

Aluminum foil

Measuring spoons & measuring cups

Air fryer basket or baking sheet

Heat resistant spatula

SPECIAL INSTRUCTIONS/DIET INFORMATION

*Cheeses should be aged over 3 months, and contain zero carbohydrates or sugars, regarding nutritional content. Pre-sliced and pre-shredded cheese will likely contain illegal ingredients to prevent the cheese from sticking and prolong shelf life. It is always best to purchase blocks of cheese, then shred, grate, crumble or slice yourself.

DIRECTIONS

1. In the air fryer, spray the butternut squash with oil and then fry the butternut squash at 400 degrees F for 20-22 minutes (fresh may require less time). Remove when the squash edges are crisp and inside tender when pierced with a fork. Set aside.

2. If using an oven preheat the oven 450 degrees F. Line a baking sheet with aluminum foil and spray with olive oil. Lay the butternut squash on the baking sheet, spray or brush the tops of the squash with oil and place on the lowest rack of the oven. Bake for 25-30 minutes (fresh may require less time), turn the butternut squash over with a spatula mid-way through the cooking process. Remove when the squash edges are caramelized and inside tender when pierced with a fork.

3. In the pan on medium heat, add onions, mushrooms, and bell peppers sauteing with olive oil. Once the vegetables are cooked, add in the leftover sliced tri tip to reheat. You can also sprinkle the cheese over the meat and vegetables to melt before serving.

4. Assemble the bowl with the butternut squash, top with beef, cooked vegetables and garnish with the recommended dressing.

Easy Oven Lemon Baked Salmon

Approximate Yield 6-10 servings	**Prep Time 15 min** **Total Time 30 min**	**Estimated Macronutrients** 12 g P • 5 g C • 11 g F

INGREDIENTS

4- 6 salmon fillets (about 5-6 oz each)
1 lemon (1/2 lemon juiced, the other half sliced in 4-6 thin rounds)
2 ½ tablespoons of olive oil
3 teaspoons minced garlic
2 tablespoons Greek Spice Rub (see recipe page 150)
Flaked sea salt and fresh ground pepper to taste
Olive oil for greasing baking dish/roaster

KITCHEN EQUIPMENT

Large glass rectangular baking dish or large roasting pan
Measuring cups & spoons
Heat resistant spatula
Meat basting brush or spoon
Meat thermometer
Small bowl or large measuring cup

DIRECTIONS

1. Preheat oven to 400 degrees F. Coat the bottom of the baking dish/roaster with olive oil.
2. Mix all the olive oil, minced garlic, Greek Spice Rub, and lemon juice in a small bowl or measuring cup.
3. Lay the salmon filets in the baking dish/roaster (skin side down if there is skin). Coat the filets with the marinade and lay a lemon slice on top of each filet.
4. Cover the entire baking dish/roaster with foil and place in oven. Roast for 12-15 minutes. Remove the foil roast for another 2-5 minutes. Continue baking until the internal temp is 145 degrees F. Remove from oven and serve hot.

Marinated Shrimp

Approximate Yield	**Prep Time 20 min**	**Estimated Macronutrients**
3-6 servings	**Total Time 60 min**	33 g P • 3 g C • 10 g F
	(To allow for marinating)	

INGREDIENTS

16 oz (or approximately 21) cooked, peeled and deveined medium to large shrimp (if using frozen defrost)

Marinade-Dressing
¼ cup olive oil
½ cup of red wine vinegar*
2 tablespoons of dijon mustard*
2 teaspoons red pepper flakes
1 teaspoon honey
1 tablespoon dried parsley or ¼ cup fresh parsley chopped
¼ cup of minced shallot or red onion
2-3 cloves finely minced garlic
Salt and pepper to taste

KITCHEN EQUIPMENT

Large bowl or container with airtight lid
Measuring spoons & measuring cups
Spatula or large spoon

SPECIAL INSTRUCTIONS

*Always confirm vinegars do not include added illegal sugars.
*There are a few commercial brands of mustard made with SCD legal ingredients. However always check ingredients carefully. Confirm with the company and determine unlisted ingredients are not being used in the manufacturing process.

DIRECTIONS

1. In a large mixing bowl, combine all dressing ingredients. Add in the shrimp, toss and coat well.
2. Cover and refrigerate for 30 minutes to an hour. Serve cold as a protein source with salad or side dish.

Bison Sloppy Joes

Approximate Yield	**Prep Time 20 min**	**Estimated Macronutrients**
6-8 servings	Total Time 55 min	19 g P • 16 g C • 11 g F

INGREDIENTS

20 oz of ground bison or lean ground beef
16 oz of frozen pepper medley or 2 cups of chopped fresh bell peppers
16 oz frozen chopped spinach
1 ¼ cup water
¼ cup of dried minced onion or ½ cup of chopped fresh onion
2 tablespoons olive oil
2 tablespoons honey
1 teaspoon granulated garlic or 1 tablespoon fresh minced garlic
¼ cup and 2 tablespoons tomato paste*
¼ cup of favorite SCD legal ketchup or use homemade Ketchup (see recipe page 117) *
1 ½ teaspoon of yellow mustard*
½ teaspoon salt
¼ teaspoon ground black pepper
Optional: 1 cup of finely diced mushrooms*

Serving Options:

6-8 "Sourdough" Buns (see recipe page 312)
12 oz steamed cauliflower rice

KITCHEN EQUIPMENT

Large skillet
Measuring spoons & measuring cups
Handheld meat chopper, mincer or heat-resistant spatula
Large heat resistant spoon or spatula

SPECIAL INSTRUCTIONS/DIET INFORMATION

*There are a couple brands manufacturing SCD legal ketchup. You can also make your own ketchup using the recipe on page 117.
*There are a few commercial brands of mustard made with SCD legal ingredients. However always check ingredients carefully. Confirm with the company and determine unlisted ingredients are not being used in the manufacturing process.
*Canned tomatoes are typically not allowed under SCD. However, there are Italian brands of canned tomatoes and tomato pastes with no artificial flavors, preservatives or additives listed as ingredients, nor used in the manufacturing process. These brands are generally sold through Wellbees and a few other stores. Read store bought canned tomato and tomato paste labels carefully. If necessary, you can make your own tomato sauce or paste using fresh tomatoes or canned tomato juice (if salt is the only other ingredient).

DIRECTIONS

1. Heat the olive oil in the pan/skillet on medium heat, then sauté the mushrooms (optional), frozen spinach and bell peppers. Stirring regularly to prevent burning of the vegetables. When all vegetables are cooked remove from the pan and set aside.

2. Using the same pan on medium heat, add the bison or lean ground beef and pour 1 cup of water over the meat. Use a meat mincer or spatula, break up the clumps of meat in the water. Allow the meat to cook, until no red or pink is seen. Replace the meat chopper or spatula with a clean one. Then add/stir in the vegetables and all other ingredients.

3. Allow the mixture to simmer and reducing the liquid in the sloppy joe sauce. Stirring well until desired thickness and both meat and vegetables are well coated in sauce. Serve warm as a sloppy joe on a bun, or over steamed cauliflower rice.

Best Darn Oven Fried Chicken

Approximate Yield 6-8 servings	**Prep Time 40 min** **Total Time 90 min**	**Estimated Macronutrients** 24 g P • 14 g C • 10 g F

This recipe provides an alternative instruction for roasting in the oven.

INGREDIENTS

1 lb. of boneless skinless chicken thighs or chicken breast tenderloins
½ cup of SCD legal pickle juice or use filtered Quick Dill Pickle juice (see recipe page 182) *
¼ cup filtered water
2 tablespoons of Best Darn Rub (see recipe page 150)
2 beaten eggs
½ cup of unsweetened cashew or coconut milk (¼ cup of SCD Nonfat Greek Yogurt can be substituted for nut milk) *
½ cup of almond flour*
2 heaping tablespoons dried/dehydrated whole egg powder

Avocado oil or virgin coconut oil if frying
Spray oil if baking

KITCHEN EQUIPMENT

Large baking pan or sheet (for oven fried chicken) or air fryer tray/basket
Medium mixing bowl
Measuring spoons & measuring cups
Heat resistant tongs or spatula

2 Large gallon size plastic zip top bag
Oven or Air fryer

SPECIAL INSTRUCTIONS/DIET INFORMATION

* SCD legal pickles should not include any sweeteners, vague ingredients, and/or additives. The pickle ingredients used in this recipe included cucumber, water, salt, distilled white vinegar, gar-lic, dill weed, dill seed, mustard seed, caraway seed, calcium chloride (a natural salt), fennel seed, mace, and turmeric. If you are unable to source SCD legal pickles use the following Quick Dill Pickles, see recipe page 182.
*You can cut the almond flour with 2 tablespoons of Yellow Split Pea Flour (see recipe page 304).
*If you are unable to eat or source dried whole egg powder you can replace with almond flour (or coconut) however the texture will be different, and there will be higher fat and less protein for the macronutrients.
*Any nut milks should only consist of nuts, water, or salt. No emulsifiers, gums, sweeteners or additives should be in the ingredient list. If you are unable to source a SCD legal nut milk you can make them easily at home (see recipe page 299).

DIRECTIONS

1. In a large gallon plastic zip top bag marinate the chicken thighs or tenderloins with the water and pickle juice. Marinate 30 min to 2 hrs.
2. If baking, preheat the oven to 450 degrees F, and line a sheet pan with parchment paper. If air frying, preheat to 375 degrees F.
3. In a large gallon size plastic bag mix well/shake the almond flour, Best Darn Rub Chicken seasoning and dried egg together. (You can also mix the ingredients in a large bowl)
4. In a medium mixing bowl beat the eggs and cashew milk (or yogurt) and set aside.
5. Dip the chicken thighs or tenderloins in the beaten egg and cashew milk, then dredge in almond flour mixture using the gallon plastic zip top bag and shake the chicken until coated. Or dredge the chicken in the large bowl, until covered in almond flour and spice mixture.
6. For oven method: Place parchment on a large baking sheet and then the coated chicken. Bake for 12 min and then flip and spray with oil for another 10-15 min or until internal temp is 165 degrees F.
7. For air frying: Line the basket or tray with parchment or foil (if using foil, spray the foil with cooking spray). Lay the chicken on the foil, and lightly spray the top of the chicken with oil. Air fry the chicken for 12 minutes then flip the chicken over, spray and cook for another 6-8 minutes.

Easy Chicken Crust Pizza

Approximate Yield	**Prep Time 10 min**	**Estimated Macronutrients**
10-12 servings	**Total Time 60 min**	**10 g P • 7 g C • 10 g F**

INGREDIENTS

1 (12.5 oz) cooked and shredded white chicken meat (if canned, drained of water) or 1 ¼ cups of leftover shredded **Roasted Chicken (see recipe page 255)** *

2 eggs (beaten)

1 tablespoon coconut or Yellow Pea Flour (see recipe page 304) *

⅛ teaspoon sea salt

½ teaspoon Italian Herb Blend (see recipe page 152)

½ teaspoon olive oil

¼ cup finely grated parmesan cheese*

KITCHEN EQUIPMENT

Parchment paper
Large baking sheet
Medium mixing bowl
Measuring spoons & measuring cups
Spatula or large spoon
Recommended: Pizza stone

SPECIAL INSTRUCTIONS/DIET INFORMATION

*Verify all ingredients and manufacturing processes for commercially canned chicken. The canned chicken used in this recipe included only chicken, salt and water.

*Parmesan cheese can be omitted if necessary, however is recommended for the best texture.

* Cheeses should be aged over 3 months, and contain zero carbohydrates or sugars, regarding nutritional content. Pre-sliced and pre-shredded cheese will likely contain illegal ingredients to prevent the cheese from sticking and prolong shelf life. It is always best to purchase blocks of cheese, then shred, grate, crumble or slice yourself.

*When in doubt of SCD legal pizza ingredients, always refer to the book, *Breaking the Vicious Cycle: Intestinal Health Through Diet,* by Elaine Gottschall or the reference sources provided in this book.

DIRECTIONS

1. Preheat oven to 450 degrees F, (preferably with a pizza stone in the oven). Cut 3 pieces of parchment paper, about the width/size of a personal pizza.
2. Mix all ingredients well in the medium mixing bowl.
3. Oil your hands with olive oil and form 2 balls of dough. Using the third sheet of parchment paper on the top of the dough, press and flatten the balls into personal pizzas on the other two pieces of paper.
4. Place the two pizza crusts with the underlying parchment paper in the oven on the pizza stone or baking sheet.
5. Bake for 15-20 min until the crusts are firm and edges are golden. Remove the crust from the oven and allow to cool for 10 minutes. This is a good point to freeze the crusts for later use; place the baking sheet with the crusts in the freezer. Once crusts are frozen, wrap the crusts in fresh parchment paper and store in airtight freezer bags.
6. When ready to eat pizza, top with favorite SCD legal pizza toppings and bake at 450 degrees F for 5-8 minutes.

Chicken and Spaghetti Squash Pizza Crust

Approximate Yield	**Prep Time 10 min**	**Estimated Macronutrients**
10-12 servings	**Total Time 60 min**	**13 g P • 12 g C • 10 g F**

INGREDIENTS

12.5 oz cooked and shredded white chicken meat (if canned, drained of water) or 1 cup of leftover shredded Roasted Chicken (see recipe page 255) *
1 cup of roasted leftover Roasted Spaghetti Squash (see recipe page 177)
2 eggs (beaten)
1 ½ tablespoons coconut flour
Pinch of sea salt
¼ teaspoon Italian Herb blend (see recipe page 153)
Optional: ½ cup of grated parmesan cheese*
½ teaspoon olive oil

KITCHEN EQUIPMENT

Parchment paper
Large baking sheet
Large mixing bowl
Measuring spoons & measuring cups
Spatula or large spoon
Recommended: Pizza stone
Oven

SPECIAL INSTRUCTIONS/DIET INFORMATION

*Verify all ingredients and manufacturing processes for commercially canned chicken. The canned chicken used in this recipe included only chicken, salt and water.
*When in doubt of SCD legal pizza ingredients, always refer to the book, *Breaking the Vicious Cycle: Intestinal Health Through Diet,* by Elaine Gottschall or the reference sources provided in this book.
*Cheeses should be aged over 3 months, and contain zero carbohydrates or sugars, regarding nutritional content. Pre-sliced and pre-shredded cheese will likely contain illegal ingredients to prevent the cheese from sticking and prolong shelf life. It is always best to purchase blocks of cheese, then shred, grate, crumble or slice yourself.

DIRECTIONS

1. Lay the spaghetti squash either in a cheese cloth or thick paper towels and squeeze out any excess water.
2. Place the spaghetti squash in the mixing bowl along with all other ingredients and stir well.
3. Preheat oven to 450 degrees F, preferably preheating a pizza stone already in the oven. Cut 3 pieces of parchment paper, about the width/size of a personal pizza.
4. Mix all ingredients well in the large mixing bowl.
5. Oil your hands with olive oil and form 2 balls of dough. Using the third sheet of parchment paper on the top of the dough, press and flatten the balls into personal pizzas on the other two pieces of paper.
6. Place the two pizza crusts with the underlying parchment paper in the oven on the pizza stone or baking sheet.
7. Bake for 15-20 min until the crusts are firm and edges are golden. Remove the crust from the oven and allow to cool for 10 minutes. This is a good point to freeze the crusts for later use; place the baking sheet with the crusts in the freezer. Once crusts are frozen, wrap the crusts in fresh parchment paper and store in airtight freezer bags.
8. When ready to eat pizza, top with favorite SCD legal pizza toppings and bake at 450 degrees F for 5-8 minutes.

Shake and Bake Chicken Tenders

Approximate Yield	Prep Time 10 min	Estimated Macronutrients
6-8 servings	Total Time 45 min	20 g P • 2 g C • 6 g F

INGREDIENTS
3 tablespoons of Best Darn Rub Chicken Seasoning (see recipe page 150)
¼ cup of dried whole egg powder
½ cup of almond flour (see notes) *
1 lb. skinless and boneless chicken breast tenderloins
Spray oil

KITCHEN EQUIPMENT
Large baking pan or sheet (for oven fried chicken)
Baking parchment paper or aluminum foil
Measuring spoons & measuring cups
1 large gallon size plastic bag
Oven
Meat thermometer

SPECIAL INSTRUCTIONS/DIET INFORMATION
*You can cut the almond flour with 1-2 tablespoons of Yellow Split Pea Flour (see recipe page 304).

DIRECTIONS
1. Preheat the oven 425 degrees F and place parchment on a large baking sheet.
2. In a large gallon plastic zip top bag pour all the ingredients in the bag, except the chicken tenderloins.
3. Add the tenderloins (a few at a time) into the dredge mixture, close and shake until the chicken is well coated. Remove the chicken from the bag and place on the parchment lined baking sheet. Spacing the chicken evenly, then giving them a light spray with the oil.
4. Bake the chicken for 20-25 min then flip the chicken over halfway through, and spray with oil. Remove the chicken when the outside is light golden and internal temp is 165 degrees F.

Loaded Turkey and Veggie Spaghetti Sauce

Approximate Yield	**Prep Time 30 min**	**Estimated Macronutrients**
10-12 servings	**Total Time 60 min**	**12 g P • 16 g C • 4 g F**

INGREDIENTS

1 (16 oz) package of lean ground turkey
2 cups of finely chopped or shredded zucchini
1 cup of baby portabella mushrooms, cleaned and chopped finely
1 cup of shredded carrots
1 (28 oz) can or 3 ½ cups of crushed San Marzano or Italian tomatoes*
1 (15 oz) can or 1 ¾ cups of tomato sauce*
1 (6 oz) can or ⅔ cups of tomato paste*
¾ cup of filtered water
¼ cup of fresh or dried minced onion
6 cloves of minced garlic
2 tablespoons olive oil
2 tablespoons honey*
2 tablespoons red wine vinegar*
½ tablespoon dried basil
2 teaspoons sea salt
1 teaspoon dried oregano
¼ teaspoon ground black pepper
⅛ teaspoon ground nutmeg
⅛ teaspoon finely ground red pepper flakes

KITCHEN EQUIPMENT

Large pot
Measuring spoons & measuring cups
Meat mincer or spatula with hard edge
Heat resistant spoon or ladle
Silicone food storage freezer trays/cubes

SPECIAL INSTRUCTIONS/DIET INFORMATION

*Canned tomatoes are typically not allowed under SCD. However, there are Italian brands of canned tomatoes and tomato pastes with no artificial flavors, preservatives or additives listed as ingredients, nor used in the manufacturing process. These brands are generally sold through Wellbees and a few other stores. Read store bought canned tomato and tomato paste labels carefully. If necessary, you can make your own tomato sauce or paste using fresh tomatoes or canned tomato juice (if salt is the only other ingredient).
*Always confirm vinegars do not include added illegal sugars.
*Honey and the acid from the red wine vinegar enhances the flavor of the tomatoes and provide depth to the sauce.

DIRECTIONS

1. In a large pot on medium to high heat, add in the olive oil, ground turkey and water. Halfway through cooking the meat (minimal pink is visible) add in the vegetables; onion, garlic, chopped mushrooms, zucchini and shredded carrots.
2. When the vegetables are cooked, add in the crushed tomatoes, sauce and paste. Continue cooking until the sauce begins to bubble, and add the remaining ingredients, stirring well to blend.
3. Allow the sauce to simmer, stirring occasionally. Then salt, pepper, red wine vinegar and honey to taste as needed. Generally, it takes about an hour for all the flavors to simmer together.
4. Serve warm with favorite SCD legal noodles or use in the Traditional Lasagna (see recipe page 248) in this book.
5. For long term storage freeze the sauce in silicone food storage freezer trays/cubes with lids.

Traditional Lasagna

Approximate Yield	Prep Time 20 min	Estimated Macronutrients
10 servings	Total Time 2 hours	25 g P • 19 g C • 17 g F

INGREDIENTS

1 tablespoon olive oil

1 egg

1 separated egg white or 2 tablespoons pasteurized liquid egg white*

1 ½ cup of SCD Nonfat Greek Yogurt (see recipe of page 298 and dripped for 24 hrs.)

½ cup of grated parmesan cheese

½ tablespoon of dried basil

½ tablespoon granulated garlic

¼ teaspoon sea salt

1 (28 oz) jar approximately 4 cups of favorite SCD legal marinara or Loaded Spaghetti Sauce (see recipe on page 247)

1 lb.- 1 ½ lb. Lean ground beef or bison (Omit if using the Loaded Spaghetti Sauce)

1 long necked large butternut squash or 1 (8oz package) of yellow pea or lentil lasagna noodles (no boil) or other SCD legal noodles

½ cup of shredded monterey jack cheese*

KITCHEN EQUIPMENT

8 x 10 or 9 x 13 glass baking dish
Medium mixing bowl
Electric mixer
Large saucepan or pot
Aluminum foil

SPECIAL INSTRUCTIONS/DIET INFORMATION

* If using liquid egg whites, be careful to read all ingredients. This should be a mono ingredient, and not contain any preservatives or additives, other than pasteurized egg whites. Note the conversion is 2 tablespoons of pasteurized liquid eggs to 1 egg white.

* Cheeses should be aged over 3 months, and contain zero carbohydrates or sugars, regarding nutritional content. Pre-sliced and pre-shredded cheese will likely contain illegal ingredients to prevent the cheese from sticking and prolong shelf life. It is always best to purchase blocks of cheese, then shred, grate, crumble or slice yourself.

DIRECTIONS

1. Preheat oven to 375 degrees F and grease the baking dish with the olive oil and set aside.

2. If not using the Loaded Spaghetti Sauce recipe, then in a large pot or saucepan on medium to high heat, break up and cook the ground beef or bison. Stir in the marinara or spaghetti sauce in with the ground beef and cook until bubbling. Remove from heat and allow to chill in the refrigerator to speed up the cooling process.

3. If using butternut squash, peel the skin off, and thinly slice the long neck of the butternut squash into discs. (Avoiding the portion with the seeds). A meat slicer or spiralizer is recommended to safely achieve thinness of ⅛-¼ inch.

4. If using SCD legal noodles, follow the cooking instructions for the noodles on the package. If the instructions indicate boiling, cook the pasta and drain off the water when the noodles are al dente in texture. Ideally do not overcook the noodles since they will continue cooking in the lasagna. Note certain noodles, specifically yellow pea lasagna noodles may not require cooking before assembling in the lasagna.

5. In a medium mixing bowl combine with an electric mixer the egg, egg white, SCD yogurt, basil, salt, and granulated garlic. Then fold in the grated parmesan and set aside.

6. When the sauce has cooled, spread 1 cup of sauce on the bottom of the pan, then arrange the butternut squash or noodles.

7. Top the butternut squash or noodles with the yogurt mixture. Spread the meat sauce over the yogurt mixture, then add noodles or butternut squash. Repeat this order of layering. Topping the remaining butternut or noodles, mixture, and sauce with a light sprinkling of monterey jack cheese or optional parmesan cheese.

8. Cover in foil and bake for 55 min. Remove the foil and sprinkle the remaining shredded monterey jack cheese and bake for an additional 5-10 minutes.

9. When cheese is melted and a knife goes through the center of the lasagna easily, remove from oven and allow to cool for 10 minutes before serving.

Butternut Squash, Sage and Chicken White Lasagna

Approximate Yield 10 servings	Prep Time 20 min Total Time 2 hours	Estimated Macronutrients 21 g P • 25 g C • 12 g F

This recipe is the author's favorite for carbohydrate loading.

INGREDIENTS

White Sauce
1 ½ cup of SCD Nonfat Greek Yogurt (recipe of page 298 and dripped for 24 hrs.)
1 egg
¼ cup pasteurized liquid egg whites*
1 teaspoon honey
1 teaspoon of granulated garlic
⅛ teaspoon nutmeg
¼ teaspoon sea salt
¾ cup of grated parmesan (½ cup for white sauce + ¼ cup for top of lasagna) *
*See notes for non-dairy white sauce alternatives

Ground Chicken or Turkey Filling
1 lb.- 1 ½ lb. Lean ground chicken or turkey
2 tablespoons Italian Sage Seasoning (recipe on page 145)
1 cup water
1 tablespoon honey

Noodles
1 8oz package of SCD legal lasagna (no boil) or penne pasta (cooked and drained per directions)
If you cannot tolerate SCD legal noodles, then use thinly sliced butternut squash as a substitute and omit the Butternut squash filling (below)

Butternut squash filling
2 (15 oz) can of butternut squash or 3 ½ lbs. of cooked butternut squash that was peeled, seeded and mashed
2 tablespoons melted butter or ghee
¼ teaspoon ground nutmeg

½ teaspoon dried ground sage or ⅓ cup loosely fresh sage leaves (coarsely chopped)
Salt and pepper to taste

Olive oil for greasing baking sheet and tossing noodles

KITCHEN EQUIPMENT
8 x 10 or 9x 13 glass baking dish depending on depth
Handheld meat chopper, mincer or heat-resistant spatula
Measuring spoons & measuring cups
2 Medium mixing bowls
Heat-resistant spoon or spatula
Electric mixer
Large pan or pot
Aluminum foil

SPECIAL INSTRUCTIONS/DIET INFORMATION
*A non-dairy version of white sauce can be made with 1 ½ tablespoon cashew butter, juice from ½ a lemon, and 3-4 cups of unsweetened cashew milk.
*Be careful to read all ingredients for pasteurized liquid egg whites. This should be a mono ingredient, and not contain any preservatives or additional ingredients. Regular separated egg whites can be used but the batter will be thicker and require many eggs.
*If using raw butternut squash to substitute the noodles then you may need to cover the baking dish with foil and bake for longer to ensure the white sauce does not burn and the squash cooks through.
*Cheeses should be aged over 3 months, and contain zero carbohydrates or sugars, regarding nutritional content. Pre-sliced and pre-shredded cheese will likely contain illegal ingredients to prevent the cheese from sticking and prolong shelf life. It is always best to purchase blocks of cheese, then shred, grate, crumble or slice yourself.

DIRECTIONS
1. Preheat the oven to 350 degrees F and grease the baking dish with the olive oil and set aside.

Ground Chicken or Turkey Filling
2. In a large pan on medium to high heat, add the ground chicken or turkey and water. Sauté and break up the ground chicken or turkey with meat mincer or spatula.
3. Stir in the honey and Italian Sage Seasoning until the meat is well coated, and simmer off any remaining moisture.

Remove from heat and allow to cool when the meat is fully cooked.

Butternut "Noodles" or Buttternut Squash Filling

4. If using butternut squash as noodles, peel the skin off, and thinly slice the long neck of the butternut squash into discs. (Avoiding the portion with the seeds). A meat slicer or spiralizer is recommended to safely achieve thinness of ⅛- ¼ inch. Toss the pieces with the butter and seasonings from the butternut squash filling (listed above, omitting the pureed butternut squash). Set aside.
5. If using SCD legal noodles, in a medium mixing bowl combine all ingredients for the butternut squash filling and stir well.
6. If using SCD legal penne, cook the noodles per the package instructions. Drain off the water and toss warm with olive oil to prevent noodles from sticking together. Set aside. (If using no boil SCD legal lasagna noodles then skip this step of cooking the noodles.)

White sauce

7. For the white sauce, in a medium mixing bowl whip with the electric mixer; the egg, egg whites, SCD yogurt, nutmeg, honey, salt, and granulated garlic. Mix the ingredients well, then stir in the grated parmesan and set aside.

Assembling the lasagna

8. In the greased baking dish, layer the bottom of the dish with butternut squash filling followed by the noodles. If using butternut squash instead of noodles, add a layer of white sauce instead and layer the butternut squash slices.
9. Then add the layer of meat, followed by white sauce. Add another layer of noodles or butternut squash, meat, and repeat the process. Until the final layer of the lasagna is white sauce and sprinkle parmesan cheese over the top.
10. Bake for 50 min, covered in foil, and then remove the foil. Bake for an additional 10- 20 minutes or until the sides are crusty and top turns golden. The no bake lasagna noodles or butternut squash should be tender when sliced with a knife.

Butternut Squash Enchilada Bake

Approximate Yield	Prep Time 20 min	Estimated Macronutrients
8-10 servings	Total Time 2 hours	21 g P • 9 g C • 14 g F

INGREDIENTS

1 large, long neck butternut squash or 2 small sized long neck butternut squash

1-2 cups of shredded monterey jack cheese (for topping) *

2 cups of ready-made defrosted SCD Enchilada Sauce, or see recipe below

Cheese Filling

1 ½ cup of SCD Nonfat Greek Yogurt (recipe of page 298 and dripped for 24 hrs.)

3 eggs

1 tablespoon of granulated garlic

1 tablespoon dried parsley

1 teaspoon dried cilantro

1 cup finely crumbled cotija cheese*

Salt and pepper to taste

Ground Beef or Bison Filling

1 lb.- 1 ½ lb. Lean ground beef or bison

1 tablespoon SCD Taco Seasoning (recipe on page 147)

1 cup water

Enchilada Sauce

1-2 cups of Chicken Bone Broth (recipe on page 255 and notes below) *

1 6 oz can or ⅔ cups of tomato paste*

¼ cup of chili powder

2 tablespoon avocado or olive oil

2 tablespoons apple cider vinegar

1 teaspoon granulated garlic

1 teaspoon ground cumin

1 teaspoon fine sea salt

½ teaspoon dried oregano

Olive oil for greasing casserole or deep baking dish

KITCHEN EQUIPMENT

8 x 10 or 9x 13 glass baking dish depending on depth
Handheld meat chopper, mincer or heat-resistant spatula
Measuring spoons & measuring cups
Medium mixing bowl
Heat-resistant spoon or spatula
Electric mixer
Medium saucepan or pot
Aluminum Foil

SPECIAL INSTRUCTIONS/DIET INFORMATION

*Using 1 cup of chicken bone broth will yield a thicker enchilada sauce.

* Cheeses should be aged over 3 months, and contain zero carbohydrates or sugars, regarding nutritional content. Pre-sliced and pre-shredded cheese will likely contain illegal ingredients to prevent the cheese from sticking and prolong shelf life. It is always best to purchase blocks of cheese, then shred, grate, crumble or slice yourself.

*Canned tomatoes are typically not allowed under SCD. However, there are Italian brands of canned tomatoes and tomato pastes with no artificial flavors, preservatives or additives listed as ingredients, nor used in the manufacturing process. These brands are generally sold through Wellbees and a few other stores. Read store bought canned tomato and tomato paste labels carefully. If necessary, you can make your own tomato sauce or paste using fresh tomatoes or canned tomato juice (if salt is the only other ingredient).

DIRECTIONS

1. In a medium saucepan on medium heat, add the ground beef or bison with the water. Breaking up the meat with spatula or mincer while cooking. When the water starts simmering, stir in the taco seasoning until the meat is well coated and cook off any remaining water. Remove from heat and allow to cool.

2. For the butternut squash peel the skin off, and thinly slice the long neck of the butternut squash into discs. (Avoiding the portion with the seeds). A meat slicer, mandolin or spiralizer is recommended to safely achieve thinness of ⅛ -¼ inch. Set aside.

3. Preheat oven to 350 degrees F and grease the baking dish with the olive oil and set aside.

4. In a medium mixing bowl, combine all the ingredients (except for the cotija cheese) with an electric mixer. Then stir in the crumbled cotija and set aside.

5. In a medium saucepan or pot, combine all ingredients for the enchilada sauce.
6. In the greased baking dish, layer the bottom of the dish with a little enchilada sauce followed by a thin layer of butternut squash.
7. Then add the layer of meat, followed by cheese mixture. Add another layer of butternut squash and repeat the process. For the final layer pour the remaining enchilada sauce over all of it and sprinkle the top with shredded monterey jack cheese.
8. Bake for 40-45 min until the sides are crusty and the cheese turns golden. If you find the cheese is getting too brown, then loosely cover with foil during the baking process. The butternut squash should be tender when sliced with a knife.

Classic Beef Pot Roast

Approximate Yield	Prep Time 20 min	Estimated Macronutrients
10-12 servings	Total Time 4-10 hours	11 g P • 14 g C • 5 g F
	(To allow for slow cooking)	

This recipe includes instructions for both oven and slow cooker.

INGREDIENTS

1 chuck roast (bone in or boneless) trimmed of excess fat (3-4 lbs.) *
1-2 tablespoons olive oil
¼ teaspoon ground black pepper
¼ teaspoon sea salt
1 yellow onion coarsely chopped
4 garlic cloves, peeled and minced
1 cup of dry red wine
¾ teaspoon dried thyme leaves
2 cups of SCD legal beef bone broth or use Beef Bone Broth or Roasted Chicken Broth (see recipes on pages 255 & 302)
4 large carrots, peeled and cut diagonally in 1-inch pieces
4 celery stalks, washed and cut diagonally in 1-inch pieces
2 tablespoons Worcestershire Sauce (see recipe page 120)
2 tablespoons tomato paste *
2 whole bay leaves
8 white or baby bella whole mushrooms, washed, destemmed and chopped into large halves or quarters
Salt & pepper to taste

KITCHEN EQUIPMENT

Large meat forks or tongs
Parchment paper
Large dishwasher safe plate or platter (large enough to fit the roast on)
Heat resistant spoon or spatula
Large 4 Qt Dutch oven with lid (check that the roast will fit in it)
Heat resistant potholders
Meat thermometer
Oven
Stovetop
Measuring spoons
Paper towels
Ladle or large spoon
Optional: Large stove top pan and crockpot/ slow cooker
Non latex food service gloves (to wear when handling raw meat) *

SPECIAL INSTRUCTIONS/DIET INFORMATION

* Bone in chuck roast bone can be used later for bone broth.
*Canned tomatoes are typically not allowed under SCD. However, there are Italian brands of canned tomatoes and tomato pastes with no artificial flavors, preservatives or additives listed as ingredients, nor used in the manufacturing process. These brands are generally sold through Wellbees and a few other stores. Read store bought canned tomato and tomato paste labels carefully. If necessary, you can make your own tomato sauce or paste using fresh tomatoes or canned tomato juice (if salt is the only other ingredient).
*Important note: Regardless of using gloves always follow best food safety practices to prevent cross contamination and food born illness when cooking with raw meat. See notes on Hygiene and General Food Safety on page 30.

DIRECTIONS

Dutch Oven Method

1. Preheat oven to 350 degrees F. Measure out ingredients and prepare vegetables ahead of time.
2. On the stovetop, heat the olive oil on medium heat in the large Dutch oven. Place parchment paper on the platter or large dish, put the roast on top of the paper and pat dry with paper towels. Salt and pepper each side of the chuck roast liberally.

3. Place the roast in the dutch oven and discard the parchment paper. Cook the roast for about 5-7 minutes and turning to brown each side. Remove the roast from the dutch oven and place on platter.

4. Add the onion and garlic to the dutch oven and sauté for 6-8 minutes or until tender. Scraping the bottom well and reduce heat to prevent burning.

5. Return the browned roast to the dutch oven. Then add the red wine, thyme, beef broth, 1 tablespoon of Worcestershire, 1 tablespoon of tomato paste, and bay leaves.

6. Bring to a simmer on the stovetop. Then cover with the lid and using potholders (since sometimes people forget how hot dutch oven handles can be) place in oven for 1 ½ hours and the roast is near tender.

7. At 1 ½ hours, add in the chopped carrots and celery, then cover and roast for another 30 minutes.

8. At the end of 30 minutes, add the mushrooms, remaining Worcestershire, and tomato paste. Bake for another 30- 45 minutes or until meat and vegetables are tender. If necessary, insert a meat thermometer into the middle of the largest piece of beef and verify the temperature is 165 degrees F or greater.

9. Remove the pot from the oven with potholders, uncover and remove the bay leaves with fork or tongs and discard. Shred the meat with the forks and/or tongs. Taste the broth and meat, then add salt, pepper and additional thyme if necessary.

10. Serve the roast with cooking liquid and vegetables alongside toasted SCD bread or Best Mashed No-Tatoes (see recipe page 211).

Stove Top & Slow Cooker Method

11. Preheat slow cooker on high. Measure out ingredients and prepare vegetables ahead of time, refrigerate til needed.

12. On the stovetop, heat the olive oil on medium heat in large pan. Place parchment paper on the platter or large dish, put the roast on top of the paper and pat dry with paper towels. Salt and pepper each side of the chuck roast liberally.

13. Place the roast in the large pan and discard the parchment paper. Cook the roast for about 5-7 minutes and turning to brown each side. Remove the roast from the pan and place in preheated slow cooker.

14. Add the onion and garlic to the pan and sauté for 5 minutes. Scraping the bottom well and reduce heat to prevent burning. Pour the cooked garlic, remaining oil and onions over the chuck roast in the slow cooker.

15. Pour in the red wine, beef broth, over the beef. Then add in the 1 tablespoon of Worcestershire, 1 tablespoon of tomato paste, thyme and bay leaves to the slow cooker.

16. Cover the slow cooker with lid and change the temperature to low heat. Cook for 6-7 hours. After 6-7 hours add the carrots, celery and mushrooms ensuring they are coated with liquid. (Add a bit of filtered water if needed.) Stir in the remaining Worcestershire and tomato paste.

17. Cook for an additional 1-3 hours until the vegetables and beef are very tender. Check for tenderness as needed with a fork.

18. Remove the bay leaves with fork or tongs and discard. Shred the meat with the forks or tongs. Taste the broth and meat, then add salt, pepper and additional thyme if necessary.

19. Serve the roast with cooking liquid and vegetables alongside toasted SCD bread or Mashed No-Tatoes (see recipe page 211).

Roasted Chicken and Simple Bone Broth

Approximate Yield	**Prep Time 20 min**	**Estimated Macronutrients**
10-20 servings	**Total Time 1-24 hours**	**12 g P • 1 g C • 8 g F**
	(To allow for simmering time)	

INGREDIENTS

1 whole young roasting chicken (4-5 lbs.) *
3 tablespoons of olive oil, ghee or softened butter
1 ½ - 2 tablespoons Greek Spice Rub (see recipe page 150)
Optional: Juice of ½ lemon

Bone Broth
8-12 cups filtered water

KITCHEN EQUIPMENT

Non latex food service gloves (to wear when handling raw meat)
Small dishwasher safe bowls or ramekins
Measuring spoons
Paper towels
Large roasting pan
Aluminum foil
Baster or basting brush
Meat thermometer
Bone Broth:
Large fine metal strainer/colander
Large crockpot/ slow cooker
Large stock pot
Ladle
Recommended: Silicone freezer containers/cubes with lids

SPECIAL INSTRUCTIONS

* If using a different sized chicken, you will need to review roasting safety guidelines and determine the appropriate roasting time based on the size of the chicken.

DIRECTIONS

Roasting Chicken

1. Preheat oven to 450 degrees F. Measure out spices, butter, and cut the lemon. Place all in small dishwasher safe ramekins nearby so as not to cross contaminate when working with raw meat. (Important note: Regardless of gloves always follow best food safety practices to prevent cross contamination and food born illness when cooking with raw meat. See notes on Hygiene and General Food Safety on page 30).

2. With gloved hands, place the young roasting chicken in the large roasting pan, and remove any innards. Pat the chicken dry with paper towels.

3. Slather the chicken in the olive oil or butter using a spoon or hands. Sprinkle the spice mix over the entire chicken. Squeeze and drizzle the optional fresh lemon juice all over the chicken. If using non latex food service gloves, discard in trash and wash hands, and all utensils immediately.

4. Cover the entire chicken with foil and place in oven. Roast for 50-80 minutes.

5. For the last 15 minutes, remove and discard the foil. Baste the chicken with the broth at the bottom on the roasting pan.

6. Remove from the oven when the internal temperature of the chicken is 165 degrees F. Allow the chicken to rest for 5-10 minutes and tent with new aluminum foil. Carve and serve or use in other recipes. Freeze shredded chicken meat with broth for longer storage, in appropriate freezer safe containers.

Bone Broth

7. With the leftover meat, bones and roasting juices, place all of it in a large crockpot.
8. Cover the meat, with filtered water ensuring its submerged.
9. Place lid on crockpot and cook on low for 24 hours. Turn off the crockpot and allow to cool.
10. Nest the metal strainer/colander in the large stock pot. Remove the pot from the crockpot and pour the bone broth, chicken meat and bones over the strainer/colander. Discard the bones and excess meat in the strainer/colander.
11. Pour or ladle the bone broth into airtight, freezer safe containers and freeze for later use.

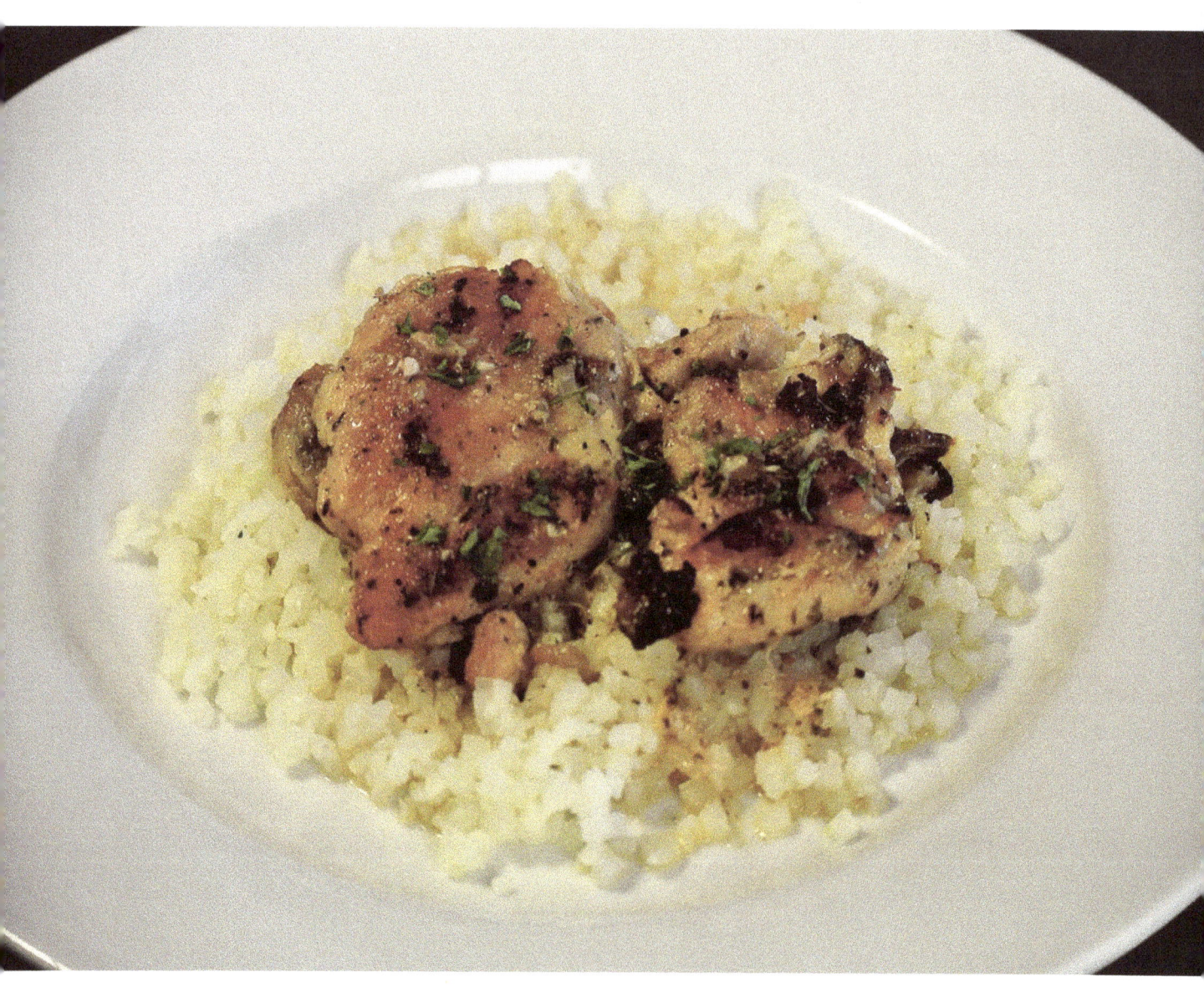

Greek Lemon Butter Crockpot Chicken

Slow Foods & Fast Freezer Meals

Slow food cooking is a method where food is cooked at a low temperature over an extended period. Slow cookers are a lifesaver. They allow busy people to simply set the appliance and forget about it, only to return to a flavorful meal with tender ingredients. This cooking technique is especially great for tenderizing tough cuts of meat and hard legumes. The benefit of slow cooking, using programmable appliances, allows the athlete more time in their day to train and recover. Freezer meals (prepped meals stored in a zip-top bag or container) make cooking even easier by simply adding them to a slow cooker. These recipes are designed to reduce preparation time and simplify meal planning.

Slow Cooker Chicken Tikka Masala

Approximate Yield	**Prep Time 20 min**	**Estimated Macronutrients**
6-8 servings	**Total Time 8 hours**	29 g P • 30 g C • 16 g F
	(To allow for slow cooking)	

INGREDIENTS

2 lbs. of boneless, skinless chicken thighs cut into 2–3-inch cubes
1 ½ cups of tomato puree or crushed tomatoes*
1 large yellow onion finely diced
1 cup of reduced fat unsweetened coconut milk*
4 cloves of minced garlic
2 tablespoon olive oil
2 tablespoons tomato paste*
1 tablespoon lemon juice
1 tablespoon of fresh grated ginger
1 tablespoon Indian red chili powder or finely ground red chili powder
1 ½ teaspoon garam masala
1 teaspoon granulated onion
1-2 teaspoon honey
½ teaspoon turmeric
¼ teaspoon ground cardamom
1 cup frozen peas
Optional: 2 cups fresh or frozen cauliflower florets (if not eating with cauliflower rice)
Sea salt and fresh ground pepper to taste

Garnishes
Fresh chopped cilantro
Dripped SCD Yogurt (see recipe page 298)
Cooked cauliflower rice or Yellow Pea Wraps (see recipe page 306)

KITCHEN EQUIPMENT
Medium bowl
Measuring spoons & measuring cups
Heat resistant tongs or spatula
Large 6 qt crockpot / slow cooker

SPECIAL INSTRUCTIONS/DIET INFORMATION
*Coconut milk cannot have emulsifiers are additives (i.e., guar gum), only water and coconut. The coconut milk should also be unsweetened.
*Canned tomatoes are typically not allowed under SCD. However, there are Italian brands of canned tomatoes and tomato pastes with no artificial flavors, preservatives or additives listed as ingredients, nor used in the manufacturing process. These brands are generally sold through Wellbees and a few other stores. Read store bought canned tomato and tomato paste labels carefully. If necessary, you can make your own tomato sauce or paste using fresh tomatoes or canned tomato juice (if salt is the only other ingredient).

DIRECTIONS
1. Place the thighs at the bottom of crockpot and if possible avoid overlapping them.
2. Whisk together all other ingredients (except peas and cauliflower) and pour over the chicken.
3. Pour the sauce over the chicken thighs. Cover crockpot with lid and heat on high for 3-4 hours or 6-8 hrs. on low. In the last 30-60 minutes of cooking, add the optional cauliflower and peas. Additional coconut milk can be added as needed during the cooking process. Salt and pepper to taste.
4. The chicken can be served with the sauce from the crockpot, over cauliflower rice or on yellow pea wraps. Garnish as needed.

Greek Lemon Butter Crockpot Chicken

Approximate Yield	Prep Time 20 min	Estimated Macronutrients
6-8 servings	Total Time 8 hours	15 g P • 11 g C • 5 g F
	(To allow for slow cooking)	

INGREDIENTS

6-8 boneless, skinless chicken thighs
1 shallot
1 tablespoon of Greek Spice Rub (see recipe page 150) *
1 teaspoon granulated onion
1 lemon, juiced and zested (approximately ½ teaspoon zest and ¼ cup juice, divided)
¼ cup butter
⅓ cup favorite SCD legal bone broth or Roasted Chicken Bone Broth (see recipe page 255)
Sea salt and fresh ground pepper to taste

Garnishes
Fresh minced parsley
Lemon slices

KITCHEN EQUIPMENT

Measuring spoons & measuring cups
Heat resistant tongs or spatula
Large 6 qt Crockpot
Optional: Large cast iron in oven or stovetop

SPECIAL INSTRUCTIONS/DIET INFORMATION

*Note the amount of spice used is to taste, you can always sprinkle with more seasoning as needed once the chicken is cooked.

DIRECTIONS

1. Place the thighs at the bottom of crockpot and if possible avoid overlapping them.
2. Sprinkle the spices, zest and lemon juice over the chicken.
3. Pour the SCD bone broth over the chicken.
4. Cut the butter into tablespoon sized squares and place over the chicken thighs in different areas of the crockpot.
5. Cover crockpot with lid and heat on high for 3-4 hours or 6-8 hrs. on low.
6. The chicken can be served moist with the sauce from the crockpot, or you can remove the thighs gently with a frying spatula and crisp up using the oven and cast-iron method.
7. If using the oven, pre heat the oven to broil (500 degrees F). Place the chicken in a well-oiled and seasoned large cast iron pan. Add a little broth/juice from the crockpot over the chicken and place the cast iron pan in the oven. Broil the chicken until they start to brown, and edges start to crisp. (Watch carefully to prevent burning.) You can also flip the thighs midway to evenly crisp them. Remove from oven when they reach desired crispness and serve.
8. If using the cast iron on the stove you can heat and melt some butter in the pan, then gently fry and brown the outside of the chicken thighs. Remove from oven when desired crispness and serve.

Slow Cooker Thai Peanut Chicken

Approximate Yield
6-8 servings

Prep Time 20 min
Total Time 8 hours
(To allow for slow cooking)

Estimated Macronutrients
32 g P • 14 g C • 23 g F

INGREDIENTS

2 lbs. of boneless, skinless chicken thighs
1 cup of reduced fat coconut milk*
½ cup of peanut butter
⅓ cup of tamari or No Soy Sauce (see recipe page 121) *
¼ cup of SCD chicken bone broth (or use recipe page 255)
1 lime juiced
4 cloves of minced garlic
2 tablespoons honey
1 tablespoon of fresh grated ginger
1 teaspoon granulated onion
1 teaspoon coarse red pepper flakes
Sea salt and fresh ground pepper to taste

Garnishes
Fresh minced cilantro
Chopped roasted and salted peanuts
Green onions chopped
Cooked cauliflower rice

KITCHEN EQUIPMENT

Medium bowl
Measuring spoons & measuring cups
Heat resistant tongs or spatula
Large 6 qt crockpot / slow cooker

SPECIAL INSTRUCTIONS/DIET INFORMATION

*Coconut milk cannot have emulsifiers are additives (i.e., guar gum), only water and coconut. The coconut milk should also be unsweetened.
* Important to note, when substituting No Soy Sauce for tamari, you may need to increase the salt and reduce the honey in the recipe.
*Note the amount of spice used is to taste, you can always sprinkle with more seasoning as needed once the chicken is cooked.

DIRECTIONS

1. Place the thighs at the bottom of crockpot and if possible avoid overlapping them.
2. In a medium bowl, whisk the tamari or No-Soy Sauce, coconut milk, bone broth, honey, peanut butter, minced garlic, ginger, spices and lime juice. (except salt and pepper)
3. Pour the sauce over the chicken thighs. Cover crockpot with lid and heat on high for 3-4 hours or 6-8 hrs. on low and chicken is cooked through. Salt and pepper to taste.
4. The chicken can be served with the sauce from the crockpot, over cauliflower rice and garnish.

Freezer Bag Chicken Curry

Approximate Yield	Prep Time 10 min	Estimated Macronutrients
6 servings	Total Time 30 min	20 g P • 17 g C • 15 g F

INGREDIENTS

1 (15 oz) can (approximately 1 ½ cups) of reduced fat coconut milk*
1 tablespoon curry powder
1 tablespoon tomato paste*
½ teaspoon sea salt
¼ teaspoon finely crushed red chili flakes
½ small yellow onion minced
2 cloves of grated garlic
16 oz boneless skinless chicken thighs or chicken breast cut in ½ inch diameter strips
1 10oz bag of frozen peas
Salt and pepper to taste
Optional: 2 cups of cauliflower florets

Garnishes and Complimentary Sides
Fresh cilantro leaves chopped
Yellow Pea Wraps (see recipe page 306)
Cauliflower rice (cooked)

KITCHEN EQUIPMENT

1–2-gallon zip top freezer bag
Non-stick or ceramic skillet
Measuring cups & spoons
Heat resistant spatula or large spoon
Optional: baking sheet

SPECIAL INSTRUCTIONS/DIET INFORMATION

*Any coconut milk should only consist of coconut and water. No emulsifiers, gums, sweeteners or additives should be in the ingredient list.
*Canned tomatoes are typically not allowed under SCD. However, there are Italian brands of canned tomatoes and tomato pastes with no artificial flavors, preservatives or additives listed as ingredients, nor used in the manufacturing process. These brands are generally sold through Wellbees and a few other stores. Read store bought canned tomato and tomato paste labels carefully. If necessary, you can make your own tomato sauce or paste using fresh tomatoes or canned tomato juice (if salt is the only other ingredient).

DIRECTIONS

1. In the zip top bag, add the coconut milk, curry, tomato paste, and sea salt. Seal the bag and shake all the ingredients well mixed.
2. For a complete meal add in the sliced chicken, onion, garlic, cauliflower, and peas. However it is recommended to store the frozen vegetables separately until the intended day of cooking. Try to remove all air from the bag before sealing (this is to help prevent freezer burn). Massage and shake the bag until the marinade covers the vegetables and chicken well. Label the bag with date and contents.
3. Place the sealed bag in the freezer. As an option, place it on a baking sheet, flattening the bag and then freezing. Once the meal is frozen the baking sheet can be removed and meal stacked in the freezer. Generally, this freezer meal should last for 6 months.
4. When ready to cook, remove the meal from the freezer and allow to thaw in the refrigerator for at least 24 hours. As a best practice, defrost the meal on a large plate or in a large bowl to prevent any bag leaks during defrosting.
5. Pour the meal into a large skillet on medium to high heat. If the frozen vegetables were stored separately, add them into the dish midway through to prevent overcooking them. Stir often until the chicken is cooked through and vegetables tender. (Approximately 12-20 minutes) Season with salt, and pepper to taste. Add additional ground red chilli flakes as needed.
6. Garnish with fresh cilantro and serve with either yellow pea wraps or on top of cauliflower rice.

Slow Cooker Pork Chili Verde

Approximate Yield	Prep Time 20 min	Estimated Macronutrients
10-12 servings	Total Time 8 hours	25 g P • 8 g C • 10 g F
	(To allow for slow cooking)	

INGREDIENTS

1 (3-4 lbs.) boneless pork shoulder trimmed of excess fat
3 tablespoons olive oil
¼ teaspoon ground black pepper
¼ teaspoon sea salt
4 cups SCD legal chicken bone broth or use Roasted
Chicken Bone Broth (see recipe page 255)

Chili Verde Sauce
2 poblano peppers (stems removed and tops cut off)
2 large onions
2 anaheim peppers (stems removed and tops cut off)
2 jalapeno peppers (stems removed and tops cut off)
6 garlic cloves, peeled
1 tablespoon dried cilantro
1 teaspoon of salt
½ teaspoon of cumin
¾ teaspoon dried oregano
Optional: 4-6 tomatillos with husks removed
¼ cup of filtered water
Drizzle of olive oil

Salt & pepper to taste
Optional Taco Seasonings (see recipe page 147)

Garnishes and Complementary Sides
Fresh cilantro
Shredded cabbage
Lime wedges
Thinly sliced radishes
Savory Black Beans (see recipe page 199)
Lime Cilantro Cauliflower Rice (see recipe page 198)
Pumpkin Street Tortillas (see recipe page 307)
Yellow Pea Wraps (see recipe page 306)
Quick Pickled Onions (see recipe page 200)
Dripped SCD Yogurt (see recipe page 298)
SCD Restaurant Style Salsa (see recipe page 137)

KITCHEN EQUIPMENT

Baking sheets/pans
Blender or handheld immersion blender and large bowl
Baking parchment paper
Large meat forks or tongs
Large stove top pan
Parchment paper
Paper towels
Large dishwasher safe plate or platter (large enough to fit the roast on)
Large crockpot/ slow cooker
Heat resistant spoon or spatula
Stovetop
Measuring spoons
Ladle or large spoon
Optional: Non latex food service gloves (to wear when handling raw meat) *

SPECIAL INSTRUCTIONS

*Important note: Regardless of using gloves always follow food safety best practices to prevent cross contamination and food born illness when cooking with raw meat. See notes on Hygiene and General Food Safety on page 30.

DIRECTIONS

1. Preheat oven at 425 degrees F. Line the baking sheet with parchment and lay the vegetables for the sauce on paper and drizzle with 1 tablespoon of olive oil. Roast the vegetables for 20-25 minutes.
2. Place the roasted vegetables and remaining Chili Verde Sauce ingredients in a blender or large bowl. Puree the vegetables and spices well. Set aside sauce.

3. Preheat the slow cooker on high.
4. On the stovetop, heat the olive oil on medium heat in large pan. Place parchment paper on the platter or large dish. Then put the pork shoulder on top of the paper and pat dry with paper towels. Salt and pepper each side of the pork shoulder liberally.
5. Place the pork in the large pan and discard the parchment paper. Cook the pork for about 5-7 minutes and turning to brown each side. Remove the pork from the pan and place in preheated slow cooker with remaining oil.
6. Pour in the chicken bone broth, and chili verde sauce over the pork shoulder.
7. Cover the slow cooker with lid and change the temperature to low heat. Cook for 8-10 hours on low or 6-8 hours on high. (Add a bit of filtered water if needed.)
8. Once cooked, shred the meat with the forks or tongs. Taste the sauce and meat, then add salt, pepper and optional Taco seasonings if necessary.
9. Serve the pork chili verde with cooking liquid alongside Lime Cilantro Cauliflower Rice, Savory Black Beans, Pumpkin tortillas or Yellow Pea Wraps. Garnish and serve.

Freezer Bag Chicken Fajitas

Approximate Yield	Prep Time 10 min	Estimated Macronutrients
6 servings	Total Time 30 min	25 g P • 11 g C • 13 g F

INGREDIENTS

¼ cup avocado oil

2 tablespoons Taco Seasonings or Pincho Seasonings (see recipes page 147 & 149)

Juice of 1 lime

1 red bell pepper, (stem and seeds removed) julienned

2 orange or yellow bell peppers, (stems and seeds removed) julienned

1 small red onion

3 cloves of chopped garlic

16 oz boneless skinless chicken thighs or chicken breast cut in ½ inch diameter strips

1 tablespoon olive or avocado oil

Salt and pepper to taste

Optional: ground cayenne or chipotle pepper

Garnishes and Complimentary Sides

Fresh cilantro leaves chopped

Pumpkin Street Tortillas (see recipe page 307)

Lime Cauliflower Rice (see recipe page 198)

KITCHEN EQUIPMENT

1–2-gallon zip top freezer bag

Cast iron skillet

Measuring cups & spoons

Metal spatula or large spoon

Optional: baking sheet

DIRECTIONS

1. In the zip top bag, add the oil, seasoning and lime juice. Seal the bag and shake all the ingredients until well mixed.
2. Add in the sliced chicken, peppers and onion. Try to remove all air from the bag before sealing (this is to help prevent freezer burn). Massage and shake the bag until the marinade covers the vegetables and chicken well. Label the bag with date and contents.
3. Place the sealed bag in the freezer. As an option, place it on a baking sheet, flattening the bag and then freezing. Once the meal is frozen the baking sheet can be removed and meal stacked in the freezer. Generally, this freezer meal should last for 6 months.
4. When ready to cook, remove the meal from the freezer and allow to thaw in the refrigerator for at least 24 hours. As a best practice, defrost the meal on a large plate or in a large bowl to prevent any spills or bag leaks during defrosting.
5. Pour the meal into a large skillet on medium to high heat. Cooking and stirring often until the chicken and vegetables are cooked through. (Approximately 12-20 minutes) Season with salt, and pepper to taste. Add additional ground cayenne or chipotle peppers as needed.
6. Garnish with fresh cilantro and serve with either pumpkin tortillas or cauliflower rice.

Freezer Bag & Slow Cooker Beef Chili

Approximate Yield	Prep Time 10 min	Estimated Macronutrients
8 servings	Total Time 7-9 hours	27 g P • 20 g C • 15 g F
	(To allow for slow cooking)	

INGREDIENTS

1 ½ - 2 lbs. of boneless chuck roast or beef brisket trimmed of fat, and cut into 1-inch pieces

1 (15 oz) can or 2 cups of crushed or pureed tomatoes*

2 cups of soaked and cooked SCD kidney beans (see recipe page 303) *

1 large red onion chopped

1 large green bell pepper seeds and stems removed, chopped

4 cloves of minced garlic

¼ cup of chili powder

2 tablespoons of tomato paste*

½ teaspoon of ground cumin

¼ cup avocado oil

Salt and ground black pepper

Cayenne or chipotle pepper for added spice

Optional: 1 tablespoon of Pincho or Taco Seasoning (see recipes page 149 & 147)

Garnishes and Complimentary Sides

Shredded cheddar cheese

Dripped, SCD Yogurt (see recipe page 298)

Fresh Cilantro

Minced white onion

Blender No-Corn Bread (see recipe page 309)

KITCHEN EQUIPMENT

1–2-gallon zip top freezer bag
Slow cooker
Measuring cups & spoons
Metal spatula or large spoon
Optional baking sheet

SPECIAL INSTRUCTIONS/DIET INFORMATION

*Canned tomatoes are typically not allowed under SCD. However, there are Italian brands of canned tomatoes and tomato pastes with no artificial flavors, preservatives or additives listed as ingredients, nor used in the manufacturing process. These brands are generally sold through Wellbees and a few other stores. Read store bought canned tomato and tomato paste labels carefully. If necessary, you can make your own tomato sauce or paste using fresh tomatoes or canned tomato juice (if salt is the only other ingredient).

DIRECTIONS

1. In the zip top bag, Layer the beef, tomato puree, tomato paste, bell pepper, onion and spices. Squeeze out the air from the bag and seal the bag well. Label the bag with date and contents.

2. Place the sealed bag in the freezer. As an option, place it on a baking sheet, flattening the bag and then freezing. Once the meal is frozen the baking sheet can be removed and meal stacked in the freezer. Generally, this freezer meal should last for 6 months.

3. When ready to cook, remove the meal from the freezer and allow to thaw in the refrigerator for at least 24 hours. As a best practice, defrost the meal on a large plate or in a large bowl to prevent mess from any bag leaks during defrosting.

4. Pour the meal into a large slow cooker and cook on low for 7 to 9 hours. Season with salt, and pepper to taste. Add additional ground cayenne or chipotle peppers as needed.

5. Garnish with fresh cilantro, shredded cheese, onion, top with a bit of yogurt. Serve with No- Corn Blender Bread.

Slow Cooker Tomato Vegetable Beef Pot Roast

Approximate Yield 10-12 servings	Prep Time 40min Total Time 8-10 hours (To allow for slow cooking)	Estimated Macronutrients 25 g P • 8 g C • 18 g F

INGREDIENTS

1 chuck roast (bone in or boneless) trimmed of excess fat (3-4 lbs.) *
1-2 tablespoons olive oil
¼ teaspoon ground black pepper
¼ teaspoon sea salt
3-4 cups of leftover Tomato Vegetable Gazpacho (see recipe page 167)
4 garlic cloves, peeled and chopped
1 cup of dry red wine
2 tablespoons Worcestershire Sauce (see recipe page 120)
1 teaspoon-1 tablespoon of grated horseradish (note this is to taste and more can be added as needed)
1 tablespoon of dijon or yellow mustard*
2 whole bay leaves
¾ teaspoon dried thyme leaves
1 chopped green bell pepper, stems and seeds removed
4 celery stalks (approximately 1 cup), washed and cut diagonally in ½ -inch pieces
3 large carrots, peeled and cut diagonally in ½ -inch pieces
Salt & pepper to taste

KITCHEN EQUIPMENT

Large meat forks or tongs
Large stove top pan
Parchment paper
Paper towels
Large dishwasher safe plate or platter (large enough to fit the roast on)
Large crockpot/ slow cooker
Heat resistant spoon or spatula
Stovetop
Measuring spoons
Ladle or large spoon
Optional: Non latex food service gloves (to wear when handling raw meat) *

SPECIAL INSTRUCTIONS

* Bone in chuck roast bone can be used later for bone broth.
*There are a few commercial brands of mustard made with SCD legal ingredients. However always check ingredients carefully. Confirm with the company and determine unlisted ingredients are not being used in the manufacturing process.
*Important note: Regardless of using gloves always follow best food safety practices to prevent cross contamination and food born illness when cooking with raw meat. See notes on Hygiene and General Food Safety on page 30.

DIRECTIONS

1. Preheat slow cooker on high. Measure out ingredients and prepare vegetables ahead of time, refrigerate until needed.
2. On the stovetop, heat the olive oil on medium heat in large pan. Line the platter or large dish with parchment paper. Then place the roast on top of the paper and pat dry with paper towels. Salt and pepper each side of the chuck roast liberally.
3. Place the roast in the large pan and discard the parchment paper. Cook the roast for about 5-7 minutes and turning to brown each side. Remove the roast from the pan and place in preheated slow cooker.
4. Add the garlic to the pan and sauté. Scraping the bottom well and reduce heat to prevent burning. Pour the cooked garlic, and remaining oil over the chuck roast in the slow cooker.
5. Pour in the red wine, and Tomato Vegetable Gazpacho over the beef. Then add in the 1 tablespoon of Worcestershire, horseradish, mustard, thyme, and bay leaves to the slow cooker.
6. Cover the slow cooker with lid and change the temperature to low heat. Cook for 6-7 hours. After 6-7 hours add the carrots, celery and bell pepper ensuring they are covered in the liquid. (Add a bit of filtered water if needed.) Stir in the remaining Worcestershire.

7. Cook for an additional 1-3 hours until the vegetables and beef are very tender. Check for tenderness as needed with a fork.
8. Remove the bay leaves with fork or tongs and discard. Shred the meat with the forks or tongs. Taste the sauce and meat, then add salt, pepper and additional horseradish if necessary.
9. Serve the roast with cooking liquid and vegetables alongside toasted SCD bread, cooked SCD pasta or Best Mashed No-Tatoes (see recipe page 211).

Easy SCD Marinades and Freezer Meals

Here are several convenient recipes to reduce time in the kitchen. Oftentimes it is best to prepare a variety in bulk, once a month, and freeze for later use. Having a protein source marinated and ready for a slow cooker is a perfect meal prep solution on a busy day. Servings and macronutrients are not provided for these recipes, as ingredients and servings can vary.

INGREDIENTS
All recipes are your choice of 1-2 lbs. of either chicken, lean beef cuts, or lean pork cuts.

Southwest Marinade
Juice and zest of 1 lime
¼ cup of olive oil
2 cloves of minced garlic
1 tablespoon apple cider vinegar
1 teaspoon chili powder
1 teaspoon granulated garlic
1 teaspoon granulated onion
½ teaspoon salt
½ teaspoon ground cumin
¼ teaspoon coarse ground black pepper

Hawaiian BBQ Marinade
¼ cup pineapple juice (not from concentrate)
2 tablespoons tamari or No Soy Sauce (see recipe page 121 and notes) *
1 tablespoon sesame oil or olive oil
2 teaspoons granulated garlic
1 teaspoon granulated onion
1 teaspoon sea salt
1 teaspoon turmeric
1 teaspoon ground ginger
½ teaspoon ground black pepper

BBQ Marinade
1 cup favorite SCD legal BBQ sauce or scratch made SCD BBQ Sauce (see recipe page 119)
2 cloves minced garlic
¼ cup olive oil
1 teaspoon chili powder
½ teaspoon smoked paprika
½ teaspoon salt
¼ teaspoon coarse ground black pepper

Honey Mustard Marinade
¼ cup of olive oil
2 tablespoons honey
2 tablespoons SCD legal dijon or yellow mustard*
3 cloves of minced garlic
1 tablespoon freshly lemon juice
1 teaspoon salt
½ teaspoon ground black pepper

Garlic and Lemon Marinade
¼ cup of olive oil
3 cloves of minced garlic
3 tablespoons fresh squeezed lemon juice
2 tablespoons honey
½ tablespoon white wine vinegar
1 teaspoon of dried dill weed
1 teaspoon of granulated onion
½ teaspoon ground mustard
½ teaspoon sea salt

KITCHEN EQUIPMENT
Large gallon size plastic zip top bag
Large bowl
Measuring cups & measuring spoons
Large glass measuring cup or small bowl
Tongs

SPECIAL INSTRUCTIONS / DIET INFORMATION
*Check the labels of the tamari, many will list rice wine vinegar and other ingredients which may be illegal when following SCD. Tamari should generally be gluten free, grain free, and sugar free. For example, tamari includes only water, organic soybeans, salt and/or organic alcohol (as part of fermentation process).
*There are a few commercial brands of mustard made with SCD legal ingredients. However always check ingredients carefully. Confirm with the company and determine unlisted ingredients are not being used in the manufacturing process.

DIRECTIONS
1. Add all ingredients to a measuring cup or small bowl. Stir and mix all ingredients well.
2. Place the meat in large bowl or plastic zip top bag. Pour the marinade over the meat and seal the bag or cover bowl with plastic wrap. Refrigerate for 1-3 hours.

DIRECTIONS (continued)

3. You can also freeze the marinades and meat together in a bag for later use. These meals can generally last a few months in the freezer.
4. When ready to cook, place the freezer meal bag in a large bowl (to prevent leaking as it defrosts). Place the bowl in the refrigerator and allow to defrost for at least 24 hours.
5. Many of these recipes can be cooked in a slow cooker or programmable pressure cooker. You may need to add water, bone broth or additional sauce (i.e. SCD BBQ other legal sauce depending on the flavors of the marinade). Generally, when placing the meat on the bottom of the slow cooker water or broth should cover the meat by 1-2 inches to prevent burning and provide adequate moisture.

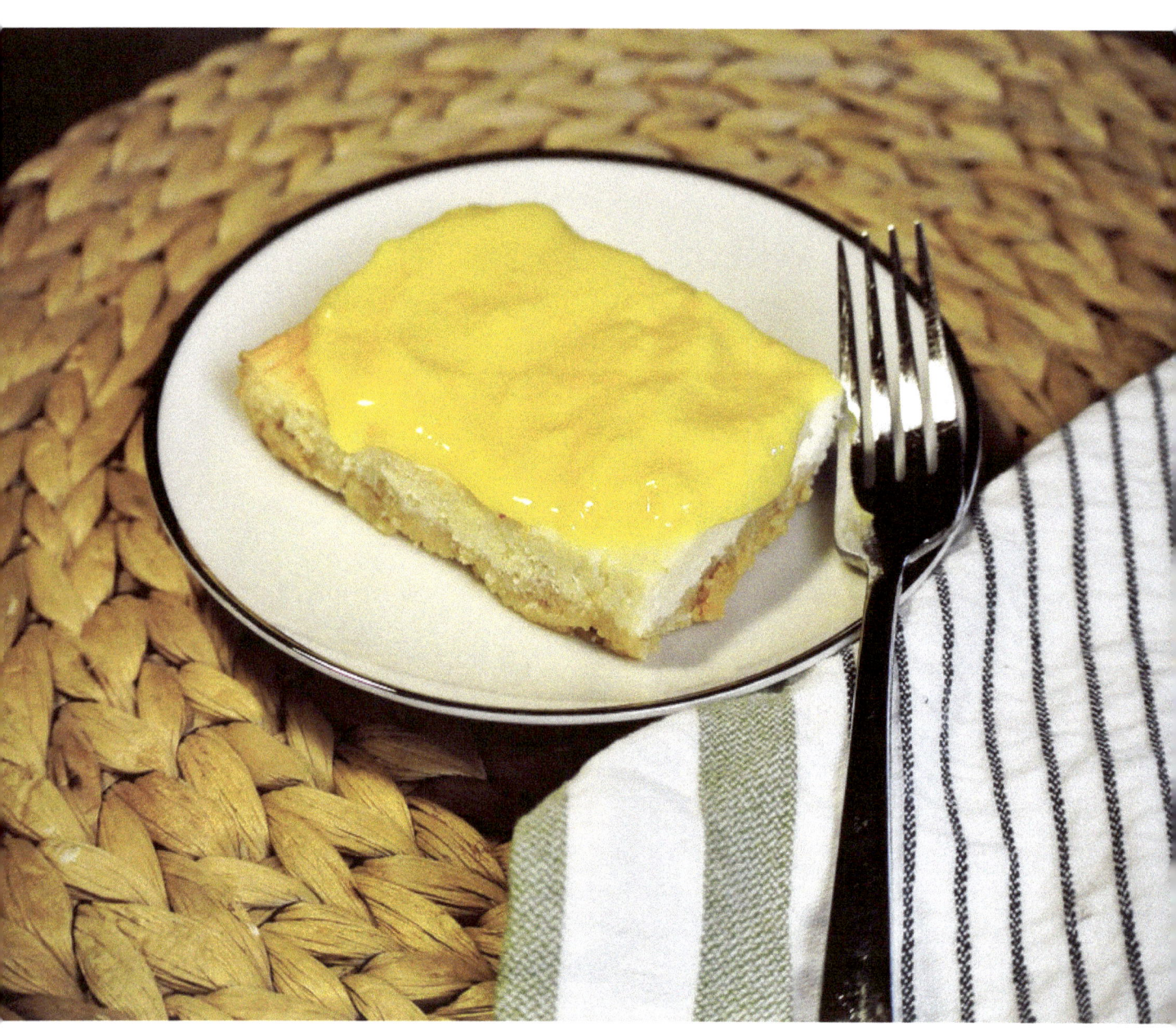

Lemon Coconut Yogurt Bars
with Honey Lemon Curd

Desserts

Desserts are often overlooked as efficient fuel and delicious protein sources. Unfortunately, their reputation of being fat laden or full of sugar demonizes them in the world of sports nutrition. However, desserts done well, with macronutrients considered and natural sweeteners (such as honey), they can be a healthy form of energy in moderation. Additionally, they can also satisfy cravings and trigger the release of serotonin.

Desserts can also be effective in purposeful weight gain if nutritionally balanced. However, we should not forget they can be a sweet treat and reward for accomplishing a major victory or goal. Desserts are commonly brought to competitions and events to celebrate the athlete's months and even years of hard work.

Cherry Swirl No-Cheese Cake

Approximate Yield **10-12 servings**	**Prep Time 20 min** **Total Time 4 hours** (To allow for refrigeration)	**Estimated Macronutrients** 13 g P • 25 g C • 9 g F

INGREDIENTS

Crust*
3 tablespoons coconut flour
¾ cup almond flour
2 tablespoons melted butter
1 tablespoon honey
1 teaspoon cinnamon

Cherry Sauce
*You can omit this step if you have Cherry Compote already prepared (see recipe page 108)
1 cup of frozen pitted cherries
2 tablespoons water

Filling
16 oz (2 cups) of SCD Nonfat Greek Yogurt (see recipe page 298)
½ cups of pasteurized liquid egg whites*
½ cup of honey
1 egg
1 teaspoon of vanilla extract
3 ½ teaspoons unflavored gelatin

KITCHEN EQUIPMENT
Immersion blender
9–10-inch springform pan
Baking parchment paper
Standing or handheld electric mixer
Spatula or large spoon
Mixing bowls
Measuring spoons & measuring cups

SPECIAL INSTRUCTIONS/DIET INFORMATION
*Note you can also substitute the almond flour, and coconut flour by using leftover Chewy Graham Crackers (Recipe on page 275) as a crust by blending them in a food processor with honey and melted butter. However macronutrient values will change.
*Be careful to read all ingredients for pasteurized liquid egg whites. This should be a mono ingredient, and not contain any preservatives or additional ingredients. Regular separated egg whites can be used but the batter will be thicker and require many eggs.

DIRECTIONS

1. Preheat oven to 350 degrees F. Line the spring form pan with parchment paper, ensuring it reaches the bottom edges. Be careful not to poke any holes or rip the parchment. Spray or brush the sides of the pan with cooking oil well.

Cherry Compote (You can omit steps 2-3 if the compote is already prepared)

2. In a medium pot with lid, combine the cherries and water. Cook the cherries on medium heat stirring to prevent the cherries from burning on the bottom. When tender pierced with a fork, lower the heat and use an immersion blender to puree the cherries into a compote. Be careful not to lift the immersion blender above the compote to prevent splatters.

3. Continue cooking on low and stirring to reduce the water in the compote. Remove from heat and place in a glass container to cool.

Crust

4. Combine the ingredients for the crust, mixing until the dough is crumbly. With greased hands spread and press the crust dough into a thin layer on the bottom of the spring form pan covered in parchment paper.

5. Bake the crust for 12 min or until golden. Remove from oven and allow to cool on a wire rack.

Filling & Assembly

6. For the filling, combine all the ingredients in a large bowl and mix with a standing or handheld electric mixer.

7. Pour filling batter into the pan over the cooled crust. Spread the batter evenly, then drizzle the cherry sauce in a circle. Using a knife or toothpick, swirl the cherry topping to create a pattern and mixing it with batter filling.

8. Bake for 50-60 min and the center is firm and does not jiggle. Then allow to cool on a wire rack for an 1-2 hrs. Place in refrigerator to chill and serve cold.

Chewy Graham Crackers

Approximate Yield	Prep Time 20 min	Estimated Macronutrients
10-12 servings	**Total Time 45 min**	**9 g P • 19 g C • 16 g F**

INGREDIENTS

Wet
2 eggs
¼ cup honey
4 tablespoons coconut oil softened or melted
2 tablespoons melted butter or ghee
2 tablespoons unsweetened cashew milk (unsweetened almond or coconut milk can be substituted) *
1 teaspoon vanilla extract

Dry
1 ½ cup almond flour
¼ cup + 1 tablespoon coconut flour
1 teaspoon baking soda
⅛ teaspoon ground cinnamon
pinch sea salt

Coconut or neutral spray cooking oil

KITCHEN EQUIPMENT

Food processor or high-powered blender
Large spoon or spatula
Measuring spoons & measuring cups
Oven
Baking sheet
Heavy cutting board
Pizza cutter/wheel or knife
Fork
Baking parchment paper

SPECIAL INSTRUCTIONS/DIET INFORMATION

*Any nut milks should only consist of nuts, water, or salt. No emulsifiers, gums, sweeteners or additives should be in the ingredient list. If you are unable to source a SCD legal nut milk you can make them easily at home (see recipe page 299).

DIRECTIONS

1. Preheat the oven to 350 degrees F. Line the baking dish with parchment paper (enough to cover the sides).
2. In the blender or food processor, add all the wet ingredients and pulse until blended.
3. Add in the remaining dry ingredients and pulse until a wet dough has formed.
4. Pour dough onto the parchment lined baking sheet.
5. Cut a second piece of parchment paper the same size of the pan and spray lightly with cooking oil. Place the oiled side of the parchment on the top of the dough. Then on the non-oiled side of the parchment lay a heavy or nonpliable cutting board and press down to flatten the dough until the dough thickness is ¼-⅛ inch. Gently remove the board and top parchment paper.
6. Spray the knife blade or pizza cutter/wheel blade with cooking oil. Cut the dough into the shape of squares or rectangles. Use the tines of a fork to press holes into each of the dough squares.
7. Place the baking sheet in the oven for 10-15 minutes depending on desired texture of crunchy or soft crackers. Remove the baked graham crackers from the oven and use the knife or pizza cutter/wheel to cut along the previous indents. Allow the crackers to cool for about 10-20 minutes.
8. These crackers freeze well wrapped in parchment paper and stored in zip top freezer bags. Use in other recipes as needed.

Monster S'mores Cookies

Approximate Yield	Prep Time 10 min	Estimated Macronutrients
6-12 servings	Total Time 30 min	13 g P • 25 g C • 19 g F

INGREDIENTS

Dry
1 ½ cup almond flour
2 tablespoons coconut flour
¼ cup of dried egg white powder*
½ teaspoon sea salt
½ teaspoon baking soda
¼ cup finely grated cacao butter (food grade)

Wet
1 egg
⅓ cup honey
½ cup butter softened
1 tablespoon vanilla extract

Optional Add ins
¼ cup pecan pieces
¼ cup shredded unsweetened coconut

Layering
6-12 SCD Coconut Marshmallows (see recipe page 284)
6- 12 Chewy SCD Graham Crackers (see recipe page 275)

KITCHEN EQUIPMENT
Mixer and beaters
Oven
Mixing bowls
Measuring spoons & measuring cups
Baking pan/cookie sheet
Spatula
Baking parchment paper

SPECIAL INSTRUCTIONS/DIET INFORMATION
*If you are unable to eat or source dried egg white powder you can replace with almond flour. However it will not rise as high, the texture will be different, and there will be higher fat and less protein for the macronutrients.

DIRECTIONS

1. Preheat oven to 350 degrees F. Line the baking sheet with parchment paper.
2. Measure out and stir together all the dry ingredients and set aside.
3. In one large mixing bowl, beat the egg and mix in all the remaining wet ingredients.
4. Add all the dry ingredients to the wet continually mixing the dough.
5. Fold the remaining ingredients into the cookie dough; pecans, shredded coconut, and grated cacao butter.
6. Place a graham cracker square on the parchment lined baking sheet. Place a large SCD marshmallow on top of the graham cracker, then scoop a very large dollop of cookie dough and cover the marshmallow and graham cracker.
7. Ensuring the cookie dough covers both the marshmallow and cracker. Continue to scoop and cover for each cookie.
8. Bake for 9- 18 minutes (depending on the size of the cookies) and the tops are golden. Remove from oven and set aside to cool.

Chewy and Soft Peanut Butter Cookies

Approximate Yield	Prep Time 10 min	Estimated Macronutrients
24 servings	Total Time 30 min	13 g P • 14 g C • 22 g F

INGREDIENTS

Wet
1 ⅔ cup peanut butter*
1 ½ cup honey
3 eggs
6 tablespoons unsalted, softened butter
2 teaspoons vanilla extract

Dry
3 cups of almond flour
¼ cup coconut flour
2 ½ teaspoons baking soda
½ teaspoon sea salt
½ teaspoon cinnamon
Optional ¾ cup of chopped unsalted roasted peanuts

KITCHEN EQUIPMENT
Mixer and beaters
Oven
1 Large mixing bowl
1 medium mixing bowl
Baking pan/cookie sheet
Spatula
Baking parchment paper

SPECIAL INSTRUCTIONS/DIET INFORMATION
*Nut butters that are SCD legal should only include the nut and possibly a legal oil and/or salt. For example, peanut butter is generally roasted peanuts and salt. There are some brands that will sweeten with honey but there are very few commercially available.

DIRECTIONS

1. Preheat oven to 350 degrees F. Line the baking sheet with parchment paper.
2. In one large mixing bowl, beat the eggs and all the wet ingredients, then set aside.
3. In the medium mixing bowl, blend the dry ingredients and set aside.
4. Slowly add the dry ingredients to the wet ingredients, mixing well with the electric mixer. If adding chopped peanuts, stir them into the dough.
5. Place large dollops of cookie dough on the parchment paper or roll the dough into balls by hand. You can also press the balls down into disks using a cup with a flat bottom or wooden cookie press.
6. Bake for 10-12 minutes (depending on the size of the cookies) and the tops are light golden. The cookies will be soft until cooled. Remove from oven and set aside to cool on the pan. You may need to work in multiple batches until all the cookies are baked.
7. These cookies freeze well when vacuum sealed or wrapped in parchment and stored in zip top freezer bags for later use.

Honey Lemon Curd

Approximate Yield 10-24 servings	Prep Time 15 min Total Time 2 hours (To allow for refrigeration)	Estimated Macronutrients 10 g P • 9 g C • 12 g F

This recipe conveniently provides the ingredients and directions for both a small and large batch of honey lemon curd.

INGREDIENTS

Large Batch (5 batches)
20 lemons zested and juiced (Meyer lemon variety are preferred) yielding approximately 3 and ⅓ cups of juice, and 5 tablespoons of fine lemon zest
20 eggs (15 yolks and 5 whole eggs) *
1 ¾ cup honey
3 sticks (1 ½ cups) unsalted butter

Small Batch (1 batch)
4 lemons zested and juiced (Meyer variety are preferred) yielding approximately ⅔ cup of fresh lemon juice, and 1-2 tablespoons of fine lemon zest
4 eggs (3 yolks and 1 whole egg) *
⅓ cup honey
4 tablespoons of unsalted butter cut into cubes

KITCHEN EQUIPMENT

Measuring spoons & measuring cups
Standing or handheld electric mixer
Large mixing bowl
Heat-resistant spoon or spatula
Medium bowl or large glass measuring cup
Large pot or medium pot that is not reactive (preferably ceramic or stainless steel)
Optional: Airtight, freezer safe silicone or plastic containers

SPECIAL INSTRUCTIONS/DIET INFORMATION

*This recipe will leave extra egg whites, and there are several recipes in this book that require multiple egg whites such as bread, tortillas, wraps, egg bake, etc. (see a few of those recipes on pages 70, 71, 310, 284, 306, 307, 308)

DIRECTIONS

1. In a bowl, separate egg yolks and set aside.
2. In the large mixing bowl, cream the honey and cubed butter with mixer.
3. Then add in the lemon juice and zest, to the butter and honey. Continue to gently mix.
4. Add the yolks and eggs slowly while mixing. The mixture will look like the butter curdled, but this is normal and will eventually become smooth when heated on the stove top.
5. Pour the lemon curd mixture into the large pot (or medium pot if making a small batch).
6. The goal is to gradually heat the eggs and melt the butter, tempering the eggs in the mix so you do not overcook and scramble them. Start with low-medium heat and continually stir for the first 10 to 15 minutes.
7. This process will take 20-40 minutes of continuous stirring; however, you will incrementally raise the heat to medium and watch for simmering bubbles.
8. The lemon curd will eventually become thicker as you stir, and a few bubbles will begin to form. Once this happens stir for 2-4 minutes and remove from heat before the bubbles increase.
9. Allow the lemon curd to cool to just above room temperature. Then divide into containers for storage. The lemon curd will freeze soft and allows for easy use in recipes.
10. The curd will generally last in the refrigerator stored in an airtight container for 7-10 days. Honey lemon curd freezes well and does not harden. Allowing you to scoop out curd as needed and defrosting in the refrigerator for later use.

Lemon Coconut Yogurt Bars

Approximate Yield 8-10 servings	**Prep Time 20 min** **Total Time 4 hours** (To allow for refrigeration)	**Estimated Macronutrients** 19 g P • 39 g C • 15 g F

INGREDIENTS

Crust*

¾ cup almond flour
¼ cup finely shredded unsweetened coconut
3 ½ tablespoons coconut flour
3 tablespoons melted butter (salted)
2 tablespoons honey
¼ teaspoon ground ginger

Filling

16oz (2 cups) of SCD Nonfat Greek Yogurt (see recipe page 298)
2 eggs
½ cup of pasteurized liquid egg whites*
½ cup of honey*
¼ cup lemon juice*
1 tablespoon lemon zest*
⅛ teaspoon ground ginger
1 teaspoon of vanilla extract
3 ½ teaspoons unflavored gelatin

Optional Topping:

1 cup of Honey Lemon Curd (see recipe page 278)
1 cup of Blueberry or Cherry Compote (see recipe page 108)
½ cup of toasted unsweetened coconut flakes

KITCHEN EQUIPMENT

Immersion blender
Large mixing bowl
Measuring spoons & measuring cups
Spatula or large spoon
Glass baking dish, 7 x 11 or 9 x 9 inch
Baking parchment paper
Standing or handheld electric mixer

SPECIAL INSTRUCTIONS/DIET INFORMATION

*Note you can also substitute the almond flour, and coconut flour by using leftover Chewy Graham Crackers (recipe on page 275) as a crust by blending them in a food processor with honey and melted butter. However macronutrient values will change.

*You can also substitute the honey, lemon zest and juice with ½ cup of Honey Lemon Curd (see recipe page 278) and 2 tablespoons of honey if more sweetness is necessary.

*Be careful to read all ingredients for pasteurized liquid egg whites. This should be a mono ingredient, and not contain any preservatives or additional ingredients. Regular separated egg whites can be used but the batter will be thicker and require many eggs.

DIRECTIONS

1. Preheat oven to 350 degrees F. Line the baking dish with parchment paper, ensuring sure it reaches above the edges, or use a well-greased baking dish.
2. Combine the ingredients for the crust, mixing until the dough is crumbled. With greased hands spread and press the crust dough into a thin layer on the bottom of the baking dish.
3. Bake the crust for 12 min or until golden. Remove from oven and allow to cool on a wire rack.
4. For the filling, beat the eggs and combine remaining ingredients (except the gelatin) in a large bowl with a standing or handheld electric mixer. Sprinkle in the gelatin and mix in well.
5. Pour the filling batter into the baking dish over the cooled crust. Spread the batter evenly.
6. Bake for 50-60 min and the center is firm and does not jiggle. Then allow to cool on a wire rack for an 1-2 hrs. Place in refrigerator to chill (at least 2 hours) and serve cold with the optional toppings.

Lemon Curd Froyo Pops

<table>
<tr><td align="center">Approximate Yield
6 servings</td><td align="center">Prep Time 15 min
Total Time 2 hours
(To allow for freezing)</td><td align="center">Estimated Macronutrients
7 g P • 22 g C • 9 g F</td></tr>
</table>

INGREDIENTS

1 cup dripped SCD Yogurt (see recipe page 298) *

1 cup of Honey Lemon Curd (see recipe page 278)

1 tablespoon light colored honey (heaping)

2 teaspoons unflavored gelatin

¼ teaspoon vanilla extract

KITCHEN EQUIPMENT

Wire whisk or handheld immersion blender

Large metal or glass mixing bowl

Measuring spoons & measuring cups

Popsicle freezer tray or mold

SPECIAL INSTRUCTIONS/DIET INFORMATION

* SCD yogurt with higher fat content will have a creamier texture when frozen.

DIRECTIONS

1. Place all ingredients in a large metal or glass mixing bowl. (Large liquid measuring cups with spout and handle work the best).

2. With the immersion blender or whisk, whisk the ingredients together until well blended and smooth.

3. Pour the froyo mixture in the popsicle molds and place in freezer to set for two hours.

4. When ready to serve remove from freezer and allow to thaw slightly before removing the pops from their molds.

Vanilla Bean "Froyo" Tacos

Approximate Yield	Prep Time 15 min	Estimated Macronutrients
3-6 servings	Total Time 2 hours	8 g P • 12 g C • 4 g F
	(To allow for freezing)	

INGREDIENTS

1 cup dripped SCD Yogurt (see recipe page 298) *
Seeds of 1 vanilla bean pod
2 tablespoons honey (heaping)
1 teaspoon vanilla extract
½ teaspoon unflavored gelatin
3-6 leftover crispy Stroopwaffels /Pumpkin Spice Sweet
Wraps (see recipe page 95)

KITCHEN EQUIPMENT

Wire whisk or handheld immersion blender
Large metal or glass mixing bowl
Measuring spoons & measuring cups
Spatula
Optional: Pastry bag
Baking sheet or freezer safe tray
Baking parchment paper

SPECIAL INSTRUCTIONS/DIET INFORMATION

* SCD yogurt with higher fat content will have a creamier texture when frozen. SCD yogurt made with heavy whipping cream will be the creamiest.

DIRECTIONS

1. Place the metal or glass mixing bowl in a freezer to chill.
2. Remove the chilled bowl from freezer and add all other ingredients, mixing with a whisk or immersion blender until smooth.
3. Place the froyo mixture in the freezer briefly to set for 5-8 minutes. Then using a spoon or pastry bag fill the wraps like a taco and lay one side down on the baking sheet or tray lined with parchment paper.
4. Place baking sheet or tray in the freezer. For a creamier froyo texture freeze the tacos halfway before serving. For long term storage, wrap the frozen tacos in parchment and foil. Be sure to also seal the taco packets in a plastic zip top bag or airtight container to prevent freezer burn.

Easy Lemon Coconut Pudding

<table>
<tr><td>**Approximate Yield**
4-6 servings</td><td>**Prep Time 15 min**
Total Time 2 hours
(To allow for refrigeration)</td><td>**Estimated Macronutrients**
8 g P • 15 g C • 31 g F</td></tr>
</table>

INGREDIENTS

¼ cup filtered water or unsweetened cashew milk*
1 lemon zested and juiced
2 tablespoons honey (heaping)
1 tablespoon unflavored gelatin
1 cup of unsweetened coconut cream (full fat) without additives or thickeners*

KITCHEN EQUIPMENT

Small saucepan
Wire whisk or whisk attachment for immersion blender
Handheld immersion blender
Large metal or glass mixing bowl (freezer safe)
Spatula
Glass or plastic storage container with airtight lid

SPECIAL INSTRUCTIONS/DIET INFORMATION

*Any nut milks should only consist of nuts, water, or salt. No emulsifiers, gums, sweeteners or additives should be in the ingredient list. If you are unable to source a SCD legal nut milk you can make them easily at home (see recipe page 299).

DIRECTIONS

1. Place the metal or glass mixing bowl in the freezer to chill.
2. In a small saucepan on medium low heat, add the honey, lemon juice, zest, water, and unflavored gelatin. When all gelatin is added mix vigorously to dissolve it. (This whole process should take about 5 minutes.)
3. Remove the chilled bowl from freezer and add the coconut cream and warm gelatin mixture, mixing vigorously with a whisk. Continue to mix vigorously until the there are no clumps and everything is combined well. (Use the immersion blender if clumps form)
4. Place bowl in fridge and whisk or blend the pudding every 15 minutes to prevent clumps and until it reaches the texture of a thick pudding.
5. Serve the pudding cold. Store in an airtight container with lid and use the immersion blender or whisk to create a smooth texture if needed before serving.

Vanilla Bean Coconut Pudding

Approximate Yield
4-6 servings

Prep Time 15 min
Total Time 2 hours
(To allow for refrigeration)

Estimated Macronutrients
8 g P • 15 g C • 31 g F

INGREDIENTS
¼ cup filtered water or unsweetened cashew milk*
Seeds of 1 vanilla bean pod
2 tablespoons honey (heaping)
½ teaspoon vanilla extract
1 tablespoon unflavored gelatin
1 cup of unsweetened coconut cream (full fat) without additives or thickeners*

KITCHEN EQUIPMENT
Small saucepan
Wire whisk or whisk attachment for immersion blender
Handheld immersion blender
Large metal or glass mixing bowl (freezer safe)
Spatula
Glass or plastic storage container with airtight lid

SPECIAL INSTRUCTIONS/DIET INFORMATION
*Any nut milks should only consist of nuts, water, or salt. No emulsifiers, gums, sweeteners or additives should be in the ingredient list. If you are unable to source a SCD legal nut milk you can make them easily at home (see recipe page 299).

DIRECTIONS
1. Place the metal or glass mixing bowl in the freezer to chill.
2. In a small saucepan on medium low heat, add the honey, vanilla extract, water, and unflavored gelatin. When all gelatin is added mix vigorously to dissolve it. (This whole process should take about 5 minutes.)
3. Remove the chilled bowl from freezer, add the coconut cream, vanilla bean seeds and gelatin mixture, mixing vigorously with a whisk. Continue to mix vigorously until pudding is clump free and everything well combined. (Use the immersion blender if clumps form)
4. Place bowl in fridge and whisk or blend the pudding every 15 minutes to prevent clumping and until it reaches the texture of a thick pudding.
5. Serve the pudding cold. Store in an airtight container with lid and use the immersion blender or whisk to create a smooth texture if needed before serving.

Coconut Marshmallows

Approximate Yield 24 servings	Prep Time 50 min Total Time 2 hours (To allow for setting and cooling)	Estimated Macronutrients 3 g P • 4 g C • 3 g F

INGREDIENTS

5 teaspoons of unflavored gelatin
½ cup cold water
1 ½ cup honey
⅓ cup water
1-2 egg white separated from yolk*
1 teaspoon vanilla extract
1 teaspoon coconut extract* (this can also be substituted with more vanilla extract)
¼- ½ cup of finely shredded coconut or coconut flour for dusting
Neutral oil spray

KITCHEN EQUIPMENT

Large pot or saucepan
Measuring spoons & measuring cups
Spatula or large spoon
Standing electric mixer or handheld*
Digital candy thermometer
Large mixing bowl
Baking parchment paper
12 x 10 rectangle glass baking or similarly large rectangle roaster

SPECIAL INSTRUCTIONS/DIET INFORMATION

*The amount of eggs in this recipe is based on egg size. Do not use pasteurized liquid egg whites as they will not whip into stiff peaks. Allowing the eggs to come to room temperature before whipping will yield the best results.

*Always verify ingredients for coconut extract if purchasing. However, you can make your own by using ¾ -1 cup of unsweetened shredded coconut, then cover ¾ – 1 cup of distilled SCD legal alcohol. (Essentially equal parts ratio of coconut and alcohol). Place in a sterilized airtight glass bottle or container (i.e. mason jar). Store in a cool dark area and let sit for several day to 2 weeks and give a shake once a day. Once the extract has reached the desired level of coconut flavor, drain the extract form the shredded coconut and store in an airtight container in the fridge.

*A standing kitchen mixer is highly recommended since the process takes time and may require additional hands when adding the honey syrup.

DIRECTIONS

1. Soften the gelatin in a ½ cup of cold water and set aside.
2. Line the baking dish with parchment paper and set aside. You may need to grease the pan with oil or butter to allow the parchment to form and stick to the sides.
3. In the large pot add the honey and ⅓ cup of water together. Heat the honey and water, stirring until the mix reaches the "soft ball" stage at approximately 235 degrees F.
4. Remove the pot from heat. Stir in gelatin until dissolved and allow the sauce to cool down 10-15 minutes.
5. In the large mixing bowl, beat the egg white to stiff peaks. Then slowly add syrup until the candy is beaten into soft peaks. (Important to note this will take a while) Then mix in the extracts.
6. Line the large rectangular dish or roaster with parchment paper. Pour the marshmallow fluff into the pan, dust with coconut flour and/or finely shredded coconut.
7. Lay a large piece of parchment paper over the top of the dish and allow to stand overnight. (Note the marshmallows will set best when the temperature is cooler.)
8. Cut into squares using a knife sprayed with neutral oil and dust the marshmallows with more coconut flour or shredded coconut. Place the marshmallow squares in airtight container and freeze for long term storage.
9. You can use the marshmallows later in other recipes like blondies, frosting and cookies.

Low Fat Caramel Apple Dip

Approximate Yield
24 servings

Prep Time 20 min
Total Time 2 hours
(To allow for refrigeration)

Estimated Macronutrients
3 g P • 7 g C • 2 g F

INGREDIENTS

1 cup of SCD Nonfat Greek Yogurt (see recipe page 298)
1 cup of SCD Coconut Marshmallow Fluff
(see recipe page 284)
½ cup Sea Salt Caramel Sauce (see recipe page 103)
1 tablespoon peanut butter softened*
Chopped shelled and roasted peanuts

Sliced granny smith apples

KITCHEN EQUIPMENT

Standing electric mixer or handheld
Spatula or large spoon
Measuring spoons & measuring cups
Large mixing bowl
Dip dish with lid or plastic wrap

SPECIAL INSTRUCTIONS/DIET INFORMATION

*Nut butters that are SCD legal should only include the nut and possibly a legal oil and/or salt. For example, peanut butter is generally roasted peanuts and salt. There are some brands that will sweeten with honey but there are very few commercially available.

DIRECTIONS

1. In the large mixing bowl, whip the SCD nonfat Greek yogurt and coconut marshmallow fluff.
2. Place in refrigerator to set.
3. Mix well the caramel sauce and peanut butter (You may need to warm the caramel sauce to soften it).
4. Pour the peanut butter caramel sauce on the marshmallow fluff dip, and sprinkle with chopped roasted peanuts. Serve with apple slices.

Caramel Apple No-Cheese Cake

Approximate Yield	Prep Time 20 min	Estimated Macronutrients
10-12 servings	Total Time 2 hours	13 g P • 37 g C • 16 g F
	(To allow for refrigeration)	

INGREDIENTS

Crust*

1 cup almond flour
4 tablespoons butter (salted)
3 tablespoons coconut flour
2 tablespoons honey
1 teaspoon cinnamon
¾ teaspoon unflavored gelatin
Pinch of salt
Neutral cooking oil or spray

Salted Caramel Sauce

1 cup of (full fat) coconut cream*
½ cup of honey
½ teaspoon sea salt
1 teaspoon vanilla

Filling

16oz (2 cups) of SCD Nonfat Greek Yogurt (see recipe page 298)
½ cup of honey
½ cup of pasteurized liquid egg whites or 6-8 egg whites separated from yolks*
1 egg
1 teaspoon of vanilla extract
1 tablespoon gelatin

Streusel Topping

3 tablespoons honey
2 tablespoons toasted unsweetened coconut coarse flakes
2 tablespoons thinly sliced almonds
2 tablespoons chopped pecans
¾ teaspoon cinnamon
¼ cup chopped, salted, roasted shelled peanuts

Apple layer

2 ½ - 3 cups of peeled thinly sliced chopped apples
2 teaspoons lemon juice
¾ teaspoon ground cinnamon
3 tablespoons Sea Salt Caramel Sauce (see recipe page 103 or below) Be sure to set aside enough to drizzle for serving

KITCHEN EQUIPMENT

Immersion blender
9–10-inch springform pan
Baking parchment paper
Standing or handheld electric mixer
Spatula or large spoon
Mixing bowls
Measuring spoons & measuring cups

SPECIAL INSTRUCTIONS/DIET INFORMATION

*Note you can also substitute the almond flour, and coconut flour by using leftover Chewy Graham Crackers (recipe on page 275) as a crust by blending them in a food processor with honey and melted butter. However macronutrient values will change.
*Coconut cream cannot have emulsifiers are additives (i.e., guar gum), only water and coconut. The coconut cream should also be unsweetened and full fat.
* If using pasteurized liquid egg whites, be careful to read all ingredients. This should be a mono ingredient, and not contain any preservatives or additives other than pasteurized egg whites. Regular separated egg whites can be used but the batter will be thicker and require many eggs. Note the conversion is 2 tablespoons of pasteurized liquid eggs to 1 egg white.

DIRECTIONS

Crust

1. Preheat oven to 350 degrees F. Line the spring form pan with parchment paper, ensuring it reaches the bottom edges. Be careful not to poke any holes or rip the parchment. Spray or brush the sides of the pan well with cooking oil.
2. Combine the ingredients for the crust, mixing until the dough is crumbled. With greased hands spread and press the crust dough into a thin layer on the bottom of the spring form pan covered in parchment paper.
3. Bake the crust for 12 min or until golden. Remove from oven and allow to cool on a wire rack.

DIRECTIONS (continued)

Salted Caramel Sauce

4. In a medium saucepan and on high heat whisk together the coconut milk, honey, and sea salt.
5. Bring the mixture to a boil and allow to bubble for 3-5 minutes before lowering the heat to medium-low.
6. Allow the sauce to simmer for 30-40 minutes, continually stirring to thicken and prevent burning.
7. Remove the sauce from heat and stir in the vanilla extract. Then allow the sauce to cool to warm and pour in a glass jar with lid to refrigerate.

Streusel Topping

8. Combine all the ingredients in a small mixing bowl ad stirring until the streusel is well mixed. Set aside.

Filling

9. For the filling, combine all the ingredients in a large bowl and mix with a standing or handheld electric mixer.
10. Pour filling batter into the pan over the cooled crust. Spread the batter evenly and set aside for assembling the cake.

Apple Topping & Assembling the Cake

11. In a mixing bowl combine all the ingredients, stirring and coating the apples well.
12. Place the apples evenly across the top of the filling.
13. Then add the streusel topping and spread evenly over the apples.
14. Preheat the oven at 325 and place foil over the cake. Bake for 30 min and remove the foil. Then bake for another 20-25 min without the foil, until the center is firm and does not jiggle. Allow the cake to cool on a wire rack for 1-2 hrs. before placing in refrigerator to chill.

Pumpkin Pie

Approximate Yield
10-12 servings

Prep Time 20 min
Total Time 4 hours
(To allow for refrigeration)

Estimated Macronutrients
18 g P • 29 g C • 14 g F

INGREDIENTS

Crust
¾ cup almond flour
3 tablespoons coconut flour
3 tablespoons hazelnut flour
3 tablespoons butter (unsalted)
2 tablespoons honey
1 teaspoon unflavored gelatin

Pumpkin Filling
1 can of pureed pumpkin (15 oz or 2 cups)
2 eggs
2 egg whites or ½ cup pasteurized liquid egg whites*
½ cup honey
1 tablespoon + 1 teaspoon Pumpkin Pie Spice (see recipe page 144)
1 tablespoon unflavored gelatin
¾ cup of SCD Nonfat Greek Yogurt (see recipe page 298)

KITCHEN EQUIPMENT
Immersion blender
9–10-inch springform pan
Mixing bowls
Measuring spoons & measuring cups
Spatula or large spoon
Baking parchment paper
Standing or handheld electric mixer

SPECIAL INSTRUCTIONS/DIET INFORMATION
*Be careful to read all ingredients for pasteurized liquid egg whites. This should be a mono ingredient, and not contain any preservatives or additional ingredients. Regular separated egg whites can be used but the batter may be thicker and require many eggs.

DIRECTIONS

Crust
1. Preheat oven to 350 degrees F. Line the spring form pan with parchment paper, ensuring it reaches the bottom edges. Be careful not to poke any holes or rip the parchment. Spray or brush the sides of the pan well with cooking oil.
2. Combine the ingredients for the crust, mixing until the dough is crumbled. With greased hands spread and press the crust dough into a thin layer on the bottom of the spring form pan covered in parchment paper.
3. Bake the crust for 12 min or until golden. Remove from oven and allow to cool on a wire rack.

Pumpkin Filling
4. For the pumpkin pie, beat the eggs with a standing or handheld electric mixer. Then combine remaining filling ingredients in a large bowl.
5. Pour the filling batter evely over the cooled crust.
6. Bake for 45 min with foil, then remove the foil to bake for an additional 15-20 min and the center is firmly set and does not jiggle. Then allow to cool on a wire rack for 1-2 hours. Place in the refrigerator to chill and serve cold.

Pumpkin Spice Bread Pudding

Approximate Yield	Prep Time 20 min	Estimated Macronutrients
10-12 servings	Total Time 55 min	30 g P • 13 g C • 6 g F

INGREDIENTS

1 bread loaf (approximately 3-4 cups cut into cubes) of leftover Cloud Bread or Cashew Bread or (see recipes page 310 & 311)

1 (15 oz can or 2 cups) pureed pumpkin or butternut squash

¾ cup unsweetened cashew milk or other nut milk*

¾ cup pasteurized liquid egg whites*

3 large eggs

¼ cup of honey

2 teaspoons of vanilla extract

¼ teaspoon cinnamon

¼ teaspoon ground nutmeg

¼ teaspoon ground cloves

Pinch of sea salt

Butter or neutral oil for greasing baking dish

KITCHEN EQUIPMENT

Large mixing bowl
Measuring spoons & measuring cups
Spatula or large spoon
Whisk or mixer and beaters
9 x 13 glass rectangular baking dish
Aluminum foil

SPECIAL INSTRUCTIONS/DIET INFORMATION

*Any nut milks should only consist of nuts, water, or salt. No emulsifiers, gums, sweeteners or additives should be in the ingredient list. If you are unable to source a SCD legal nut milk you can make them easily at home (see recipe page 299).
*Be careful to read all ingredients for pasteurized liquid egg whites. This should be a mono ingredient, and not contain any preservatives or additional ingredients. Regular separated egg whites can be used but the batter will be thicker and require many eggs.

DIRECTIONS

1. Preheat oven to 350 degrees F. Spray or brush the glass baking dish with cooking oil well including the sides of the dish.
2. Cut the bread into cubes and lay in the baking dish.
3. In a large mixing bowl, beat the eggs, pumpkin and all other ingredients.
4. Pour the batter over the cubed bread. Cover with foil and place in oven.
5. Bake for 40-45 min. Remove the foil and bake for another 15-20 minutes. Insert a toothpick or knife into the center and if it comes out clean the bread pudding is done.

Marbled Pumpkin No-Cheese Cake

Approximate Yield	Prep Time 20 min	Estimated Macronutrients
10 servings	**Total Time 55 min**	**14 g P • 13 g C • 1 g F**

INGREDIENTS

Crust
3 tablespoons coconut flour
3 tablespoons hazelnut flour
¾ cup almond flour
3 tablespoons butter (unsalted)
2 tablespoons honey
1 teaspoon unflavored gelatin

Pumpkin Filling
1 can of pureed pumpkin (15 oz or 2 cups)
1 egg
2 egg whites or liquid egg
½ cup honey
1 tablespoon Pumpkin Pie Spice (see recipe page 144)
1 tablespoon unflavored gelatin
Optional: ⅓ cup of Nonfat SCD Greek Yogurt for additional protein

No Cheesecake Filling
16oz (2 cups) of SCD Nonfat Greek Yogurt
(see recipe page 298)
1 egg
½ cup of honey
1 teaspoon of vanilla extract
1 tablespoon unflavored gelatin
½ cup of pasteurized liquid egg whites*

KITCHEN EQUIPMENT
Immersion blender
Large mixing bowl
Measuring spoons & measuring cups
Spatula or large spoon
9–10-inch springform pan
Baking parchment paper
Standing or handheld electric mixer
Oven

SPECIAL INSTRUCTIONS/DIET INFORMATION
*Be careful to read all ingredients for pasteurized liquid egg whites. This should be a mono ingredient, and not contain any preservatives or additional ingredients. Regular separated egg whites can be used but the batter will be thicker and require many eggs

DIRECTIONS

Crust

1. Preheat oven to 350 degrees F. Line the spring form pan with parchment paper, ensuring it reaches the bottom edges. Be careful not to poke any holes or rip the parchment. Spray or brush with cooking oil well the sides of the pan.
2. Combine the ingredients for the crust, mixing until the dough is crumbled. With greased hands spread and press the crust dough into a thin layer on the bottom of the spring form pan covered in parchment paper.
3. Bake the crust for 12 min or until golden. Remove from oven and allow to cool on a wire rack.

Pumpkin Filling

4. For the pumpkin filling, combine all the ingredients in a large bowl and mix with a standing or handheld electric mixer. Set aside in the refrigerator while combining the remaining cake filling.

No-Cheese Filling

5. For the No-Cheesecake filling, beat the eggs and add the remaining ingredients, mixing with a standing or handheld electric mixer.

6. Pour the No-Cheesecake filling batter into the pan over the cooled crust evenly.
7. Then pour the pumpkin filling over the No-Cheesecake batter evenly. Using a knife or toothpick, swirl the pumpkin to create a marbled pattern and mixing it with batter filling.
8. Bake for 45 min with foil, then remove the foil to bake for an additional 20-25 min and the center is firmly set and does not jiggle. Then allow to cool on a wire rack for an 1-2 hrs. Place in refrigerator to chill and serve cold.

Raisin Bread Pudding with Vanilla Sauce

Approximate Yield	Prep Time 20 min	Estimated Macronutrients
10-12 servings	Total Time 55 min	28 g P • 56 g C • 29 g F

INGREDIENTS

1 loaf (approximately 3-4 cups cut into cubes) of leftover
SCD Cinnamon Raisin Bread (see recipe page 66)
3 large eggs
1 teaspoon of vanilla extract
¾ cup unsweetened cashew milk or other nut milk*
¾ cup pasteurized liquid egg whites*
¼ cup of honey
¼ teaspoon cinnamon

Butter or neutral oil for greasing baking dish

Optional Vanilla Sauce
2 tablespoons coconut butter
½ cup honey
1 cup unsweetened cashew milk
1 tablespoon vanilla extract
Dash of cinnamon
Dash sea salt

KITCHEN EQUIPMENT

Large mixing bowl
Measuring spoons & measuring cups
Spatula or large spoon
Whisk or mixer and beaters
9 x 13 glass rectangular baking dish
Aluminum foil

SPECIAL INSTRUCTIONS/DIET INFORMATION

*Any nut milks should only consist of nuts, water, or salt. No emulsifiers, gums, sweeteners or additives should be in the ingredient list. If you are unable to source a SCD legal nut milk you can make them easily at home (see recipe page 299).
*Be careful to read all ingredients for pasteurized liquid egg whites. This should be a mono ingredient, and not contain any preservatives or additional ingredients. Regular separated egg whites can be used but the batter will be thicker and require many eggs.

DIRECTIONS

1. Preheat oven to 350 degrees F. Spray or brush the glass baking dish with cooking oil well including the sides of the dish.
2. Cut the bread into cubes and lay in the baking dish.
3. In a large mixing bowl, beat the eggs, and all remaining ingredients together.
4. Pour the batter over the cubed bread. Cover the baking dish with foil and place in oven.
5. Bake for 40-45 min. Remove the foil and bake for another 15-20 minutes. Insert a toothpick or knife into the center and if it comes out clean the bread pudding is done.

Optional Vanilla Sauce

6. Melt the coconut butter in a glass bowl over a small pot of boiling water. Then add the honey and remaining ingredients. Drizzle the vanilla sauce over the warm bread pudding before serving.

PB & Coconut "Blookie" Cake

Approximate Yield	Prep Time 20 min	Estimated Macronutrients
12-16 servings	Total Time 90 min	23 g P • 46 g C • 35 g F

A blookie, is a blondie and cookie, arranged in layers and baked into a cake. After a competition, many athletes celebrate with decadent desserts. Athletes often undergo months (even years) of dedicated training and regimented nutrition in pursuit of athletic goals. This recipe is considered a decadent and celebratory dessert to be shared with family and friends once a competition is over or you've experienced a major athletic achievement.

INGREDIENTS
Pecan Coconut Chip Cookies
Wet
1 egg
½ cup butter softened
⅓ cup honey
1 tablespoon vanilla extract

Dry
1 ½ cup almond flour
¼ cup of dried egg white powder*
2 tablespoons coconut flour
½ teaspoon sea salt
½ teaspoon baking soda

¼ cup pecan pieces
¼ cup shredded unsweetened coconut

Blondies
Wet
8 oz of peanut butter*
½ cup honey
1 egg
1 teaspoon vanilla extract

Dry
⅓ cup of dried egg whites or ¼ cup of egg white protein powder*
¼ cup finely shredded coconut
½ teaspoon fine sea salt
½ teaspoon baking soda

Coconut Vanilla Cake
Wet
½ cup honey
¼ cup full fat unsweetened coconut milk or coconut cream
¼ cup ghee or softened butter
2 large eggs
2 tablespoons vanilla extract
Seeds of 1 vanilla bean pod
1 ½ tablespoons vanilla extract

Dry
½ cup coconut flour
½ cup dried egg white powder*
4 tablespoons grated cacao butter
¼ teaspoon baking soda
¼ teaspoon salt
¼ cup finely shredded unsweetened coconut

KITCHEN EQUIPMENT
Mixer and beaters
Measuring spoons & measuring cups
Spatula or large spoon
Fine grater
Oven
Large 9x13 inch glass baking dish
3-6 Medium to large mixing bowls (Generally you can reuse mixing bowls as you make the various batters. Reusing one medium bowl for the dry ingredients to save time cleaning.)
Baking parchment paper

SPECIAL INSTRUCTIONS/DIET INFORMATION
*If you are unable to eat or source dried egg white powder you can replace with almond flour. However it will not rise as high, the texture will be different, and there will be higher fat and less protein for the macronutrients.
*Nut butters that are SCD legal should only include the nut and possibly a legal oil and/or salt. For example, peanut butter is generally roasted peanuts and salt. There are some brands sweetened with honey but there are very few commercially available.
*If there is excess/leftover cake batter, bake separately in a muffin tin lined with parchment paper liners or a greased small cake pan. However, bake separately and after the Blookie Cake is baked.

DIRECTIONS
1. Preheat oven to 350 degrees F. Line the 9 x 13 baking dish with parchment paper.

2. For the Pecan Chip Cookies, in one large mixing bowl, beat the egg and mix in all the wet ingredients for the cookies. Slowly adding in the dry ingredients (except the shredded coconut and pecans). Once the dough has formed, stir in the shredded coconut and pecans. Set the dough aside in the refrigerator for assembly later.
3. For the Blondies, in a second large mixing bowl, beat the egg and mix in all the wet ingredients. Add in the dry ingredients, until a wet, gooey batter forms and set aside.
4. For the Vanilla Coconut Cake, in the third mixing bowl, add all the wet ingredients together and mix well. Slowly add in the dry ingredients and set aside the wet batter.

Layering

5. First scoop and press the pecan chip cookie dough into the bottom of the 9x 13 pan creating a crust on the parchment.
6. Next pour the blondie batter over the pecan chip cookie dough, smoothing the top well with the spatula.
7. For the final layer, pour the vanilla cake batter over the blondie batter carefully. Gently smoothing the top. If there is extra cake batter see notes*
8. Bake for 50-60 minutes until tops are golden and a knife or toothpick when inserted in the center comes out clean. Do not open the oven until 40 minutes has passed. When fully baked, remove from oven and set aside to cool.
9. For long term storage, refrigerate the blookies first and allow them to chill before cutting them into squares. Then freeze in airtight freezer bags or freezer safe containers for enjoyment on a later date.

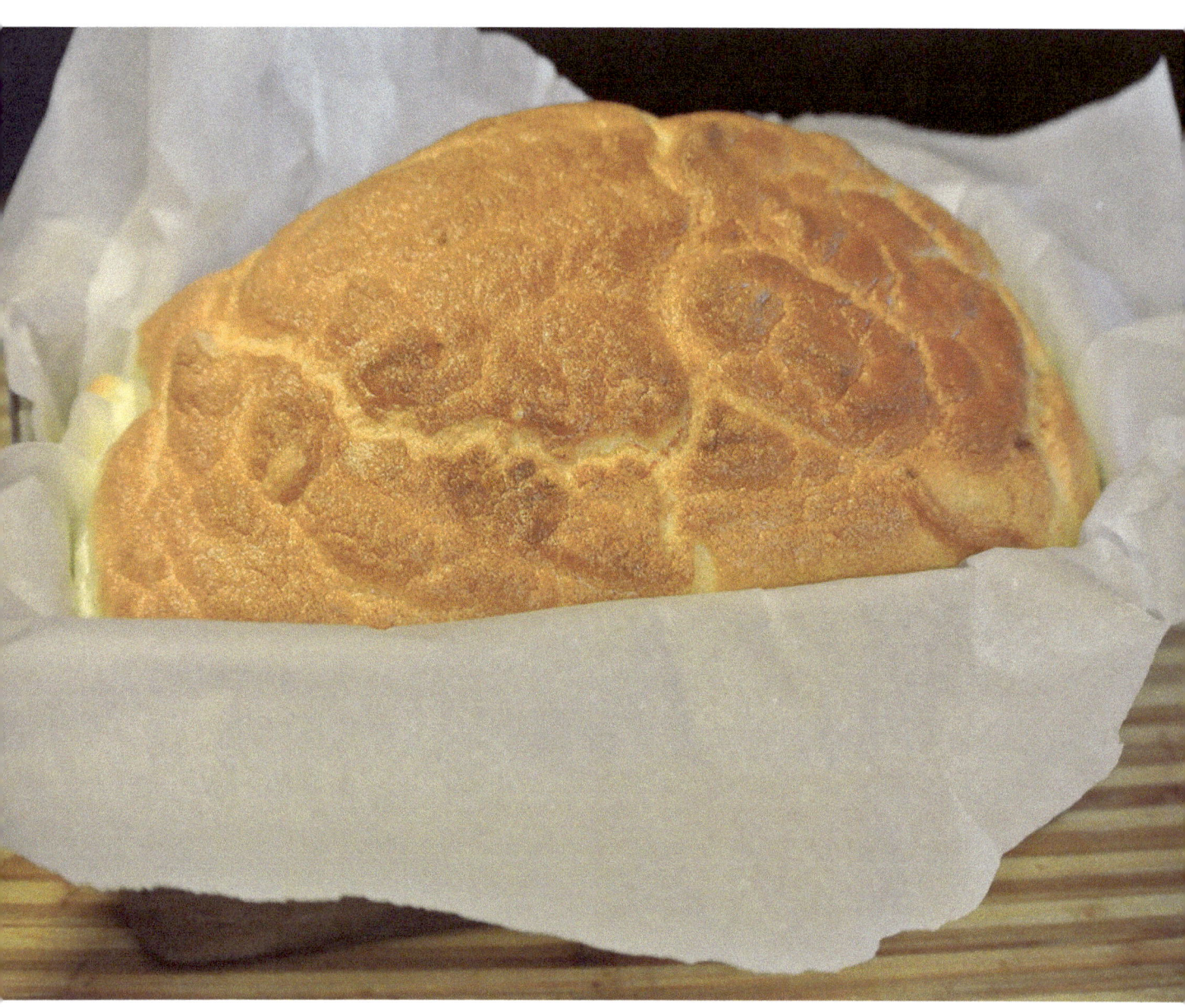

SCD Cloud Bread

Basics & Staples

As a busy athlete you don't have time to spend days in the kitchen preparing daily meals. Weekly and monthly meal preparation is key to reducing "cooking fatigue." Also, certain foods which take time to soak, marinate or slow cook should be cooked in large batches. For example, foods such as yogurt, legumes, breads, and wraps are frequently used in various recipes throughout the cookbook. Many of these foods can be prepared ahead and frozen for later use.

Easy Instant pot SCD Yogurt

Approximate Yield	Prep Time 15 min	Estimated Macronutrients
8-12 servings	**Total Time 26 hours**	**8 g P • 6 g C • 0 g F**
	(To allow fermenting & cooling)	

INGREDIENTS
1 half gallon of choice of milk or cream*
⅛ teaspoon SCD legal granulated yogurt starter or 2 tablespoons prepared plain yogurt with SCD legal cultures*

KITCHEN EQUIPMENT
Large half gallon or 2 qt sized yogurt strainers with lids
Whisk
Measuring spoons
Programmable pressure cooker/Instant pot
Sterilized large jars with lids or airtight containers for storage
Freezer silicone ice cube trays or cubes with lids

SPECIAL INSTRUCTIONS/DIET INFORMATION
*Throughout the cookbook SCD yogurt of varying fat contents are used for different recipes. The higher the fat content the recipe will generally yield a higher volume of yogurt and thicker in texture. Dripping the yogurt beyond 12 hours will yield thicker yogurt and is a good substitute for cream cheese or soft cheese in recipes. SCD Nonfat Greek Yogurt is made with nonfat milk and dripped for 12-24 hours depending on the desired thickness. Note, nonfat will also yield the least amount of yogurt since nonfat milk has minimal fat content and a high-water content.
* The recommended cultures in the Elaine Gottschall's book, Breaking the Vicious Cycle, are lactobacillus bulgaricus, L. acidophilus, and S. thermophilus. She recommended avoiding cultures with bifidus as they have been known to cause digestive issues.

DIRECTIONS
1. Pour the half gallon of non-fat milk, half and half, low fat or whole milk into the programmable pressure cooker such as an Instant pot.
2. Whisk the milk vigorously and secure the lid of the cooker. Then set the Instant pot to boil by using the yogurt function and raising the temperature from med to high. The digital indicator will say boil.
3. This will roughly take an hour. Ensuring there is enough room in the refrigerator to store a hot metal pot and lay a heat-resistant protective barrier on the surface of the shelf if needed.
4. When finished boiling the Instant pot will chime and indicate finished. Remove the metal internal pot, whisk the milk vigorously again, place foil over the top of the pot, then place in the refrigerator to cool. This will remain in the refrigerator for a minimum of 2 hours.
5. When ready to start the yogurt, put the internal pot back in the Instant pot and whisk in vigorously ⅛ teaspoon of granulated yogurt starter or 2 tablespoons of plain yogurt with cultures as a starter.
6. Secure the lid of the Instant pot, select yogurt then lower the temperature back to medium. Change the time to 24 hours and press the start button.
7. After 24 hours, ladle the yogurt into the yogurt strainers, and cover them with lids. Place yogurt in the refrigerator, straining the yogurt for 12 hours. The longer you strain the yogurt, the denser it will become.
8. Spoon the yogurt from the strainers and place in storage containers in the refrigerator.
9. The yogurt can generally be stored in a covered airtight container, refrigerated for up to one week. You can also freeze the yogurt in silicone ice cube trays or cubes, then store frozen yogurt in zip top freezer bag for later use in recipes.

Simple Cashew Milk and Other Unsweetened Nut Milks

Approximate Yield	Prep Time 15 min	Estimated Macronutrients
2-8 servings	Total Time 12 hours	4 g P • 6 g C • 9 g F
	(To allow for soaking)	

Many commercially available nut milks are made with ingredients considered illegal under the Specific Carbohydrate Diet. These ingredients often include emulsifiers, sweeteners, artificial flavors, and other additives. However, nut milk is very simple to make at home and takes very little time. Nut milk makers make the process convenient and quick, but fresh nut milk can be achieved with minimal tools.

INGREDIENTS
1 cup of raw unsalted cashews (or other kind of nut such as almonds, macadamia, etc.)
2 cups of filtered water

KITCHEN EQUIPMENT
Bowl or glass storage container with lid
Fine mesh colander or strainer
Food processor or blender with opening in lid
Measuring cups
Yogurt strainer with lid*
Sterilized large wide mouth mason jar with airtight lid (preferably with a pour spout)

SPECIAL INSTRUCTIONS/DIET INFORMATION
* Some yogurt strainers have a pressure mechanism that can be used to expedite the straining process, but not recommended for fine plastic/fabric yogurt strainers.

DIRECTIONS
1. Place the cashews in the bowl and cover with water to soak overnight.
2. Drain the cashews in the colander and rinse thoroughly with water.
3. Place the cashews in the food processor or high-speed blender and add the 2 cups of filtered water. Blending and processing at high speed until the cashews are completely ground up. This takes about 2-3 minutes.
4. Pour the nut pulp into the yogurt strainer and cover. Allowing it to drip and strain out the milk. This may take 1-2 hours in the refrigerator.
5. Pour the strained nut milk into the mason jar with airtight lid. The nut milk can generally be stored in the refrigerator for several days.
6. Leftover nut pulp can be used in various baked goods or dishes.

Simple Cashew Cream Butter

Approximate Yield
8-12 servings

Prep Time 15 min
Total Time 12 hours
(To allow for soaking)

Estimated Macronutrients
5 g P • 6 g C • 13 g F

If you are unable to source cashew butter without any additives or ingredients other than raw cashews, use this recipe. Nut butters are very simple to make at home and takes very little time. For the smoothest consistency, a high-powered food processor is the best tool for ensuring creamy cashew butter. Also you are not limited to cashews as this recipe can be used with a variety of nuts. However their textures and fat content will vary.

INGREDIENTS
2 cups of raw unsalted cashews
Optional: avocado oil for thinning

KITCHEN EQUIPMENT
Large food processor (7-11 cup size)
Spoon or spatula
Airtight container with lid

DIRECTIONS
1. Place the cashews in the food processor, and process for 10-20 minutes.
2. You will need to stop every 3 -4 minutes and scrape the sides of the processor, since cashews have a low-fat content. You can drizzle a tiny bit of avocado oil to lubricate and thin as needed. However, you will likely need to break up clumps and keep processing until the cashew butter has the smooth consistency of frosting and is no longer stiff.
3. Spoon the butter into an airtight container with lid. The cashew butter can generally be stored in the refrigerator for several days to be used in various baked goods or dishes.

Rustic Apple Sauce

Approximate Yield
2-6 servings

Prep Time 15 min
Total Time 3-6 hours
(To allow for slow cooking)

Estimated Macronutrients
1 g P • 25 g C • 0 g F

This recipe includes two different ways to make rustic apple sauce. One is by small batch and on the stovetop, while the other is large batch and in a crockpot.

INGREDIENTS

Small batch Stovetop Method
1-2 green or pink apples (peeled, cored, and sliced thinly)
Juice of one small lemon
2 tablespoons water
½ teaspoon cinnamon

Large Batch Crockpot Method
8 green or pink apples (peeled, cored, and sliced thinly)
¼ cup lemon juice
¼ cup water
1 tablespoon ground cinnamon

KITCHEN EQUIPMENT
Medium pot with lid
Optional: Handheld immersion blender
Measuring spoons & measuring cups
Heat-resistant spoon or spatula
Slotted spoon
Crockpot / slow cooker
Sterilized large mason jars with lids or silicone ice cube trays to freeze

DIRECTIONS

Stovetop Method
1. In the medium pot, add all ingredients and heat on medium – low heat with the lid on.
2. Stir the ingredients every 2-5 minutes to ensure the apples are not burning on the bottom. Lower the heat as needed.
3. The apples should be soft after 10-15 minutes. If you want to puree the apples you may need to add a couple tablespoons of water.
4. Allow to cool a bit before puree with an immersion blender.

Crockpot Method
5. Place the washed, cut and peeled apples in the crockpot. Then add the cinnamon, lemon juice and water.
6. Cover and cook 2-6 hours on low.
7. Either remove the apples or discard all water except ¼ cup for puree. Using a handheld immersion blender puree the apples.
8. The apple sauce can generally be stored in a covered airtight container, refrigerated for up to 7-10 days. You can also place in silicone ice trays to freeze into cubes and use for later.

Beef Bone Broth

Approximate Yield	Prep Time 60 min	Estimated Macronutrients
10-20 servings	Total Time 24 hours	6 g P • 5 g C • 1 g F
	(To allow for slow cooking)	

INGREDIENTS

2-4 lbs. of beef bones*
2 carrots cleaned, peeled and cut into 1–2-inch pieces
3 celery sticks, cleaned and cut into 1–2-inch pieces
5 cloves of peeled garlic
1 teaspoon of salt
3-4 quarts filtered water
2 tablespoons Worcestershire sauce (see recipe page 120)
3 whole bay leaves
¼ teaspoon dried thyme or 3 sprigs of fresh thyme
Optional:
2 tablespoons of red wine vinegar
⅛ teaspoon black pepper

KITCHEN EQUIPMENT

Oven
Baking sheet with sides or shallow large baking dish
Baking parchment paper
Large fine metal strainer/colander
Large slow cooker / crockpot
Measuring cups & measuring spoons
Large stock pot
Ladle or large spoon
Recommended: Silicone freezer containers/cubes with lids

SPECIAL INSTRUCTIONS/DIET INFORMATION

* Note if a simple beef bone broth is needed, you can omit the vegetables, herbs, sauce, vinegar and spices. Following the same directions, Roast the bones with salt, place in slow cooker and cover with water. Cook on low for 24 hours and discard the bones before storing

DIRECTIONS

1. Preheat oven to 375. Line the baking sheet or baking dish with parchment paper.
2. Place the beef bones, vegetables, and garlic on the parchment paper, sprinkle with a ¼ teaspoon salt and bake for 45-50 minutes.
3. Remove from the oven and place all beef bones, and vegetables in a large slow cooker.
4. Cover the meat and vegetables, with filtered water ensuring they are submerged. Then add in the Worcestershire sauce, bay leaves, dried thyme, remaining salt, optional red wine vinegar and black pepper.
5. Place lid on crockpot and cook on low for 24 hours. Turn off the crockpot and allow to cool.
6. Nest the metal strainer/colander in the large stock pot. Remove the pot from the crockpot and pour the bone broth, bones, and vegetables over the strainer/colander. Discard the bones and excess remnants from the strainer/colander.
7. Pour or ladle the bone broth into airtight, freezer safe containers and freeze for later use.

SCD Cooked Lentils & Legumes

Approximate Yield	Prep Time 15 min	Estimated Macronutrients
6-10 servings	Total Time 24 hours	2 g P • 5 g C • 1 g F
	(To allow for soaking & cooking)	

This recipe includes both slow cooker and stove pot cooking options.

INGREDIENTS

2 ½ cups red lentils, navy "white" beans, lima beans or black beans
½ teaspoon baking soda
8-12 cups of filtered water
½ teaspoon salt

Savory Option:

2 cups of bone broth or use recipes pages 302 & 255
1 tablespoon of any desired spice mixes, adjusting salt as needed

KITCHEN EQUIPMENT

Fine mesh colander
Large bowl or storage container with lid
Measuring spoons & measuring cups
Large pot with lid or large slow cooker
Heat-resistant spoon or spatula
Freezer safe plastic storage container with lids or silicone soup containers with lids to freeze

DIRECTIONS

1. Pour the red lentils, navy "white" beans or black beans in the fine mesh colander and rinse well with water. Remove any non-bean grit or processing residual from the beans.
2. Place the lentils or beans in the large bowl or storage container and cover with filtered water.
3. Stir in the baking soda and cover with lid. Place in refrigerator to soak. Important to note the beans or lentils will expand when soaking so ensure your container is large enough.
4. The beans or lentils will need to soak 12- 24 hours, and you will want to change out the water and baking soda halfway through the process.
5. If using a slow cooker, once the beans or lentils are soaked and drained of water, place the beans in the slow cooker. They will need to be covered with water and/or bone broth by about two inches. Add favorite spices if you are making savory beans or lentils.
6. Based on time constraints the beans can be cooked on high for 4-5 hours or low 6-8 hours. Lentils will take approximately 2-4 hours on high or 4-6 hours on low. Please note you should test the beans or lentils for tenderness regularly to prevent over cooking them.
7. If using a stove pot, once the beans or lentils are soaked and drained of water, place the beans in the large pot. They will need to be covered with water and/or bone broth by about two inches. Add favorite spices if you are making savory beans or lentils.
8. Bring to a boil and then reduce the heat to simmer and cover the pot with the lid. Generally, beans should take 45 minutes, and lentils should take 20-30 minutes.
9. To know they are done, the beans or lentils should be tender but firm, and you can check for doneness by smashing one.
10. It's important to not overcook lentils as it may be hard to strain off the water and they become mushy.
11. When the lentils or beans are done (for either slow cooker or stove top) Drain them from the liquid in a fine mesh colander or strainer. They can be used for other dishes that week or freezing them by storing in airtight containers for up to 3 months. Silicone soup trays or cubes are ideal. You may want to keep the beans covered with either broth or water to maintain moisture.
12. Puree or mash them when warm and still moist, then freezing is ideal for use in some recipes.

Easy SCD Slow Cooker Yellow Peas and Flour

Approximate Yield
8-12 servings

Prep Time 15 min
Total Time 24 hours
(To allow for soaking & cooking)

Estimated Macronutrients
12 g P • 35 g C • 13 g F

INGREDIENTS
2 ½ cups dried yellow split peas
½ teaspoon baking soda
8-12 cups of filtered water + more as needed

KITCHEN EQUIPMENT
Fine mesh colander
Measuring spoons & measuring cups
Large bowl or storage container with lid
Large crockpot/slow cooker (preferably 6 quarts) *
Sterilized plastic storage container with lids or silicone soup containers with lids to freeze
Optional: Handheld blender

For Flour:
Oven and baking sheets or food dehydrator and mesh trays
Baking parchment paper
Airtight BPA free food storage containers
High-speed, high-powered blender or grinder
Flour sifter
Optional: 1 gram food safe desiccant packets to prevent moisture

SPECIAL INSTRUCTIONS/DIET INFORMATION
* Certain alternative flours, such as vegetable or pea flours are recommended only in small quantities (i.e., cutting the amount of nut flours in baked goods, and for dredging meats before frying or baking) Vegetable and pea flours are generally dehydrated foods and without proper rehydration may cause gastric discomfort. It is best to increase the moisture content in various recipes if lentil, pea or squash flour is used.
*A programmable pressure cooker can be used however the cooking time will be significantly shortened. Cook times may vary based on how old the peas were, how long they soaked for, high mineral content in the water, the addition of salt etc. Program the cook time on high at 15 minutes, allow for pressure to build and release with the expected total cook time of 45 minutes. Always test the peas by squeezing a couple for tenderness.

DIRECTIONS
1. Pour the dried yellow split peas in the fine mesh colander and rinse well with water. Remove any non-pea grit or processing residual from the beans.
2. Place the split peas in the large bowl or storage container and cover with filtered water.
3. Stir in the baking soda and cover with lid. Place in refrigerator to soak. Important to note, the peas will expand when soaking so ensure your container is large enough.
4. The peas will need to soak 12-24 hours, and you will want to change out the water and baking soda halfway through the process.
5. Once the peas are soaked and drained of water, place them in the crockpot. They will need to be covered with water by about two inches.
6. Turn the crockpot on high for 4-6 hours and low for 8 hours. Check for doneness towards the end of those times. If the beans are old, they will take longer to cook and so be prepared for an extended cooking time. The peas should be tender but firm, and you can check for doneness by smashing one. It is important to not overcook the peas as it may be hard to strain off the water and they become mushy.
7. When the peas are done, turn off the crockpot to allowing them to cool a bit, then drain off the liquid (pour them over a fine mesh colander in case the peas tip out of the crockpot).
8. To make pea flour, remove excess water by straining with a fine mesh colander for an hour and allow the peas to cool. (Follow instructions for yellow split pea flour below)
9. If you intend to mash the peas, reserve some water, and using the handheld immersion blender puree the peas. Ideally, puree or mash the peas when warm and still moist.

DIRECTIONS (continued)

10. They can be used for other dishes that week or freeze by storing them in airtight containers for up to 3 months. Silicone soup trays or cubes is ideal. If you did not mash them, you may want to keep the peas covered with either broth or water to maintain moisture.

For Yellow Split Pea Flour

Oven Method:

11. If using an oven, preheat at 150- 200 degrees F (this is dependent on humidity and type of oven, for example some ovens cannot be turned lower than 200 degrees F).
12. Line the baking sheets with baking parchment paper. Evenly lay the cooked split peas on the paper, providing space for air to circulate. (This may require multiple baking sheets.)
13. Bake the peas for 2-6 hours, shaking and rotating the peas every hour to prevent overcooking and ensuring enough air is circulating. However dehydrating time varies based on humidity and oven temps. Check the peas for moistness and soft textures as this generally indicates the peas are not fully dehydrated.
14. Once the peas are dehydrated, turn off heat and allow to slowly cool to room temperature in oven.
15. Pour the dehydrated split peas into a high-speed grinder or blender. Grind the peas into a powder. Pea flour generally doesn't grind fully into a fine powder and has a medium coarseness like corn meal.
16. Store the flour in an airtight storage container. A cool, dry, dark cupboard is ideal for storage, and optionally add a 1-gram desiccant packet to allow the flour to last longer. Be careful to remove the desiccant packet before using or consuming the flour.

Dehydrator Method:

17. If using a dehydrator, line the mesh trays with parchment paper and evenly lay the cooked split peas on the paper, providing space for air to circulate. (This may require multiple dehydrator trays.)
18. Dehydrate the cooked split peas at 120-130 degrees F for 6-8 hours. Large cube dehydrators with fans generally allow for quicker drying times.
19. Check the peas for moistness and soft textures as this generally indicates the peas are not fully dehydrated.
20. Once the peas are dehydrated, turn off heat and allow to slowly cool to room temperature.
21. Pour the dehydrated split peas into a high-speed grinder or blender and grind the peas into a powder. Peas generally don't grind fully into a fine flour and a flour sifter may be needed to separate the larger pieces. You can regrind the medium to larger bits of pea or separate and use in recipes like corn meal.
22. Store in airtight storage container. A cool, dark cupboard is ideal for storage and optionally add 1-gram desiccant packet to allow the flour to last longer. Be careful to remove the desiccant packet before using or consuming the flour.

Yellow Pea Wraps

Approximate Yield	Prep Time 10 min	Estimated Macronutrients
10-20 servings	Total Time 40 min	5 g P • 13 g C • 1 g F

INGREDIENTS

1 cup of Yellow Split Pea Mash (see recipe page 304) *
1 tablespoon coconut flour
1 ½ cup egg whites or pasteurized liquid egg whites
1 teaspoon salt
1 teaspoon granulated garlic
Neutral oil

KITCHEN EQUIPMENT

Pizzelle or waffle cone maker
Heat resistant fork, tongs or spatula
Spoon or spatula
Medium bowl
Measuring spoons & measuring cups
Optional: Heat resistant brush & small bowl for oil

SPECIAL INSTRUCTION/DIET INFORMATION

*If using pasteurized liquid egg whites, be careful to read all ingredients. This should be a mono ingredient, and not contain any preservatives or additives, other than pasteurized egg whites. Regular separated egg whites can be used but the batter will be thicker and require many eggs. Note the conversion is 2 tablespoons of liquid eggs to 1 egg white.

DIRECTIONS

1. Preheat the pizzelle or waffle cone maker per the manufacturer's instructions. Then brush or spray the maker with coconut oil.
2. In a bowl place mix all the ingredients, stirring well to blend them together.
3. Ladle approximately 2 tablespoons of batter onto the waffle cone iron maker and press the lid down.
4. Each wrap should take approximately 3-4 minutes and remove the wraps from the maker when golden. Cool on parchment.
5. Wraps store for up to 3 days in a refrigerator and can be frozen for later use.

Pumpkin Street Tortillas

Approximate Yield
10-12 servings

Prep Time 10 min
Total Time 40 min

Estimated Macronutrients
5 g P • 10 g C • 3 g F

INGREDIENTS

1 (15 oz) can of pumpkin puree (or approximately 2 cups roasted pumpkin puree) *
1 cup pasteurized liquid egg whites*
3 tablespoons coconut flour
1 teaspoon granulated garlic*
1 teaspoon sea salt
1 teaspoon cumin
Neutral oil

KITCHEN EQUIPMENT

Pizzelle or waffle cone maker
Heat resistant fork, tongs or spatula
Spoon or spatula
Medium bowl
Measuring spoons & measuring cups
Optional: Heat resistant brush & small bowl for oil

SPECIAL INSTRUCTION/DIET INFORMATION

*Fresh pumpkin can be cooked and pureed as an alternative to canned.
*Be careful to read all ingredients for pasteurized liquid egg whites. This should be a mono ingredient, and not contain any preservatives or additional ingredients. Regular separated egg whites can be used but the batter will be thicker and require many eggs.

DIRECTIONS

1. Preheat the pizzelle or waffle cone maker per the manufacturer's instructions. Then brush or spray the press with coconut oil.
2. In a bowl, mix the pureed pumpkin, egg whites, coconut flour and spices together until smooth.
3. Ladle approximately 2 tablespoons of tortilla batter onto the waffle cone maker (or 1 tablespoon per each pizzelle) and press the lid down.
4. Each tortilla should take approximately 3-4 minutes and remove the tortilla from the maker when golden. Cool on parchment.
5. Tortillas store for up to 3 days in a refrigerator and can be frozen for later use.

Asian Style Green Onion Wraps

Approximate Yield	**Prep Time 10 min**	**Estimated Macronutrients**
12-20 servings	**Total Time 40 min**	**4 g P • 9 g C • 1 g F**

INGREDIENTS

3 green onions washed, and finely sliced
1 can of butternut squash (15 oz or approximately 2 cups roasted butternut squash puree)*
1 cup pasteurized liquid egg whites*
3 tablespoons coconut flour
1 teaspoon sea salt
½ teaspoon granulated garlic or 1 clove of finely grated garlic
Neutral oil

KITCHEN EQUIPMENT

Pizzelle or waffle cone maker
Immersion blender
Heat resistant fork, tongs or spatula
Spoon or spatula
Medium bowl
Measuring spoons & measuring cups

Optional: Heat resistant brush & small bowl for oil

SPECIAL INSTRUCTION/DIET INFORMATION

*Fresh butternut squash flesh can be pureed and cooked as an alternative to canned.
*Be careful to read all ingredients for pasteurized liquid egg whites. This should be a mono ingredient, and not contain any preservatives or additional ingredients. Regular separated egg whites can be used but the batter will be thicker and require many eggs.

DIRECTIONS

1. Preheat the pizzelle or waffle cone maker per the manufacturer's instructions. Then brush or spray the maker with coconut oil.
2. In a bowl place the sliced green onions, and butternut squash, then using the handheld immersion blender, puree them together well. Then stir in the remaining ingredients.
3. Ladle approximately 2 tablespoons of batter onto the waffle cone maker and lay the lid down.
4. Each wrap should take approximately 3-4 minutes and remove the wraps from the maker when golden. Cool on parchment.
5. Wraps store for up to 3-5 days in a refrigerator and can be frozen for later use.

Blender No-Corn Bread

Approximate Yield	Prep Time 20 min	Estimated Macronutrients
6-8 servings	Total Time 60 min	9 g P • 26 g C • 14 g F

INGREDIENTS

Wet

3 eggs

½ cup + 2 tablespoons unsweetened cashew milk
(unsweetened almond or coconut milk can be substituted) *

¼ cup melted butter or ghee

3 tablespoons honey

Dry

¼ cup almond flour

¼ cup Yellow Split Pea Flour (see recipe page 304) *

¼ cup coconut flour

¼ teaspoon baking soda

¼ teaspoon sea salt

KITCHEN EQUIPMENT

Food processor or blender

Large spoon or spatula

Measuring spoons & measuring cups

Oven

9x9 or 8x8 baking dish

Baking parchment paper

SPECIAL INSTRUCTIONS/DIET INFORMATION

*The yellow pea flour can be substituted with 2 tablespoons coconut flour and 2 tablespoons almond if necessary. However, the macronutrients and texture will be different.

*Any nut milks should only consist of nuts, water, or salt. No emulsifiers, gums, sweeteners or additives should be in the ingredient list. If you are unable to source a SCD legal nut milk you can make them easily at home (see recipe page 299).

DIRECTIONS

1. Preheat the oven to 350 degrees F. Line the baking dish with parchment paper (enough to cover the sides)
2. Mix all the dry ingredients in a small mixing bowl and set aside.
3. In the blender or food processor, add all the wet ingredients and pulse until well blended.
4. Add in the remaining dry ingredients until a wet dough has formed. Allow the dry ingredients to absorb the wet, and the pea flour to rehydrate. This should take about 10-15 minutes.
5. Pour batter into the parchment lined baking dish and bake for 35-40 minutes.
6. Remove from oven when the top is lightly golden, and when an inserted knife comes out clean, allow to cool for 5-10 minutes before serving warm.

SCD Cloud Bread

Approximate Yield **10-12 servings**	**Prep Time 20 min** **Total Time 70 min** (To allow for baking)	**Estimated Macronutrients** **10 g P • 1 g C • 0 g F**

Two variations, based on size of loaf and availability of ingredients.

INGREDIENTS

Variation 1

1 cup egg white powder
1 cup water
½ cup of thick, dripped SCD Nonfat Greek Yogurt (see recipe page 298)

Variation 2

4 egg whites*
1 cup of dried egg white powder*
1 cup of thick, dripped SCD Nonfat Greek Yogurt (see recipe page 298) or SCD legal farmers cheese*
¾ - 1 cup of water
1 teaspoon baking soda

KITCHEN EQUIPMENT

Standing electric mixer or handheld mixer
Measuring spoons & measuring cups
Large mixing bowls
Baking parchment paper
Standard bread loaf pan (approximately 8 ½ x 4 ½ in.)
Spatula or large spoon

SPECIAL INSTRUCTIONS/DIET INFORMATION

*Do not use liquid egg whites. You will need to separate the yolks which can later be used in the following recipes such as mayonnaise page 112 or bison fried rice page 302
*If you are unable to eat or source dried egg white powder you can replace with almond flour. However it will not rise as high, the texture will be different, and there will be higher fat and less protein for the macronutrients.
*If using farmers cheese, use a food processor or handheld immersion blender to whip the farmers cheese smooth

DIRECTIONS

1. Preheat oven to 350 degrees F. Line the loaf pan with parchment paper, ensuring it lines the sides and edges of the pan. Be careful not to poke any holes or rip the parchment.
1. Separate the egg whites from the yolks in two small bowls, prevent any shell fragments from falling in the egg whites.
2. Pour the egg whites into a large mixing bowl and beat the egg whites until stiff whipped peaks form.
3. Add in the remaining ingredients and beat until thoroughly mixed.
4. Pour into the parchment lined loaf pan and bake for 30-40 min. Insert a toothpick or knife into the center and if it comes out clean the bread is done. Allow to cool on a wire rack or cutting board.

Dairy Free Cashew Bread & Buns
(Large Batch)

Approximate Yield	Prep Time 20 min	Estimated Macronutrients
6-18 servings	**Total Time 90 min**	**14 g P • 33 g C • 15 g F**

*Use this recipe when you have excess egg whites from other recipes such as avocado mayonnaise or lemon curd.

INGREDIENTS
Wet
9 egg whites*
3 egg yolks*
14 oz (approximately 1 ¼ cup) of raw cashew butter*
½ cup unsweetened cashew milk or other nut milk*
3-4 tablespoons honey (depends on sweetness preference)
1 tablespoon apple cider vinegar

Dry
½ cup of coconut flour
¼ cup + 1 tablespoon of dried egg white powder or ¼ cup of egg white protein powder*
2 teaspoons baking soda
1 teaspoon sea salt

KITCHEN EQUIPMENT
2 large mixing bowls
Small mixing bowl
Electric mixer and beaters
Measuring spoons & measuring cups
Spatula or large spoon
Oven

3–4-inch diameter 6 bun silicone or non-stick pan
Standard bread loaf pan (approximately 8 ½ x 4 ½ in.)
Baking parchment paper

SPECIAL INSTRUCTIONS/DIET INFORMATION
*Egg whites need to be separated and not liquid in a carton as they will not whip into peaks
*Any nut milks should only consist of nuts, water, or salt. No emulsifiers, gums, sweeteners or additives should be in the ingredient list. If you are unable to source a SCD legal nut milk you can make them easily at home (see recipe page 299).
*If you are unable to eat or source an egg white protein powder with legal ingredients, or dried powdered egg whites, you can substitute with almond flour. However, it will not rise as high, the texture will be different, and there will be higher fat and less protein for the macronutrients.
*You will have extra egg yolks remaining however these can be used in another recipe i.e. Avocado Mayonnaise, Quick Moo Shu Pork or in the Bison Fried Cauliflower Rice recipe (see recipes pages 112, 229, 202)
*Nut butters that are SCD legal should only include the nut and possibly a legal oil and/or salt. For example, peanut butter is generally roasted peanuts and salt. There are some brands that will sweeten with honey but there are very few commercially available.

DIRECTIONS
1. Preheat oven to 325 degrees F. Line the bread loaf pan with parchment paper and grease the bun pan. Set both aside
2. Mix all the dry ingredients in a small mixing bowl and set aside
3. In a large mixing bowl, beat the egg whites until stiff peaks form (a standing mixer is recommended as this can take time) and set aside.
4. In the second large mixing bowl, beat the remaining wet ingredients. Then slowly add in the dry ingredients until a wet dough has formed.
5. Fold the whipped egg whites into the wet dough gently.
6. Pour dough into the parchment lined bread loaf pan, and greased bun pan.
7. Bake for 50-60 minutes until tops are golden and when an inserted knife or toothpick in the center comes out clean. Do not open the oven until 40 minutes has passed, the buns may be done baking after 40 minutes, but the bread may not be done and top fall limp.

Sourdough Bread or Buns

Approximate Yield	Prep Time 20 min	Estimated Macronutrients
6-12 servings	Total Time 90 min	27 g P • 23 g C • 12 g F

INGREDIENTS

Wet

3 eggs (yolks and whites separated)

¼ cup raw cashew butter*

1 ¼ cup of SCD Nonfat Greek Yogurt (see recipe page 298)

1 ½ tablespoons apple cider vinegar

¼ cup unsweetened cashew milk or other nut milk*

2 tablespoons honey (depends on sweetness preference)

Dry

½ cup of dried powdered egg whites*

⅓ cup of coconut flour

1 teaspoon baking soda

1 teaspoon sea salt

KITCHEN EQUIPMENT

Mixer and beaters

Measuring spoons & measuring cups

Spatula or large spoon

Large mixing bowls

Oven

Standard bread loaf pan (approximately 8 ½ x 4 ½ in.) or 3–4-inch diameter 6 bun silicone or non-stick pan

Baking parchment paper

SPECIAL INSTRUCTIONS/DIET INFORMATION

*Egg whites need to be separated and not pasteurized in a carton as they will not whip into stiff peaks needed for the recipe.

*If you are unable to eat or source egg white protein powder with legal ingredients or dried egg white powder, you can replace with almond flour. However it will not rise as high. The texture will be different, and it will have higher fat and less protein in macronutrients.

*Nut butters that are SCD legal should only include the nut and possibly a legal oil and/or salt. For example, peanut butter is generally roasted peanuts and salt. There are some brands that will sweeten with honey but there are very few commercially available. If you are unable to source raw cashew butter, see recipe page 300.

*Any nut milks should only consist of nuts, water, or salt. No emulsifiers, gums, sweeteners or additives should be in the ingredient list. If you are unable to source a SCD legal nut milk you can make them easily at home (see recipe page 299).

DIRECTIONS

1. Preheat the oven to 325 degrees F. Line the bread loaf pan with parchment paper, and grease the bun pan. Set both aside.
2. Mix all the dry ingredients in a small mixing bowl and set aside.
3. In a large mixing bowl, beat the egg whites until stiff peaks form (a standing mixer is recommended as this can take time).
4. In another large bowl beat together the egg yolks and the add in the remaining wet ingredients. Slowly mix in the dry ingredients until a wet dough has formed.
5. Fold the egg whites into the wet dough and beat briefly with the mixer.
6. Pour the bread batter into the parchment lined bread loaf pan, or bun pan.
7. For a bread loaf, bake for 50-60 minutes. Do not open the oven until 50 minutes has passed, or the bread will fall. The bread generally will take 60-70+ minutes. Remove from oven when the top is golden and when a knife or toothpick inserted in the center comes out clean.
8. If baking buns, they may be done baking after 35-40 minutes. Do not open the oven until 30 minutes has passed to ensure the buns rise. Remove from oven when the top is golden and when a knife or toothpick inserted in the center comes out clean.

Sourdough Bread and Buns
(Large Batch)

Approximate Yield	Prep Time 20 min	Estimated Macronutrients
6-18 servings	Total Time 90 min	24 g P • 25 g C • 10 g F

INGREDIENTS

Wet

9 egg whites*
3 egg yolks*
1 cup of raw cashew butter*
1 cup of SCD Nonfat Greek Yogurt (see recipe page 298)
1 tablespoon apple cider vinegar
½ cup unsweetened cashew milk or other nut milk*
3 tablespoons honey (depends on sweetness preference)

Dry

½ cup of coconut flour
¼ cup of egg white protein powder or ¼ cup of dried powdered egg whites*
1 teaspoon sea salt
2 teaspoons baking soda

KITCHEN EQUIPMENT

Mixer and beaters
Measuring spoons & measuring cups
Oven
3–4-inch diameter 6 bun silicone or non-stick pan
Standard bread loaf pan (approximately 8 ½ x 4 ½ in.)
Spatula or large spoon
Baking parchment paper

SPECIAL INSTRUCTIONS/DIET INFORMATION

*Egg whites need to be separated and not pasteurized in a carton as they will not whip into stiff peaks needed for the recipe.

*If you are unable to eat or source egg white protein powder with legal ingredients or dried egg white powder you can replace with almond flour. However it will not rise as high, the texture will be different, and there will be higher fat and less protein for the macronutrients.

*You will have extra egg yolks remaining however these can be used in another recipe i.e., Mayo, custard ice cream or in the breakfast bison cauliflower recipe (see recipes pages 202)

*Nut butters that are SCD legal should only include the nut and possibly a legal oil and/or salt. For example, peanut butter is generally roasted peanuts and salt. There are some brands that will sweeten with honey but there are very few commercially available.

*Any nut milks should only consist of nuts, water, or salt. No emulsifiers, gums, sweeteners or additives should be in the ingredient list. If you are unable to source a SCD legal nut milk you can make them easily at home (see recipe page 299).

DIRECTIONS

1. Preheat the oven to 325 degrees F. Line the bread loaf pan with parchment paper, and grease the bun pan. Set both aside.
2. Mix all the dry ingredients in a small mixing bowl and set aside.
3. In a large mixing bowl, beat the egg whites until stiff peaks form (a standing mixer is recommended as this can take time).
4. Add in the remaining wet ingredients until mixed together with egg whites. Slowly add in the dry ingredients until a wet dough has formed.
5. Pour into the bread loaf pan and bun pan.
6. Bake for 50-60 minutes until tops are golden and when a knife or toothpick inserted in the center comes out clean. Do not open the oven until 40 minutes has passed, the buns may be done baking after 40 minutes. However, the bread may not be fully baked, and it will not rise properly if the oven is opened too soon. The bread generally takes a full 60 minutes.

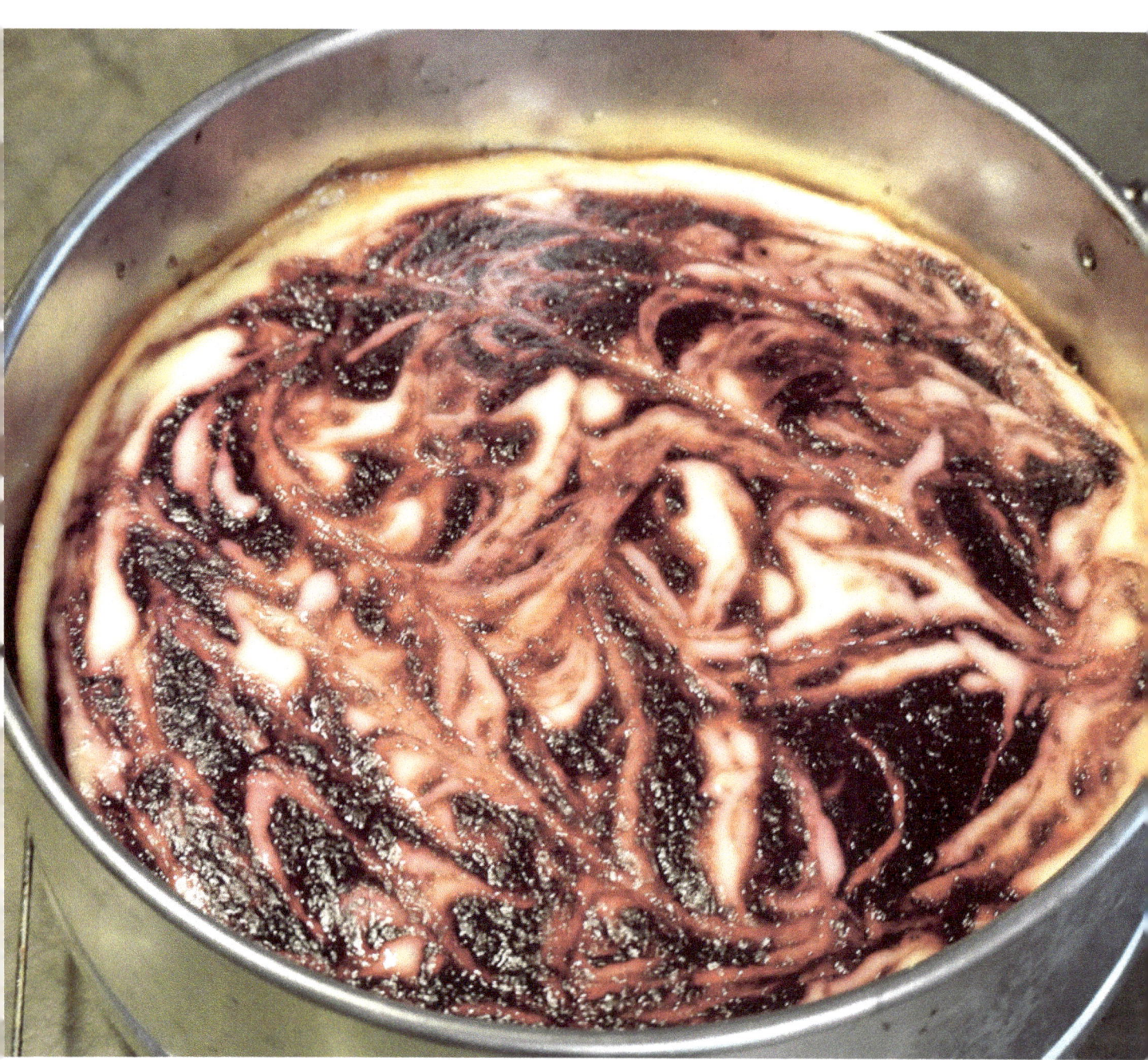

Cherry Swirl No-Cheese Cake

Recipe "Stacking" Reference

This guide reduces the guesswork of what to do with leftovers, as many of the recipes in this cookbook are intentionally created for large portions and freezing. It's important to note that this reference guide is not all-inclusive, as many of the recipes in the cookbook are intended to be combined in various ways.

Recipe	Other Recipe Uses
Roasted Chicken	Southwest Bean Salad Thai Coconut Chicken Soup SCD Enchilada Soup Asian Chicken "Noodle" Salad SCD Chicken Paella Goi Ga (Vietnamese Chicken Salad) Pesto Chicken Salad Easy Chicken Crust Pizza
Sage and Turkey Sausage	SCD Paleo Zuppa Toscano Portable Baked Pasta Stuffed Breakfast Squash
SCD Cooked Lentils, White Beans or Black Beans	SCD Enchilada Soup Southwest Bean Salad Minestrone Soup Greek White Bean, Cucumber and Tomato Salad Freezer Bag Beef Chili Red Pepper Hummus Dip Refried Beans Mediterranean Hummus Dip Dill Pickle Hummus Dip
Electrolyte Vegetable Juice	Tomato Vegetable Gazpacho Slow Cooker Tomato Vegetable Beef Pot Roast
Easy Oven Lemon Baked Salmon	Salmon and Dill Pasta Salad
Roasted Spaghetti Squash	Yakisoba Style Spaghetti Squash Easy Chicken and Spaghetti Squash Crust Pizza Singapore Style Spaghetti Squash SCD Lasagna

Recipe	Other Recipe Uses
Cowboy Candy	Sweet & Spicy Cowboy Chicken
Habanero Mango Lime Cod	Cod Ceviche
Best Darn Tri Tip	California Cheesesteak Bowl Beef Bahn Mi Bowl
Bulgogi Beef Marinade and Glaze	Beef Bahn Mi Bowl
SCD "Sourdough"Bread Cashew Buns Cloud bread Dad's Zucchini Bread Walnut Cranberry SCD Cinnamon Raisin Bread Loaded Pumpkin Bread	French Toast Cakes Blender Bread Balls SCD Portable Shepherd Pies Crustless Sandwich Pies Portable Pie Variations SCD Raisin Bread Pudding with Vanilla Sauce Pumpkin Spice Bread Pudding
Loaded Turkey and Veggie Spaghetti Sauce	Portable Baked Pasta SCD Lasagna
SCD Creamy No-Tato Chicken Soup	Cheddar Biscuit Dumpling Chicken Pot Pie
Honey Lemon Curd	Lemon Curd Froyo Pops Lemon Coconut Yogurt Bars Lemon Poppyseed Sheet Pan Protein Pancakes
SCD Enchilada Sauce	SCD Beef Pozole Rojo SCD Enchilada Soup Butternut Squash Enchilada Bake
SCD Harissa Paste (Mild)	Harissa Honey Carrots Sriracha Mayo
Habanero Mango Sauce	Habanero Mango Lime Cod Cod Ceviche Habanero Mango Coleslaw Beef Bahn Mi Bowl

Recipe	Other Recipe Uses
Korean Easy Pickled Vegetables Salad	Vietnamese Grilled Pork with Salad Korean Ground Beef Korean BBQ Chicken Tacos
Pumpkin Street Tortillas	Portable Pie Variations Slow Cooker Pork Chili Verde Freezer Bag Chicken Fajitas Ground Turkey Tacos
SCD Asian Style Wraps Yellow Pea Wraps	Korean BBQ Chicken Tacos Quick Moo Shu Pork (or Chicken) Portable Pie Variations Slow Cooker Chicken Tikka Masala Gyro or Döner Meat
Walnut Pesto	Walnut Pesto Pasta Salad Pesto Chicken Salad

Measurements & Conversions

Volume Conversions		
U.S. Standard	Imperial	Metric
3 tsp = 1 tablespoon 4 tblsp = 1/4 cup 8 tblsp = 1/2 cup 16 tblsp = 1 cup	1 tablespoon = 1/2 fl oz 1 cup = 1/2 pint = 8 fl oz 2 cups = 1 pint = 16 fl oz 4 cups = 1 quart 2 pints = 1 quart 4 quarts = 1 gallon	1 teaspoon = 5 ml t tablespoon = 15 ml 1/4 cup = 60 ml 1/2 cup = 125 ml 3/4 cup = 175 ml 1 cup = 250 ml 1 pint = 480 ml 1 quart = 1 liter

Weight Conversions
1/2 oz = 15 grams
1 oz = 30 grams
2 oz = 60 grams
4 oz = 115 grams
8 oz = 225 grams
1 lb = 450 grams
2 lbs = 900 grams

Substitutions

Honey

There are a few options that can substitute for honey. Dates are the only option with a one-to-one ratio for honey. Other substitutions need to be doubled and may impact the dish either by flavor or texture. Fruit purees generally have a lower sugar content and therefore require more. Baked goods recipes are generally forgiving when using fruit purees. However, keep in mind you may need to offset the ratio of dry ingredients such as adding more nut flour or dried egg white powder.

Honey	
1 tablespoon of honey	1 tablespoon of minced dates
	1 tablespoon date syrup
	1/4 cup of unsweetened apple sauce
	2 tablespoons of minced rehydrated raisins
	2 tablespoons of minced rehydrated prunes or plum puree
	1/4 cup of persimmon puree

Vanilla Extract

Some people may have sensitivity to the alcohol in extract, therefore the seeds of the vanilla bean can be used instead. You can also add ¼ - ½ teaspoon of honey with the vanilla seeds to create a sweetened paste.

Vanilla Extract	
1 tablespoon of vanilla extract	Seeds from 1 vanilla bean
1 teaspoon of vanilla extract	1/4 of the seeds of 1 vanilla bean + 1/4 teaspoon honey (for paste)

Baking Powder

Baking powder is illegal under the Specific Carbohydrate Diet due to anti-caking properties and the starch content. However, it is easy to replicate using baking soda and an acidic compound.

Baking Powder	
1 teaspoon of baking powder	1/2 teaspoon baking soda + 1/2 tsp of white vinegar
	1/2 teaspoon baking soda + 1/2 tsp of lemon juice
	1/2 teaspoon baking soda + SCD legal yogurt

Cream of Tartar

Cream of Tartar is considered an illegal ingredient under the Specific Carbohydrate Diet. Generally its used in recipes for stabilizing the proteins, and as a leavening agent. Therefore substitutions are necessary and are very recipe dependent.

Cream of Tartar	
1/2 tsp of cream of tartar	1 teaspoon lemon juice
	1 teaspoon white vinegar
	1 tablespoon- 1/4 cup of plain SCD yogurt (note this is recipe dependent)

Nut Butter

Nuts are generally a staple under the Specific Carbohydrate Diet. However, many nut butters can be replaced with seed butters for a 1:1 ratio. In many recipes nut butters are used as fat sources, binders and thickeners. The alternatives below can be good substitutes depending on the recipe as they may change the taste.

Nut Butter	
Any amount of nut butter	Any amount of seed butter
	(Important note, soy, flax and chia seed butters are illegal under SCD)
	Palm shortening
	Full fat dripped SCD yogurt
	Avocado or avocado butter

Eggs

Eggs are one of the foods that people have a sensitivity to. Therefore having alternative ingredients to replace eggs in recipes is key. Egg protein acts as a binder and source of moisture in recipes and very hard to replicate. Just keep in mind several of the options listed (especially fruit) will change the flavor of the dish. Important to note, some people have less sensitivity to eggs from other fowl such as duck and geese. Just keep in mind when calculating quantities in a recipe 1 goose egg equates to 3 chicken eggs.

Eggs	
1 egg	1 tablespoon of unflavored gelatin dissolved in 3 tblsp of warm water
	1/4 cup of mashed ripe banana
	2 tablespoons of full fat, dripped SCD greek yogurt
	1/4 cup pureed prunes
	1/4 apple sauce
	1/4 cup persimmon puree

Common Culinary Terms Guide

Chop: Using quick and heavy blows of a knife or cleaver to cut food into bit size pieces. A food processor or vegetable chopping tool can also be used to chop foods. Chopped foods are coarsely cut and larger pieces compared to minced foods.

Bloom: To moisten gelatin in a small amount of water before adding it to a hot liquid or sauce to dissolve.

Mince: To cut foods into very small pieces, and less than bite sized. For reference, a finely minced ingredient is generally the size of the gap between the tines of a standard dinner fork. There are presses and mincing tools specifically for vegetables available if you do not have the skills.

Blanching: To quickly dip or plunge food in boiling water, then shock in an ice water bath to stop the cooking process.

Fold or folding: A technique used to gently combine a lighter mixture or ingredient with a heavier one. Using a spatula or spoon lay the heavier ingredient over the lighter ingredient and repeat gently. Folding differs from stirring, as the objective is to combine the ingredients but not lose the integrity of the lighter ingredient.

Sauté: To cook food quickly over medium to high heat, oftentimes using fat or oil. (Similar to pan-frying.)

Reduce/reduction: To boil a liquid rapidly until the volume is reduced by evaporation and changes the consistency of the sauce or dish. This technique often thickens the dish and may intensify the flavor.

Baste: To moisten food with a liquid and/or fat to keep it flavorful and moist while in the cooking process.

Julienne: To cut foods lengthwise, often in thin sticks or referred to as a "matchstick."

Parboiling/parcook: To partially cook or boil a food briefly, and commonly used for ingredients that may be denser or take longer to cook.

Broil: To cook food under direct heat, generally a term used for foods cooked in an oven. This technique is used to brown or crisp a food.

Crisscross Cut, Roll Cut or Oblique Cut: A term for cutting a carrot or long vegetable at 45-degree angles, while rotating the vegetable to create a visually appealing rounded piece, with more surface area, which speeds up the cooking process.

Puree: Any food finely mashed, generally at high speed to a thick and smooth consistency. Food processors and blenders are commonly used for this technique.

Al Dente: A term used to describe a food or pasta that is cooked to slight resistance when bitten, to prevent the food from being soft or overdone.

Strain or drain: To use a kitchen utensil such as colander or strainer used to remove excess liquid from the food. These utensils are commonly perforated, have a mesh bottom or sides. Cheesecloth and other fabric strainers are generally used for cheeses and yogurts to drain excess liquid.

Resources

WEBSITES	
The SCD Athlete	thescdathlete.com
NiMBAL	nimbal.org
Pecanbread	pecanbread.com
SCD Recipe	scdrecipe.com
Specific Carbohydrate Diet Association	specificcarbohydratedietassociation.org
Wellbees	wellbees.com

SOURCES
NASM
NIH News
UCLA Health
The Management of Celiac Disease, Sidney Haas, MD
Breaking the Vicious Cycle: Intestinal Health Through Diet, by Elaine Gottschall

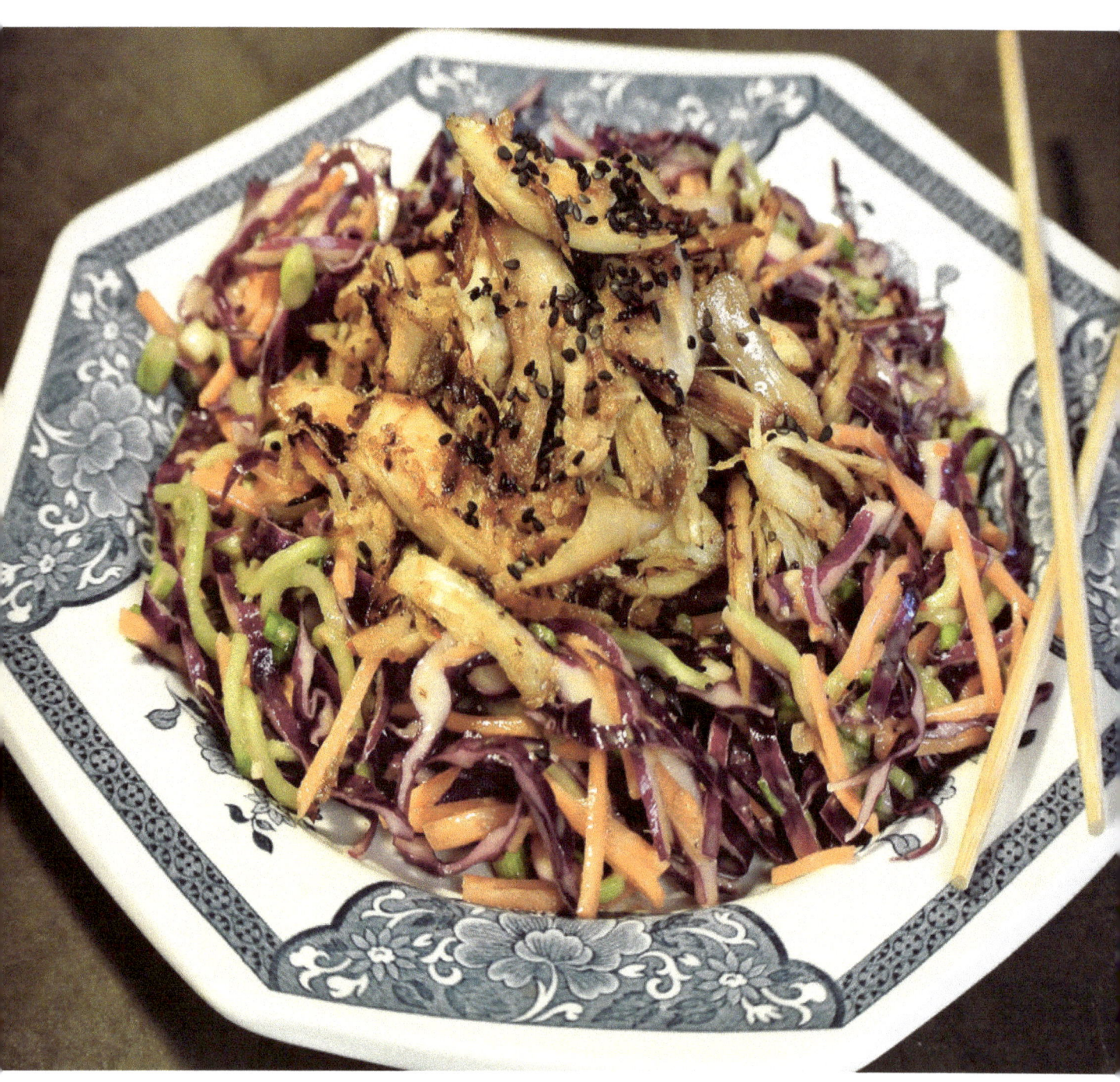

Asian Chicken "Noodle" Salad

Recipe Index

Z

Acknowledgments

To my husband, my forever sous chef, dishwasher, personal grocery shopper, and fledgling cook. This book could not have been written without your never-ending love and support.

About the Author

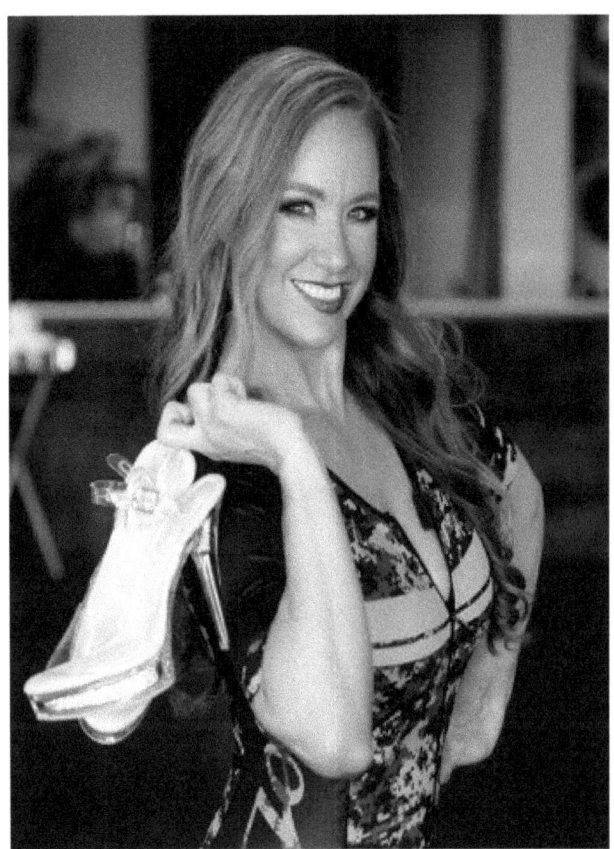

T.L. Wright is a writer, athlete and cookbook author. When diagnosed with Crohn's disease, she found the Specific Carbohydrate Diet. As a cook she experimented with recipes to help fuel her endurance and competitive sports. These recipes helped her gain a natural pro bodybuilding title, as well as fuel marathon, and triathlon training. She continues to help other athletes reach their athletic and performance goals through nutritious recipes and working with fellow coaches. You can find more information and latest news at TheIBDAthlete.com

www.ingramcontent.com/pod-product-compliance
Lightning Source LLC
Chambersburg PA
CBHW041135120626
46547CB00020B/3004